Raising the Dead

Raising the Dead

ORGAN TRANSPLANTS, ETHICS, AND SOCIETY

Ronald Munson

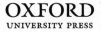

OXFORD
UNIVERSITY PRESS

Oxford   New York
Auckland   Bangkok   Buenos Aires
Cape Town   Chennai   Dar es Salaam   Delhi   Hong Kong   Istanbul
Karachi   Kolkata   Kuala Lumpur   Madrid   Melbourne   Mexico City   Mumbai
Nairobi   São Paulo   Shanghai   Taipei   Tokyo   Toronto

Copyright © 2002 by Ronald Munson

First published by Oxford University Press, Inc., 2002
198 Madison Avenue, New York, New York 10016
www.oup.com

First issued as an Oxford University Press paperback, 2004
ISBN 0-19-517801-7

Oxford is a registered trademark of Oxford University Press

The Library of Congress has cataloged the cloth edition as follows:
Munson, Ronald, 1939–
Raising the dead : organ transplants, ethics, and society / Ronald Munson.
p. cm.
Includes bibliographical references and index.
ISBN 0-19-513299-8
1. Transplantation of organs, tissues, etc. —Moral and ethical aspects.
2. Transplantation of organs, tissues, etc.—Social aspects.
3. Medical ethics.
I. Title.
RD120.7.M86 2001
174'.25—dc21   2001036119

9 8 7 6 5 4 3 2 1
Printed in the United States of America
on acid-free paper

To

MIRIAM
who makes it all possible

and

REBECCA
who is what it's all about

And when he thus had spoken, he said with a loud voice,
Lazarus, come forth. And he that was dead came forth, bound
hand and foot with graveclothes . . .

JOHN 11: 43

Contents

A Modern Lazarus

Robby Benson's Heart

The first time I saw Robby Benson alone he was stretched out in a beige plastic lounge chair in a pint-sized single room at William Osler Hospital. His hands were folded over the copy of Time in his lap, and he was staring into the distance. His face was tense and his jaw clenched. He was breathing oxygen through a clear plastic tube clipped to his nostrils.

"How are you feeling?" I asked.

I held a visiting appointment at the medical school associated with Osler, and when I mentioned to a surgeon I wanted to talk with a patient waiting for a heart transplant, he suggested I get in touch with Robby Benson.

I had introduced myself to Robby and his wife Marge a couple of days later. I talked with them a while, then asked their permission to follow Robby through the transplant process. I explained this would include granting me access to his medical information and allowing me to talk openly with people involved in his care.

"I've got nothing to hide," Robby had said. "That's the first thing I learned in the hospital." He gave a laugh, but it didn't have much vitality.

Marge gave her permission as well. "Maybe it'll help somebody else get through this ordeal." She squeezed Robby's shoulder gently. "It was all new to us."

We hadn't discussed the possibility that Robby could die before getting the heart he needed. It was too obvious and too distressing to mention.

"Weak as lunch-counter coffee," Robby said, answering my question. "But I'm a lot better with this gizmo than before."

Robby touched the thick plastic tube inserted into his abdomen on the left side. The tube's other end was connected to a small pump that hung around his waist and was powered by battery packs in the pockets of the black fabric vest he wore over a short-sleeved shirt. The pump was a left-ventricular assist device (LVAD) that gave Robby's blood a boost as it exited his heart to circulate to the rest of his body.

Robby spoke softly, making it hard to catch his words over the noise of the LVAD. It gave off a strident *whish* each time it ejected another squirt of blood. *Whish*-pause-*whish*-pause-*whish* . . . in a steady rhythm that mechanically mimicked a beating heart.

"I was in sorry shape before Dr. Rivelstein hooked me up," Robby said. He paused, catching his breath. "I couldn't walk the twenty feet from the front room to the kitchen without getting winded and so lightheaded I'd worry I was going to faint."

I knew from Robby's hospital chart that he was 48 years old. He was solid, without being fat, wide-shouldered, and, at five feet eight, about average height. He had a plump, boyish face, but his curly dirty-blonde hair was grey at the temples. Except for terrycloth slippers and the black vest, he was dressed in street clothes—a pale yellow shirt and floppy baby-blue wash pants. A shirt button was open, and I glimpsed a bandage surrounding the incision where the LVAD tube entered his body.

"You live your life taking breathing for granted," Robby said. "But I got to where I couldn't breathe when I lay down at night." He touched the oxygen tube at his nose, pushing it into place. "I couldn't get air into my lungs. It was like when you're swimming underwater and think your lungs are going to burst. I'd take a breath, but it wouldn't do much for me." He shrugged, looking puzzled. "I started sleeping propped up straight as a board."

Robby was a construction superintendent. With only a high school education, he'd worked as a carpenter for nearly twenty years, then he had become a foreman and eventually, after taking some community college courses, a job superintendent. He'd never smoked, and had never been sick, except for the usual aching muscles and bouts of flu, until twenty-two months earlier.

"I began to put on weight," Robby said. "I thought it was middle-aged spread, and when I started finding it hard to catch my breath, I believed it was the extra pounds I was lugging around. I told Marge I was going to cut back on the ice cream. I don't drink, so I couldn't give up alcohol."

"How long did you wait before seeing a doctor?"

"About two months. It got to where going to work was pointless. I couldn't hardly get out of the office to see what was happening on the site, and I didn't seem able to concentrate. I was tired all the time, no matter how much rest I got, and my feet and ankles swelled up like balloons. I felt bloated, too. Marge was worried about me and made an appointment with Dr. Fuller. Then at supper one night she informs me I've got to call in sick, because, by God, I'm going to the doctor."

Dr. Howard Fuller, a specialist in internal medicine, listened to Robby's story, examined him, took blood and urine samples for analysis, then referred him to Dr. John Atkins, a cardiologist at Osler. Dr. Atkins ordered a series of tests. Robby was given, in addition to more blood and urine tests, an electrocardiogram, an echocardiogram, a sonogram, and a CT-scan so Dr. Atkins would have more information about how Robby's heart was functioning.

The data confirmed Dr. Atkins's initial impression, and he arranged for Robby to have a cardiac angiogram. In a special facility in the hospital, a contrast agent was injected into Robby's coronary arteries through a catheter snaked into his heart from an artery in his groin. Radiologists then made x-ray videotapes of the blood moving through his heart. Snippets of tissue were taken from his heart for microscopic analysis by a hospital pathologist.

The additional data led Dr. Atkins to diagnose Robby's problem as idiopathic dilated cardiomyopathy. The muscle of Robby's heart was dying, with the result that his heart was losing its pumping effectiveness. The resulting low blood pressure explained why fluid had accumulated in his feet, ankles, and abdomen. The CT-scan and the sonogram showed Robby's liver was swollen and his heart expanded to three times normal size. Fluid bubbled in his lungs.

Robby was in congestive heart failure.

Cardiomyopathy can result from an infection or genetic factors. But Robby couldn't recall any illness near the time he started experiencing his first symptoms, nor could he remember anyone in his family ever having a heart problem. His disease was thus labeled "idiopathic," meaning "of unknown origin."

"I've always kept myself in pretty good shape," Robby said. "So hearing I had heart trouble surprised me. Dr. Fuller had mentioned the possibility, so when Dr. Atkins told me it was definite, I figured, 'Shoot, they'll do a bypass, and I'll be all right.' I know six or eight people who've had it done."

Robby paused, sniffing at the oxygen. The *whish-whish-whish* of the LVAD made the silence seem longer. "Then I was really floored. Dr. Atkins said he could help with my symptoms, but he couldn't cure me. He said the numbers were against me."

Once the signs of heart failure from dilated cardiomyopathy become obvious, I learned, up to 50 percent of those with the disease die within the first year. Within five years, more than 75 percent are dead.

"Dr. Atkins told me my only hope was to get a transplant." Robby frowned. "That sounded like a fairy tale to me. But I'm a gambler, and I told him I was ready to swap my busted ticker for a new model whenever he was ready." He slumped, his energy gone. "What choice did I have?"

Dr. Atkins sent Robby downstairs to Osler's Cardiac Transplantation Unit to be evaluated for a transplant. Robby soon discovered that getting a new heart wasn't so easy.

I decided to find out how the evaluation procedure worked at Osler. Robby had already been accepted as a transplant candidate, so I would be looking at a stage he'd already passed through. I would then follow him forward, talking to the key players in the heart transplantation process.

Robby was going to be my index case, the one that would serve as a reference in my thinking about organ transplantation and the ethical and social issues associated with it. His case couldn't illustrate all of them, but it would be a touchstone to keep me oriented. It would also give me a chance to find out how the transplant system worked, the social mechanics of it all.

Most important, knowing about Robby would make sure that when I thought about the abstract issues, they would have a human face associated with them. I never wanted to lose sight of the hard fact that decisions about organ transplantation are life-and-death decisions about people.

Rosemary Rangle, CSW

Rosemary Rangle was a clinical social worker and a key member of the Heart Transplantation Unit's evaluation committee. She had interviewed Robby and Marge at length, obtaining information crucial to the committee's deliberations. She'd presented the case at a meeting, briefing all five members.

I found Rangle in a tiny, cluttered office along the hallway leading to the cardiac catheterization lab. She was in her early 50s and had a quick smile. Dressed in a loose white blouse, a blue denim skirt, her graying brown hair tied back, she could have been mistaken for a high school English teacher.

"Each center sets its own criteria for selecting patients," she said. "There are 261 transplantation centers in the country, and 142 of them have heart programs. UNOS—the United Network for Organ Sharing—suggests guidelines, but in the last analysis, it's the centers' responsibility to select patients.

"The first consideration is medical appropriateness. Not only does the patient have a heart problem, but could he benefit from a transplant? That was an easy decision in Mr. Benson's case, because he's relatively young and, except for his heart, healthy. If he'd been eighty and in kidney failure, we might have said no."

"Because of his age?"

"We don't discriminate on the basis of age, sex, or race." Rangle smiled, as if pleased to deliver the news. "But age is relevant as an indicator. Elderly people don't cope with surgery and general anesthesia as well as younger ones.

"Also, we eliminate those with a serious medical condition that a transplant can't help, such as cancer, pulmonary hypertension, morbid obesity, AIDS, liver disease—anything life-threatening. We want to save lives, but to do that, we sometimes have to say no to some patients so we can give the heart to somebody more likely to benefit. We can't waste organs."

"Does being famous or rich help in getting approved?"

"Yes and no." Rangle glanced down. "Being a big shot won't get you a heart faster. But we can't approve you for transplant unless you have the means to pay the $250,000 to $300,000 it's going to cost. The famous are usually rich, and the rich have the money. But other people may not."

"So it's no pay, no play?"

"It sounds brutal, but that's essentially it. You have to have insurance or cash, and we take Medicare and Medicaid assignments. We work with patients and do everything to find a source of payment, but we're not always successful. Some with insurance find their policies don't cover transplants. Others have policies that don't pay enough to cover expenses, but the people earn too much to qualify for an entitlement program.

"We've got some funds we can draw on to help, but we can't pay everybody's bills. And it's not just the surgery and hospital bills either. The aftercare, monitoring, and drug regimen can cost another $40,000 to $50,000 a year. Sadly, we've got to turn away patients who could benefit from a transplant, because they don't have enough money."

Rangle looked embarrassed, as if confessing a personal failing. It wasn't, of course, but I understood her feeling. Both of us were aware of the irony that in the richest and most medically advanced country in the history of the world it was possible for a child to die because her parents couldn't come up with enough money to pay for a transplant.

"So if somebody needs a transplant and can pay for it, will he or she be approved by your committee?"

"Not necessarily. We consider other factors too. Health habits are number one. We don't accept alcoholics or drug abusers, unless they can demonstrate abstinence for a six-month minimum. We don't just take their word either. We monitor them with urine and blood tests to make sure they stay clean. We do the same with smokers. We won't give a heart to somebody we aren't convinced is going to stay off cigarettes."

"Robby said he had to go through a psychological screening."

"Everyone has to have a psychiatric interview with Dr. Charles Dimmer. He's been on the committee as long as I have, which is eight years, and he's quick to detect psychopathologies or behavior problems that would make it difficult for a patient to meet the demands of living with a transplant." Rangle raised a hand as if blocking an objection. "This doesn't mean patients with psychiatric diagnoses are automatically excluded. We only want to be sure they're able to take their meds on schedule, avoid harmful behaviors, and keep their appointments."

"What about the families of candidates?"

"Getting a family involved is a definite plus for a patient. A social network with everybody in the family pulling can get a recipient over some of the rough spots. A transplant is associated with lots of stress. Recipients have to learn a new way of living and new ways of taking care of themselves. People close to them have to adjust their expectations and relate in new ways. Everyone, particularly the recipient, is aware that death is always lurking in the background."

I asked whether patients without families were excluded.

"Having a supportive family is only one factor. Lacking one could count negatively, but we never make it decisive. We don't have a point system like the University of Pittsburgh, but we take into account a variety of factors. We're careful not to discriminate against people because their lifestyle is statistically out of the norm. Being gay or lesbian wouldn't exclude somebody, for example. Nor would being single or divorced or even over 65."

"Can people appeal your committee's decision not to accept them as a transplant candidate?"

"Sure, they can ask us to take a second look. And maybe something has changed, like they've made a decision to quit drinking, and they want to tell us about it."

"If you continue to turn them down, though, there's nothing they can do?"

"They can go to some other program. Some have looser rules, and some have stricter. Some centers, for example, exclude all alcoholics, period."

"So people can choose which program to apply to."

"They can even apply to several and get evaluated, if they've got the money. And if they get approved for a transplant, they can wait and see which center comes up with an organ first."

"Does that happen often?"

"It happens." Rangle nodded. "I don't think it's fair, but I don't make the rules."

Marge Benson

Robby had already spent two weeks in the hospital waiting for a transplant. Marge had driven him in from their suburban Maryland home on a Monday morning.

"He didn't seem himself that morning," she told me during one of our meetings over coffee in the hospital cafeteria. A petite woman with short red hair swept back at the sides in a ducktail, Marge bristled with energy. Unable to remain still, she tapped her fingers against the coffee cup.

"When he got out of bed, he seemed confused, like he was drunk. He asked where Karen was. That's our daughter. She's 24 and lives in Belmont, California. She's an executive assistant to somebody in publishing. She moved out there three years ago, but Robby didn't seem to remember any of that.

"He was having trouble getting his breath too, even though he was standing up. He'd pant like a dog, take a couple of breaths, then go back to panting." Marge put her hands flat on the table. "It scared me so much, I walked him to the car and took him right to the emergency room."

Robby, it turned out, had slipped into Class 4 heart failure. Patients in Class 1 experience symptoms after strenuous exercise, while those in Classes 2 and 3 develop them after such moderate-to-mild exercise as walking a block or crossing the room. Class 4 patients have symptoms even while sitting down or propped up in bed. Their hearts are not doing enough effective work to supply their tissues with oxygen and carry off the carbon dioxide in their blood. Class 4 patients thus feel fatigued and confused. They are also likely to die.

John Atkins, M.D., Cardiologist

"The heart loses its pumping effectiveness with heart failure," Dr. Atkins told me when I asked him about Robby's disease. "In patients with heart failure, every pumping action of the heart puts out only 30 milliliters of the normal 150-milliliter capacity. That's the stroke volume, meaning the ejection fraction is only 20 percent. The normal heart has a 60-percent ejection fraction. So to get more blood out, the sick heart has to expand. If it grows to hold 300 milliliters of blood, even a 20-percent fraction will yield a 60-milliliter stroke volume. Better, but still not normal."

Dr. Atkins was a slender, silver-haired man in his 60s. Under his starched white lab coat he wore a blue and white striped shirt with a rounded white collar. His maroon tie was secured by a tiny heart-shaped gold pin.

"The body is quite marvelous, really," he said. "The heart can grow so large it all but fills the thoracic cavity. *Dilated* means *enlarged*, and in dilated cardiomyopathy, that's what the heart does." Dr. Atkins spread his hands, fingers splayed, over his chest. "Other compensations also occur. The kidneys slow down output to keep up blood volume and various hormones are released to slow fluid loss. High fluid levels are important to stretch the heart muscle to maintain the stroke volume. The heart may also beat faster to keep up the pressure."

He wagged a finger like an admonishing preacher. "These compensatory mechanisms exact a price. Retained fluid causes swelling in the legs, feet, and abdomen. Fluid also builds up in the lungs, which increases the chance of pneumonia or other infections. Hormones like epinephrine make blood vessels constrict to keep up blood pressure, but that increases resistance, and the weakened heart has to pump even harder."

Dr. Atkins explained that Robby was treated in the ER with drugs to strengthen his heartbeat, increase his urinary output, and reduce the volume of retained fluid. He was given oxygen and muscle relaxants to ease his breathing.

"Mr. Benson was on the verge of kidney failure, and we recognized he wasn't going to make it if we didn't take some bold steps. I consulted with Dr. Rivelstein, and we decided Mr. Benson could benefit from going on the pump."

Mark Rivelstein, M.D., Cardiac Transplant Surgeon

I met Dr. Rivelstein in the reception area of the heart transplant office as he was coming out of surgery. He was a compact man with gray-streaked black hair and a friendly, courteous manner. His shoes were still covered with blood-flecked paper booties.

"It's only been in the last several years that we've had much to offer to people in heart failure who have to wait for a transplant," he said. "Eventually the LVAD may become completely implantable and maybe patients can rely on it for years. Right now, though, we're using it only for a few days or weeks to keep them going until they can get a graft."

Dr. Rivelstein ushered me into his office. Plaques and framed awards hung on the walls. Papers and medical journals were stacked in neat piles on a low table.

"Here's a pump we use for teaching." He handed me a flat, circular device resembling an oversized metal hamburger with sockets to connect to tubes. "Plastic and titanium. It looks big, but it fits nicely under the rib cage. It's got a rough inner surface that gets lined with blood cells and proteins. That makes it slick and keeps blood clots from forming. If they form, they break off and cause stokes. That was the big problem with the original artificial heart."

"So what's the procedure now for Mr. Benson?"

"He's got to wait, and we've got to keep him in good shape," Dr. Rivelstein said. "If you want to know how things go from here on, I recommend you talk to the cardiac transplant coordinator."

Carol Lee Phillips, R.N., Transplant Coordinator

"I love this job," Carol Lee Phillips told me. She was a willowy African-American woman in her late thirties, wearing black trousers with a short white lab jacket. A red enameled heart pin was clipped to the lapel of her jacket. "I'd almost do it for nothing, if I didn't have two kids to help support."

I'd found her on the fourth floor, checking on patients in the coronary intensive care unit. She was carrying a clipboard and a short stack of manila folders. We sat down in one of the family waiting areas at the end of the hall.

"I do what the job title says," she said. "I coordinate all the elements and people needed to make the transplant happen. I'm in constant touch with the patients and their families. I make sure the patient is waitlisted with the United Network for Organ Sharing. I'm also in touch with our local Organ Procurement Organization, and when they call and say they've got a heart, I've got to make sure my patient is available. I've got to get that patient into the hospital, if he's not already there, and notify the surgical team, so they can be ready to swing into action to transplant the heart."

"When did Robby Benson pop up on your radar?"

"When Dr. Atkins first evaluated Mr. Benson last year, he submitted his chart to the heart transplant committee. I was present at the discussion, and when Mr. Benson was accepted as a patient, we listed him with UNOS as Status 2."

A Status 2 patient, Phillips explained, was one in chronic heart failure who was capable of functioning outside the hospital, even if restricted in activities and sustained by a variety of medications.

"When he showed up in our ER having trouble, we bumped him up to Status 1A. Even with his LVAD, he's critically ill and may not survive longer than a month. Status 1B patients have a life expectancy of more than a month. With Mr. Benson, getting a heart really is a race against the clock."

"Does Robby Benson have any special characteristics that might make it hard for him to get a heart?"

"Not really." Phillips put the folders on the chair beside her and flipped through the pages on her clipboard. "He's got type A blood, which makes it easier to get a compatible donor. We also need a heart that's proportional to the size of his body. Mr. Benson's a good-sized man, and a heart from a small person wouldn't be up to the demands he'd place on it."

"Blood type and size have to be right. Anything else?"

"The heart's got to be healthy, without infection or significant damage. If the coronary arteries are clogged, we can't use the organ. It would make zero sense for us to subject somebody to the risks of major surgery to replace one sick heart with another sick heart."

"What about tissue matching?"

"That's only for kidneys," Phillips said. "Blood type, size, condition—all three have to come together for hearts."

"And what are Robby's chances?"

"UNOS posts its statistics, and more than 5,000 people are waiting for a heart. Only 2,000 are going to get one, if experience is a guide. The rest will go on waiting, but about 1,000 will die and never get a heart."

"The numbers don't sound good."

"They're not." Phillips shrugged. "But organs are distributed to the local area first, and since we're in a big city with only a couple of transplant programs, Mr. Benson's got a reasonable chance of getting a heart before he crashes. I'm surprised one hasn't become available yet." She shrugged. "But that's the way it is."

"It's unpredictable."

"That's why it's so hard on patients and their families. They can't settle down, because they're always listening for that other shoe to drop."

Robby and Marge

Marge was propped up in Robby's bed reading a thriller called *Fan Mail* I had given her. Robby was watching an interview show on the wall-mounted TV, but he switched it off.

I asked them about the waiting.

"Carol Lee gave me a beeper so I can go out of the hospital and take care of business without worrying about something happening without me knowing about it," Marge said. "That helps a whole lot. But waiting for a heart isn't something you can ever put out of your mind. It nags at you like a sore tooth."

"I think it's easier for me than it is for her," Robby said. "Maybe because I breathe so much better than I did, and I'm here where they can take care of me. But, yeah, I can't keep my mind focused on anything else."

"I believe he worries about other people more than himself," Marge said.

"I want a heart, but I don't want somebody to have to die for me to get it," Robby said. "I know it's necessary, but I don't want to hope somebody's going to get killed today."

"I think of getting a heart as something good coming out of something bad," Marge said. "We don't want somebody to die, but that's going to happen anyway, whether Robby gets a heart or not."

"I might just peg out before a heart comes along," Robby said. "I try not to dwell on it, but I know a woman down the hall died last Tuesday. She was a Status 1B and had been waiting a month."

"I'm not going to let that happen to you, sweetie." Marge crossed to Robby's chair and put a hand flat against his cheek.

We all felt awkward, because we knew neither Marge nor anybody else had that sort of power.

Donor

Two days later, around five in the afternoon, I got a call at home from somebody who identified himself as Tom, one of Carol Lee Phillips's assistants.

"Carol Lee wanted you to know it looks like we've got a heart for Mr. Benson," Tom said. "It's coming from a local hospital, and the transplant should take place tonight. We've got to get him prepped, so we're aiming for eight."

I got to the hospital half an hour later and went to Phillips's office. She was sitting at her desk in front of her computer.

"Ten minutes ago we got a call from Dr. Vaughn, the surgeon leading the organ recovery team at St. Sebastian's Hospital. He's arrived at the hospital and seen the donor but hasn't assessed the heart yet. He'll be calling us back a couple of times, maybe more, depending on what he finds and how things go."

"Do you know anything about the donor?"

"He's a 37-year-old caucasian high school football coach who sustained a head injury in an SUV rollover early this morning. Paramedics got to him fast, but by the time they put him on a ventilator at the hospital, there was nothing anybody could do. The brain damage was too extensive. They assessed him neurologically, then declared him dead. They called UNOS, the way the law says you have to do when you've got a brain-dead patient who's a potential donor."

"But somebody still had to give permission?"

"His wife knew he wanted to be a donor and brought up the matter herself. A short time later, I got the call from the OPO, and I paged Mrs. Benson and broke the news to Mr. Benson." She smiled. "I get a thrill out of that. Everybody's like, 'I can't believe it, I can't believe it.'"

Robby and Marge

I'd never seen Robby in bed before. He wasn't lying flat, but was propped up against the raised mattress.

"I'd rather be in a chair." He looked apprehensive, and the *whish-whish-whish* of the LVAD was loud. "But they made me lay down, because they're coming to take me away and get me ready for the surgery." He scowled. "I'm hungry, too. They haven't let me eat all day, and I've had to suck on ice instead of drinking water. They said I might breathe something into my lungs during the operation."

"I thought they'd be here by now." Marge squeezed her hands into fists. She walked to the door and looked down the hall. "They warned us something might go wrong and they'd have to cancel the transplant. But I know everything's going to be all right. I just feel it."

"Karen's flying in from San Francisco." Robby sounded pleased. "I hope for her sake they don't cancel the plane."

"If they do, she can get another," Marge said. She realized whose sake the hope was for. "It's not such a big deal."

Two male nursing assistants in green scrubs came through the door with a wheeled stretcher. With expertise, they maneuvered it alongside the bed.

"Sir, we need for you to lay flat a second so we can transfer you to the stretcher," one of them said.

"I'm not going that way." Robby swung his legs over the side of the bed and was standing up before the assistants realized what he was planning. Robby walked around the foot of his bed, moving slowly and keeping a hand on it.

"Sir, we need for you to cooperate," the assistant said.

"I'm doing what you want." Holding onto the rail, Robby hoisted himself up and sat on the stretcher.

"You are stubborn as a mule." Marge sounded more proud than angry. "But don't be telling the doctors how to operate."

She walked beside the stretcher, her hand on Robby's arm, while the attendants wheeled it down the hall.

Mark Rivelstein, M.D.

Thanks to directions from Carol Lee Phillips, I caught up with Dr. Rivelstein in the surgeon's lounge. He was drinking a cup of tomato soup from a paper cup. It was his dinner, he explained.

"I got a call from Bob Vaughn a couple of minutes ago," Dr. Rivelstein said. "He's opened the donor's chest and assessed the heart. It looks like it's got some bruising, probably from the car accident. But it's got good contractility, and Bob doesn't think the damage is serious enough for us to turn it down."

"What's happening with Robby Benson now?"

"He's getting shaved, cleaned up, and draped. He's mildly sedated to keep him calm and breathing easier, and unless Bob calls me back and tells me something's wrong, I'm going to go down to the operating suite and tell Tom Breyer, the anesthesiologist, to put him under.

"We'll open up Mr. Benson's chest and get his ribs spread, but we're not going to monkey around with his heart. I'll wait and make sure everything's okay on the other end. St. Vincent's is four miles down a straight road, so we don't have to worry about storms and flight delays."

"What's the donor team going to be doing?"

"Bob's already opened the chest and the pericardium. He'll now free the superior vena cava and the aorta, then separate the aorta and the pulmonary artery to get ready to crossclamp. He'll call me before he does that, so I can get Mr. Benson ready.

"Once Bob has crossclamped, he'll pour a cold saline solution over the heart, let it beat four or five times to empty it, then fill it with a cardioplegia solution. He'll cut through the inferior vena cava, lift up the heart, resect the four pulmonary veins, the aorta, and the two pulmonary arteries."

"Then he'll take out the heart?"

"Exactly. He'll give it a good looking-over to make sure he didn't miss something, then put it in a container of cold saline. He'll ice down the container in a cooler."

"That'll preserve it?"

"It'll help. An organ starts to die as soon as it loses its blood supply, and the sooner we get it into Mr. Benson, the better shape it's going to be in. The time between removing the heart and hooking it back up is what we call the cold ischemic time, and the shorter it is the better."

Transplant

Dr. Rivelstein was scrubbed and gowned by the time the third phone call came from Dr. Vaughn. They were about to crossclamp. This was the signal for Dr. Rivelstein to go ahead with getting Robby prepared to get his new heart.

Robby was already on the operating table surrounded by the surgical team when Dr. Rivelstein walked in. Robby's body was draped, except for the large area of his chest that was painted a dull orange with a disinfectant. Around the perimeter of the area, crinkly plastic wrap covered his skin as an additional protection against contaminating the surgical wound. The endotracheal tube, taped into place, was connected to a ventilator that was already breathing for him.

Dr. Breyer, the anesthesiologist, was at the head of the table behind a screen separating him from the operative field. He was keeping his eyes on an array of dials and monitors. A perfusionist was making adjustments on the heart-lung machine that would be used to keep Robby alive until his new heart was in place.

Dr. Rivelstein watched as Dr. Allen Cummar, a surgical fellow, made the first incision down the center of Robby's chest. A bright line of blood appeared as the knife cut through the skin. Dr. Clara Wrightman, a surgical resident, helped Dr. Cummar by sealing off bleeding blood vessels with an electrocautery and suctioning out any accumulating blood.

Carol Lee Phillips came into the operating suite, standing at the edge of the room to avoid compromising the sterile field. "Dr. Vaughn says the heart is in transit," she called over to Dr. Rivelstein. "Arriving in about ten minutes."

"Thank you," Dr. Rivelstein said. "Did you hear that, Allen?" he asked Dr. Cummar. "No need to stop."

"Great." Neither Dr. Cummar nor Dr. Wrightman looked up. Dr. Cummar continued to cut through the layers of fat, muscle, and connective tissue to expose Robby's breastbone.

Dr. Cummar was using an electric saw to split the sternum some twenty minutes later when a man in surgical scrubs brought in a red and white plastic Igloo picnic cooler and put it down on a metal stand outside the sterile area. Dr. Cummar continued to work, using a stainless steel retractor to pull back the ribs and hold them in place. Dr. Wrightman rubbed bone wax on the cut edges of the sternum to seal off the bleeding.

One of the operating room nurses opened the cooler and removed a deep plastic container that looked like it had been designed for refrigerator storage. She pried off the lid, then stood aside. Dr. Rivelstein lifted the heart out of the container and placed it in a metal bowl. The heart was a mottled gray and surprisingly large. Streaks of yellowish fat and a glistening membrane covered the outside.

"Let's wash it off with some saline," Dr. Rivelstein told the nurse. She poured the liquid over the heart, while he turned it from side to side. He then put it in a second bowl of saline.

Dr. Cummar moved down the table to allow Dr. Rivelstein to take his place. Dr. Rivelstein examined Robby's heart, which seemed to occupy the entire chest cavity. "Ready to go on bypass?" he asked, looking over at the perfusionist.

"Whenever," she said.

Dr. Rivelstein attached three lines from the heart-lung machine. Robby was already being given heparin so his blood wouldn't clot as it passed through the tubing. The machine, in addition to oxygenating Robby's blood, would also cool it to 78 degrees before pumping it back into his body. The lower temperature would help protect all his organs by reducing their need for oxygen.

"Get ready to go on bypass," Dr. Rivelstein said. He secured the lines in place with a couple of stitches. "Switch when you're ready."

"On bypass," the technician said. Blood swirled through the transparent plastic tubes.

Dr. Rivelsetein stood motionless for a while, searching for leaks and making sure the heart-lung machine was doing its job. He checked Robby's blood pressure, oxygen saturation, and heart rate with Dr. Breyer.

Satisfied, Dr. Rivelstein clamped off the aorta, and a nurse put a knife into his outstretched hand. "Most people think we just cut through the blood vessels of the old heart," he said. "But that's not the way it works." He began to dissect with deft, definite strokes. Dr. Cummar moved the suction wand around, keeping the operative field clear of blood.

"Using a technique developed by Norman Shumway at Stanford, we cut through the top of the heart—the right and left atria, the aorta, and the pulmonary arteries—and leave a sort of cuff behind. An advantage is that this makes attaching the graft heart much easier and faster."

Dr. Rivelstein worked quietly and quickly. He lifted Robby's heart out of his chest and placed it in a stainless bowl. It was massive and misshapen, hardly like a human organ at all. Dr. Cummar quickly suctioned up the blood that had poured from the severed connections.

Dr. Rivelstein picked up the donor heart, drained it, and held it over the gaping hole in Robby's chest. He was like a sculptor deciding how much stone to chisel away. Using blunt scissors and a knife, he trimmed off excess material. Several times he compared the altered heart to the cuff of Robby's old heart. Satisfied at last, he sutured the new heart into place.

"Get ready to start weaning him off bypass," he told the technician. "Bring up the temperature."

Dr. Rivelstein unclamped the aorta. The gray heart began to change color, turning soft pink, then redder. A quarter of an hour passed . . . half an hour. Another ten minutes. The heart was warming, coming out of its induced hibernation.

Dr. Rivelstein began to massage the heart gently. Nothing happened for a long moment. Then the heart quivered and started to beat, delicately at first, then with increasing vigor. Eventually, when Dr. Rivelstein was satisfied the heart was going to keep on beating, he ended the weaning process and removed the tubes of the heart-lung machine. He gave an order to administer a drug that would counteract the effects of heparin. Dr. Cummar would attach the leads of a pacemaker and implant the device.

"Now that's very satisfying," Dr. Rivelstein said. "You're more likely to get this result when you've had a short ischemic time like today's." He stepped away from the table. "I'm leaving it all up to you now, Allen."

The operation had taken more than four hours.

Postoperative

Robby was awake and alert the next afternoon. Marge had stayed with him in the coronary intensive care unit, and by five o'clock, he was propped up in bed talking to their daughter Karen, who'd come directly from the airport to the hospital.

"I can't believe how great he looks," Karen told her mother over dinner in the cafeteria. She had her mother's red hair and vivacity and emphasized her words. "He seems better than he did when he had his own heart. His color is rosy, instead of grey."

"Dr. Atkins said his body is finally getting the blood it needs for the first time in two years," Marge said. She looked tired, and her hair was ruffled at the back where she'd slept in a lounge chair. But she was beaming and making wide gestures with her hands.

Robby was out of the hospital in three weeks. But his course hadn't been entirely smooth. Five days after the transplant, he developed a low-grade fever and slightly irregular heartbeat. The pacemaker kept his heartbeat under control, but his doctors had to find out what was wrong.

Dr. Atkins and Dr. Rivelstein thought it was possible Robby's body was rejecting the heart or that he had an infection. The heart itself, despite all the precautions, might be infected, but an episode of rejection seemed most likely. They biopsied Robby's heart through a catheter and took blood and urine samples to check for signs of infection.

The ordered pattern of heart cells and the relatively few inflammatory cells in the biopsied tissue the pathologists saw under the microscope didn't support the rejection hypothesis, so even before the laboratory studies were completed, Robby's doctors treated him with a course of IV-administered antibiotics. The treatment worked.

Robby's temperature went down, and the irregular rhythm disappeared. His heart beat steadily and well. They never discovered the location of the infection.

Goodbye

I said goodbye to the Bensons the day Robby checked out of Osler. I thanked them for permitting me to meet with them during a difficult time and wished them the best of luck.

"Did anybody ever tell you about the donor?" I asked him.

"Not really." Robby frowned. "Just that it was a man about my size but younger. I'm sorry for him. Sorry for his family. But I'm grateful too, and I hope I can live up to what they've given me."

"I'm going to write a letter and thank his family for what they did," Marge said. I'd heard from Carol Lee Phillips that transplant recipients or their spouses always said that but, for whatever reason, almost never did it.

Robby's life was definitely improved. He was no longer incapacitated by his heart, and he was still alive when he might reasonably have been expected to be dead. Seventy percent of heart transplant recipients return to their jobs, and Robby was already eager to get back to work.

But Robby was also sure to have some hard times ahead of him. Transplant recipients don't get a new organ, then simply go back to being the way they were before they started having problems. As Rosemary Rangle had said, Robby was exchanging an acute illness for a chronic one. Getting a new heart isn't like changing the battery in your wristwatch.

Side Effects

Robby's new illness, his transplant, will require him to take a bewildering number of kinds and combinations of drugs to control his immune response and prevent his body from rejecting the donor heart.

These drugs, with their science-fiction names, become as familiar to transplant recipients as the presidents are to American historians: prednisone, FK506, cyclosporine, azathioprine, OKT3, antithymocyte globulin, antilymphocyte globulin, Cellcept, Fluconazole. A few of these (or ones from a much longer list) Robby will need to take all the time. Others he'll take only to combat episodes of rejection or when some can't be tolerated or aren't working effectively.

The drugs are powerful and have powerful side effects. Depending on the combination prescribed by his doctors, Robby will be at risk for mood swings, agitation, weight gain, osteoporosis, hand tremors, sleep disturbance, elevated blood pressure, depressed bone-marrow function, seizures, nausea, fatigue, kidney scarring, liver damage . . . and this is only a sample of potential problems.

Robby will be given other drugs to combat the worst side effects of the immunosuppressive therapy. Among those that might be prescribed are medications to lower blood pressure, increase the production of red blood cells, combat nausea, control seizures, prevent bone demineralization, fight depression, lower anxiety, and treat infections.

Robby isn't likely to have such a range of side effects as to require all these drugs. But every recipient takes some of the antirejection drugs and each has some unwelcome side effects. It's not unusual for a transplant recipient to end up taking from a dozen to two dozen doses of medication a day.

Risks

If drugs aren't given to cripple the immune system, a transplanted organ will be rejected in a matter of days. Unfortunately, taking the drugs also has serious long-term consequences. For reasons not yet clear, either the drugs themselves, or the compromised immune response they produce, make Robby and other transplant recipients ten times more likely than other people to fall ill with a lethal form of cancer. Thus, in five or six years, Robby might develop leukemia, lymphoma, or some other type of cancer.

This threat has to be kept in perspective, of course. While the risk of cancer lies in the future, for people like Robby the need for a heart—or kidney, lung, or liver—is immediate. They must get a transplant to live long enough even to have a long-term risk.

A function of the immune system is to protect the body from such invading micro-organisms as bacteria, viruses, and fungi. Thus an immune system damped down by drugs to prevent rejection is also no longer as effective in preventing infection. The danger is greatest immediately after transplantation and in the following few weeks, because the immune response is then most heavily suppressed. Yet although the suppression is relaxed after about six months, it's never ended. Robby is thus going to have to live with the constant danger of acquiring an infectious disease that might destroy his new heart or threaten his life.

In addition to adopting such generally good practices as exercising to keep fit and eating a healthful diet, Robby will have to be more cautious than the rest of us. He should stay away from crowds during flu season, keep his distance from people with pneumonia or mononucleosis, and take precautions to avoid coming into contact with the herpes virus. And becoming intimate with somebody with a sexually transmitted disease can be as daredevil an act as base-jumping off the Chrysler Building.

Sword of Damocles

Within a few weeks of Robby's leaving the hospital, chances are he'll have the episode of acute rejection his doctors suspected was occurring when he developed a fever soon after his transplant.

The unfortunate fact is that the immunosuppressive drugs, for all their side effects and risks, don't work perfectly. When Robby has a rejection episode, his doctors will use different drugs, a new combination, or higher doses to try to bring it under control. Most likely they'll succeed. But there's no guarantee, and Robby might die or require another transplant, if his heart is seriously damaged.

Even if Robby survives one or more episodes of acute rejection, his troubles aren't necessarily over. Rejection remains a constant possibility, a damocletian sword hanging over him. His heart may function well for six months or even six years, then start failing. Biopsies may show it's deteriorating. This phenomenon is called chronic rejection, and it's responsible for 10 to 20 percent of all heart-transplant deaths. No one knows exactly why it happens or how to prevent it.

A swift medical response, such as switching Robby to different immunosuppressive drugs or increasing the doses of the ones he's taking, may preserve his heart. It's possible, though, nothing will help, and his body will reject his heart. In which case, he may die or require another transplant.

I REALIZED when I said goodbye to Robby and Marge in the parking lot of Osler that Robby still had a rough road to travel. Transplant recipients don't get a free ride.

Yet Robby had been given his life back. He was no longer teetering on the edge of the slough of death, likely at any moment to fall over and sink below the dark water.

Able to breathe easily and go about life's normal activities without gasping or becoming dizzy and confused, he was feeling better than he had for a couple of years. He was on his way to becoming the active, vibrant, confident person he had been. With a bit of luck and good medical care, Robby would be among the 70-plus percent of heart transplant recipients who would still be alive in five years.

He was a modern Lazarus.

Raising the Dead

Organ transplantation was one of the major accomplishments of the last half of the twentieth century. Thanks to the persistence of a generation of committed researchers, we are as a matter of routine able to snatch people like Robby Benson from the grasp of death by replacing their hearts or lungs, giving them new livers, or furnishing them with working kidneys.

To say organ transplantation raises the dead exaggerates its power. But not by much, because people rescued by transplants are all but dead and wholly out of medical options. They are called back to life by the skills of physicians and surgeons using organs donated by people wishing to benefit others.

The benevolence and generosity of these people must not be slighted. Some literally give of themselves by becoming living donors and contributing a kidney or a segment of liver or lung. Some direct that at the time of their death their organs be taken and used. Others make something good come out of tragedy and sadness by donating the organs of a child, a wife, a husband, a brother or sister.

Without organ donation, there would be no organ transplantation. While Marge or Robby may never get around to writing a letter thanking the woman who donated her husband's heart, organ recipients and their families are aware of how much they owe. Perhaps they seldom write thank-you letters because they feel unequal to the task of expressing so much gratitude.

Saving Lives

Each year some 25,000 Americans like Robby have their lives extended or improved by receiving new vital organs. This is a number greater than the population of Falmouth, Massachusetts. It's more than twice the annual enrollment, graduate and undergraduate, of Stanford University.

The number is particularly striking, considering that hardly more than thirty years ago virtually all those now saved would have been dead. Among those raised from the dead, maybe one person's liver was destroyed by a fast-acting virus. Or an inherited disease caused another's kidneys to shut down. Or a congenital heart defect confined someone else to her death bed.

But whatever the cause, in each case medicine three decades ago would have reached the end of its treatment possibilities. No matter how healthy the rest of a person's body might have been, without a functioning kidney, liver, or heart, death would have been the outcome.

Transplants, as Robby would learn, aren't secular miracles worked by science. If they were perfect, giving somebody a new organ would be successful in the way treating an infectious disease was during the golden age of antibiotics—hit a staph infection with a course of penicillin, and the infection disappears. The treatment made the problem go away, and the patient was as good as new and no worse for wear.

Transplantation, in contrast with antibiotic elegance, is a second-rate technology. A hand-cranked adding machine compared to a computer, a mimeograph machine compared to a Xerox copier. It's a crude, stop-gap measure to keep people from dying.

Really successful transplantation would solve the problem it's intended to solve without generating others. It would give Robby a new heart without turning him into a patient with a chronic illness. It would restore him to health and be so free of negative fallout it would resemble magic.

But let's not forget, organ transplants save lives. Twenty-five thousand last year, 100,000 every four years. One Falmouth, Massachusetts every twelve months, the equivalent of the population of a small city like Oak Park, Illinois every forty-eight.

Transplants work.

Losing Lives

Yet as impressive as the number of lives saved may be, every year about 5,000 people on the waiting list die without getting the organ they need to stay alive.

Consider what this means.

On December 2, 1988, when Pan American Airlines Flight 103 bound for New York was flying above Lockerbie, Scotland, a terrorist bomb hidden in its cargo hold exploded. The blast shattered the plane and it crashed, killing 270 people.

The destruction of Pan Am 103 was one of the major disasters in aviation history. Those who die waiting for donor organs depart quietly, becoming private family tragedies without a public face. Yet the total of their deaths is equivalent to the crash of twenty Pan Am 103s a year.

Twenty a year—every year.

About 75,000 people are on the waiting list for a donor organ at any given time in the United States. Some aren't as sick as others and wait for months or even years. Others get an organ within a few days or weeks. Some need an organ desperately and eventually get one.

Then there are those who die while waiting, those 5,000. They, like organ donors, are children, husbands, wives, mothers, fathers, brothers, sisters . . . friends and relatives. They die not because they can't be saved—their lives might have been extended for years, even decades—but because the organs needed to save them aren't available.

Twenty Pan Am 103s every year.

The waiting list is also growing at a rapid rate. A new name was added every eighteen minutes in 1998, every sixteen minutes in 1999, and every fourteen minutes at the beginning of 2001. The list will grow ever longer ever faster, given our aging population.

What's more, the 100,000 people a year who've had transplants, are waiting for one, or died while waiting are only those who got so far as to be evaluated by a transplant center and get their names on the UNOS list. No one knows for sure how many people might benefit from a transplant but never get evaluated. It could be another 100,000.

The need for organs is constant, pressing, and escalating. It's probably greater than can ever be met, even assuming complete efficiency in obtaining organs from those recently dead. Yet no matter how many people fail to get a transplant, every organ transplanted translates into a life extended. The ultimate measure of transplantation's success, therefore, must be the number of lives it has preserved.

Robby, unlike Lazarus, isn't unique. He belongs to a multitude who've been given a new lease on life. A multitude unlucky in needing a transplant, lucky in getting one.

Conjoined Problems

Transplantation is a successful treatment for dozens of what doctors call end-stage organ diseases. These are illnesses like cardiomyopathy, polycystic kidneys, and liver cirrhosis that destroy vital organs and so take the lives of their unfortunate sufferers. Transplantation is able to prevent this only when donor organs are available, and the life of a particular person (somebody like Robby) can be saved only when he or she is fortunate enough to receive one.

Thus, lying at the core of transplantation, as closely related as conjoined twins, are the gnarled and twisted problems of allocating and acquiring organs. Because the demand for organs always exceeds the supply by a wide margin, their distribution is invariably controversial. Efforts to ease the allocation crunch and save more lives by procuring additional organs only provoke additional controversies.

Policies and proposals designed to cope with these two problems often grate against our established opinions about what is fair, right, or even morally legitimate. When this happens, in the way that a knife held to a grindstone shoots off sparks, fiery ethical and social questions pepper the air.

Cases and Discussions

I set out in the following chapters to explore, explain, and (to the extent I can) resolve a handful of these questions. I begin each chapter as I began this one—by presenting a case showing how various ethical and policy issues about transplantation arise out of the circumstances.

The cases aren't all of a kind. Most are factual narratives of actual cases, but a few are pure fiction. The fiction is necessary, because one case is an account of an activity currently illegal, while two others portray a possible future. Another couple of cases are based on actual ones but are composites, compounding people and details from several sources. But no apples are put forward as oranges, and the status of each fictionalized or amalgamated case is explicitly indicated.

Why mess around with cases at all? Why not just state the basic questions up front, then deal with them? Because issues about transplants are issues about people and how we're going to treat them. Cases thus remind us not to forget the personal and emotional dimension underlying the often arid discussions of the abstract issues of transplant ethics.

"Should younger people be given priority in organ distribution?" becomes more real and pressing when we remember Robby and Marge sitting in a hospital room, the LVAD thumping, racing against the clock to get the heart needed to save Robby's life. Robby is 48 years old, old enough that many younger candidates would take precedence over him. But is he less entitled to a chance at extending his life than somebody half his age? Maybe or maybe not, but we have to keep Robby in mind.

Cases also remind us that the world is a factually complex and morally enigmatic scene of action. Issues don't come neatly packaged but must be mined out of the factual mire, then framed in a way they can be usefully addressed.

Do the good intentions of researchers justify their decisions about how to treat their patients? The answer depends on the specifics and circumstances of particular cases. Good intentions may count, but when they are a substitute for good medical judgment, they most certainly don't justify actions. While principles are crucial, details are necessary to apply them. Cases provide details and allow subtlety and shading.

I offer in the second part of each chapter a discussion of the major issue raised in the introductory case. The discussion isn't tendered as a commentary on the case. Rather, the case prompts and motivates an analysis of the questions, policies, and problems that I discuss afterward.

I present in the discussion opposing viewpoints and relevant factual information, including any necessary medical, scientific, or historical background. But I don't try to provide a textbook review of all aspects of a problem. Nor do I restrict myself to a journalistic on the one hand-and-now-on the other approach. I focus attention on a central issue in each chapter, take a position on it, and do my best to make my view convincing.

I'd like to see some changes made. Sometimes the only changes I want are in people's attitudes, but in most instances I favor altering some accepted practice or adopting a new policy regulating organ transplantation.

A Handful of Claims

I argue for a handful of claims in this book, not for a single thesis. The thread that strings the chapters together is a concern for people.

Those sick from the end-stage diseases whom we have the power to cure by a transplant deserve our deepest concern. We have a prima facie obligation to shape policies and practices to save their lives. We must make sure we don't let our discomfort in talking about death or our squeamishness about bodies keep us from securing organs that could save lives.

Yet we must do what we can to help the sick without taking advantage of the weak. We must protect the family member who agrees to be a kidney donor only because she thinks the family expects her to. We need to make sure a researcher's enthusiasm doesn't produce false hope and lead a desperate parent to consent to a pointless treatment.

The trick we must pull off in our practices and policies is to find ways of protecting people from exploitation, while also doing our best to save the lives of those who will die without an organ transplant.

I'VE WRITTEN the following chapters as if I were having a series of conversations with an intelligent and interested person—the reader. Thus they're written for bakers and bricklayers as much as for ethicists and attorneys, stockclerks and stockbrokers, surgeons and scientists. I've thus made it a point to avoid jargon and to provide only enough technical information to make issues clear.

The topics generated by the realities and possibilities of organ transplantation are, I believe, inherently compelling. I've tried to frame them in interesting and helpful ways. But I've never assumed readers would need to agree with the views I defend in order to enjoy the book.

2

Mickey Mantle's Liver, Part 1

The Case

Mickey Mantle telephoned his son David from his north Dallas home on the morning of May 28, 1995, and asked David to drive him to Baylor Medical Center on the east side.

Mantle was 63 years old and had been suffering severe stomach pains for weeks. The previous five days he'd spent doubled up in bed, convulsed by nausea and dry heaves, and feeling too sick to move.

Pain and illness weren't new experiences for Mantle. As a teenager in the 1940s he'd been kicked in the left shin during football practice and had developed chronic osteomyelitis, an infection of the bone. His leg abscessed, swelling to a grotesque size and turning blackish purple. His temperature soared to 104 degrees, and the hospital doctors wanted to amputate his leg. His mother refused to authorize the surgery and transferred him to a second hospital, where he was treated with the new drug penicillin.

The infection eventually cleared, but Mantle's leg was permanently weakened, and it bothered him throughout his career. He was also kept in constant pain by damage to both knees, as well as suffering over the years from a hip infection, recurrent stomach ulcers, an injured left shoulder, and an inguinal hernia. But this time was different.

The pain and nausea were unremitting, and his abdomen was swollen to twice its normal size, distended like an overinflated beach ball. His skin had also changed color, turning a deep yellowish-orange, the shade of a overripe pumpkin. Even his eyes had taken on a yellow tinge.

David Mantle realized his father was a very sick man.

Sports Hero

Mickey Mantle in 1995 was a baseball icon. One of the immortals of the game, he was in the pantheon that included Babe Ruth, Joe Dimaggio, Jackie Robinson, Stan Musial, and Willie Mays. He'd become a sports superstar before the word had been invented, and he maintained that status for more than four decades. If anything, his stature had grown over the years.

Leaving Commerce, Oklahoma, in 1951 and moving to Manhattan to join the New York Yankees, with two shirts and a pastel sports coat packed in a cardboard suitcase, Mantle was the embodiment of the country boy coming to the big city. But far from making him a figure of fun, his rural background and unpretentious ways endeared him to millions of fans. When his talent began to shine, his naiveté and natural modesty became part of his charm.

Mantle's achievements in baseball were stunning. In 1956, when only 24, he led the American League in batting average (.353), home runs (52), and runs batted in (130), winning him the League's Triple Crown. The first Yankee player to hit more than fifty home runs since Babe Ruth, he was voted Most Valuable Player in 1956 and again in 1957.

Mantle and his teammate Roger Maris competed in 1961 to break Babe Ruth's single-season record of sixty home runs. Mantle was sidelined for two weeks by a hip infection and finished with fifty-four. Maris, on the last day of the season, hit his sixty-first homer. Mantle had been the public's favorite to break the record, but he downplayed his own disappointment and expressed nothing but delight at Maris's success.

Such generosity toward his teammates characterized Mantle's sports career. "If I could have one thing on my tombstone," he once said, "I wouldn't want, 536 home runs. I'd rather have, 'He was a great friend and teammate.'"

Mantle flared out like a lightning flash in the Yankee lineup when baseball was extending its audience in the 50s and 60s. The flickering images of black and white television made Yankee Stadium, Ebbets Field, and Fenway Park as familiar as the local ballpark throughout the country, and players were welcomed into the nation's living rooms. Reading newspaper accounts of games by Ring Lardner or listening to radio commentaries by Red Barber had been engaging, but nothing could compete with the primal power of seeing things for yourself. Watching a player's every move and facial expression on the field was both more involving and more personal.

Television made Mantle accessible, and his self-deprecating, easygoing manner made his fans feel he was a friend. His blond, boyish good looks deepened his appeal. A steady stream of interviews, gossip pieces, and even cameo roles in movies further strengthened the bond fans established with him.

Mantle retired from baseball in 1968 and was elected to the Baseball Hall of Fame in 1974. He never really left baseball, though, and his fans didn't forget him. He never felt he deserved the tremendous affection they lavished on him, and only toward the end of his life did he even value it.

Like Elvis Presley, James Dean, Marilyn Monroe, and a handful of others, Mantle helped define what it meant to grow up in the 1950s and 1960s. He was a part of the excitement of adolescence and of the promise of what adulthood might bring. Even the name *Mickey Mantle* and the nickname *the Mick* hinted at escaping from boredom into a world of fun and excitement. But kids weren't the only ones who lived some of their dreams by associating them with sports celebrities. Mantle's spirit of careless freedom appealed to everybody.

Mantle entered Baylor Hospital without publicity. But once the public learned he was sick, every change in his condition and every decision of his doctors became a matter of intense concern. Some of that concern, as information about his condition and treatment emerged, was transformed into outright hostility, however. For the first time in his career, Mantle became the target of a surprising amount of anger and disapproval.

Diagnosis

The doctors at Baylor immediately began to investigate Mantle's condition. Daniel DeMarco and Kent Hamilton, both gastroenterologists, recognized that the yellowing of Mantle's skin and eyes was jaundice caused by the failure of his liver to metabolize bilirubin, a breakdown product of red blood cells. The swelling of his abdomen resulted from the accumulation of fluid called ascites, another telltale sign of a poorly performing liver.

A kidney function test showed Mantle's failing liver was also affecting his kidneys. Urea and other waste products ordinarily cleared from the blood by the kidneys had been slowly accumulating, and he was on the verge of slipping into a coma.

Mantle was diagnosed as having end-stage liver disease.

Sobriety

A year and a half earlier, in January 1994, Mantle had signed himself into the Betty Ford Clinic in Palm Springs, California and spent the next thirty-two days working through the clinic's twelve-step program for ending alcohol addiction. Inspired by the success of his son Danny at the clinic, he'd been determined to quit drinking, and he'd succeeded.

The treatment put an end to a forty-three-year love affair with alcohol. His drinking career had long been punctuated by episodes of reckless driving, car wrecks, quarrels, and embarrassing public scenes. But over the preceding decade his drinking had also come to be accompanied by confusion, memory loss, and complete blackouts. Then came the abdominal pains, nausea, ascites, and jaundice.

Mantle's private physician, Dr. Arthur DeLarios, had cautioned him several times that his drinking was ruining his liver, but Mantle failed to sense urgency in the warning. He always figured he'd cut back later. But the physicians who tested him at Betty Ford were more emphatic and explicit than DeLarios.

They told him he'd already developed alcoholic cirrhosis so advanced he was likely to need a liver transplant within a few years. "I'm not going to lie to you," one doctor said. "The next drink you take may be your last."

Mantle heeded the warning and stopped drinking. He succeeded in staying completely alcohol free. But by the time he stopped, it was too late to reverse the damage to his liver that his decades of drinking had caused.

Worse News

Bad as it was for Mantle to learn he had end-stage liver disease, he was to get even worse news. A CT scan revealed a tumor in the center of his liver. More tests were performed. CT scans, MRIs, and ultrasound examinations were made of his chest and abdomen, then a complete bone scan was performed. While the liver tumor was assumed to be malignant, none of the tests yielded evidence suggesting the presumed cancer had spread.

A blood test for alphafetoprotein (AFP), a substance produced in the fetal liver but made also by liver cancers, was compatible with this conclusion. Mantle's AFP level measured 2,400 micrograms per liter, and any level above 400 is considered abnormal. But cirrhosis and hepatitis C can also cause AFP levels to rise. Thus, the finding of an elevated AFP level was too unspecific for Mantle's doctors to conclude that if he had cancer, it had metastasized.

The imaging studies showed the growing tumor in Mantle's liver had compressed his common bile duct, the tube carrying the secretion to the upper end of the small intestine. The close association of the tumor and the duct made DeMarco and Hamilton suspect the tumor was a cancer that might have invaded the tissues. Using a fiber-optic instrument and x-ray tests, they looked into Mantle's bile duct but found no signs of cancer. What they did discover was that his bile duct was infected with bacteria and fungi. Its blockage by the tumor had turned it into a dead-end tube, thus making it a protected breeding ground for micro-organisms. Prompted by this finding, DeMarco and Hamilton performed a follow-up CT scan and discovered Mantle's liver was riddled with pockets of pus. As if this were not enough, they also found it was infected with the Hepatitis C virus. Mantle may have acquired the infection decades earlier from a transfusion with contaminated blood during one of the several operations performed on his knees.

Chronic hepatitis C infections are known to be a risk factor in the development of liver cancer. Mantle's infection "probably isn't lifestyle," Hamilton said later. "It's bad luck." His suggestion was that Mantle's years of drinking may have had little to do with his developing liver cancer. Yet critics of the decisions made by the Baylor group soon pointed out that alcoholic cirrhosis also predisposes people to liver cancer.

Listed for Transplant

Mantle was in bed and barely conscious when DeMarco and Hamilton informed him that his medical condition was so serious that a liver transplant offered the only possibility for extending his life.

Mantle remained silent a moment as he listened to the news. He then lifted his head from his pillow and pulled himself together. "I'm a fighter," he told his doctors. "I want to do whatever we have to do. It goes back to my days as a ballplayer. I never give up."

On June 6, 1995, Mantle's doctors contacted the United Network for Organ Sharing (UNOS) and supplied the information about Mantle's medical condition necessary to enter his name on the waiting list for a donor liver. UNOS, according to its policy, then assigned Mantle a numerical ranking determined by the medical urgency, his blood group, and time on the waiting list.

Mantle was classified as Status 2, the second highest rank in the priority ordering. Patients in this category were those hospitalized and undergoing treatment to keep them stable. The only ones ranked higher were those requiring intensive care, on life-support, and expected to die within a week without a transplant. Mantle's doctors believed he could be stabilized for two or three weeks.

Factors other than the medical condition of the patients on the waiting list would also play a role in determining who would get the next donor liver when it became available.

Unlike kidneys, livers aren't matched by tissue types, but they must have a blood type compatible with the recipient's. They must also be of the proper physical size. So a donor liver that is ABO blood group-incompatible or a poor size match for an intended recipient will be offered to the next candidate on the list.

Similarly, because organs begin to deteriorate when they lose their blood supply, there's a limit to how long a liver remains useable after it's removed. Preservation techniques can extend, but not eliminate, this limit, which is about twelve hours at the outside. Thus, if a donor is so far away from the intended recipient that the transport time would compromise the quality of the organ, the liver will go to a patient closer at hand, even if the patient's medical condition isn't as urgent or the patient hasn't been waiting as long.

Because transplantable vital organs are both potentially life-saving and extremely scarce, the guiding principle behind distribution policies is to avoid wasting them.

Baylor

The liver transplant program at Baylor Medical Center in 1995 was the third largest in the nation. It was also one of the most successful. Some 85 percent of its recipients survived for at least one year after transplant, and 70 percent survived for at least five years.

The head of the program was Dr. Goran Klintmalm, a 44-year-old Swedish-American recognized internationally for his surgical skills and research soundness. Educated at the prestigious Karolinska Institute in Stockholm, he received specialty training in surgery at the University of Pittsburgh under the direction of Thomas Starzl, who pioneered the development of liver transplants.

Klintmalm returned to Sweden, but in 1984 he received a call from Starzl asking if he was interested in heading a new liver transplant program being established at Baylor in Dallas. Klintmalm accepted the position, and the Baylor unit, the first in the Southwest, quickly became one of the world's leading liver transplant centers.

Klintmalm didn't become Mantle's transplant surgeon, though. That job fell to the program's Assistant Director, Robert Goldstein. In Baylor's rotation scheme, Goldstein was scheduled to take the next patient accepted for transplant, and that patient happened to be Mantle. Klintmalm, however, along with other members of the group, participated in making decisions about Mantle's care.

Goldstein violated the stereotype of the austere academic surgeon. The son of a wealthy Tennessee textile manufacturer, he was a college dropout who eventually returned to become an honors student. Planning to pursue his passion for plants by studying for a Ph.D. in botany at the University of Wisconsin, he decided at the last minute to go to medical school. When his chosen specialty of pediatrics became boring, he turned to surgery.

Goldstein was selected to become a surgical fellow under Starzl at Pittsburgh, but when the promised position didn't materialize, Starzl shipped him off to Baylor to work with Klintmalm. Goldstein found his calling at last in transplant medicine, and he soon established a reputation as an outstandingly skillful surgeon who operated almost as fast as Klintmalm himself.

Goldstein also broke the medical dress code. As well as letting his curly brown hair grow to shoulder length, he wore open-toed sandals and avoided neckties. Until his marriage, he had played the role of hospital heartthrob, partying whenever possible and driving around in a black Lexus with fuzzy pink dice hanging from the rearview mirror. When working, he kept his long hair tied back in a ponytail. "I'm not sure why," Mantle's wife Merlyn later wrote, "but . . . I found that sign of independence reassuring."

June 6

Six days after Mantle entered Baylor, the hospital held a press conference to report on his condition. But Mantle's physicians weren't free to be completely candid in their statements. They could say he needed a transplant but not that he had liver cancer. Mantle had made clear he didn't want anyone but his family and close friends to know how very sick he was. A sports hero for so long, he couldn't stand becoming the object of public pity. He also didn't want reporters mounting a death watch at the hospital, anticipating bulletins chronicling his declining condition.

"If he doesn't get a liver in a couple or three weeks, he's going to die," gastroenterologist Kent Hamilton announced to reporters. "The alcohol and the hepatitis C were a witches' brew" that destroyed his liver.

Robert Goldstein told the press that Mantle might last three to four weeks, but "his condition could change at any time." Even with a liver transplant, Goldstein said, "it will be very difficult for him, but I feel comfortable he will survive."

The physicians' public remarks hardly reflected unbridled optimism, but the reality was worse. Even while the press conference was taking place, Mantle was slipping into a coma. Some of his doctors thought that without a new liver, he might not live another forty-eight hours. From being stable, he might suddenly crash, plunging into kidney and heart failure.

Alcoholism

Mantle's physicians were forthright about the contribution made by his decades of drinking to his liver problems. "There is no doubt that his lifestyle has played a part in his condition today," Goldstein said. "Maybe people should reconsider their drinking habits, as Mickey has pointed out."

Goldstein was referring to the newly abstinent Mantle's recent efforts to motivate people to get help with their alcohol problems. Before he got sick, in interviews in front of the television cameras Mantle would jerk a thumb at himself and say, "Here's a role model for you. Don't be like me."

Mantle had tried to come to some understanding of his own alcoholism in a journal he kept at the Betty Ford Clinic. For most of his life, he wrote, drinking "was part of the camaraderie, the male bonding thing."

It was also something people did to have fun. Mantle came of age in the postwar era of the 40s and 50s, a time when people out on the town often drank until they staggered, became incoherent, or even passed out and had to be carried home. It was a time when hard drinking was an even bigger part of partying than now. "I drank because we were having a good time," Mantle said.

Mantle's drinking increased every year he was with the Yankees, even though it rarely affected his performance. It was after he retired at the end of the 1968 season and his life seemed to have lost its purpose that his alcohol consumption soared and became an essential part of his daily life. "When he stopped hitting home runs, the only time he had any self-esteem was after a drink or two," Merlyn wrote in a family memoir.

Mantle, by the late 80s, would start drinking at lunch and continue into the night. "The weeks, months, and years began to blur," he wrote in his rehab journal. With age, he lost his resilience, and his hangovers lasted two or three days. His health deteriorated. He developed stomach ulcers and became malnourished, the result of a poorly balanced diet.

While Mantle felt more relaxed when he drank, he wasn't a mellow drunk. He turned loud, obnoxious, and rude. During his ballplaying career, he disliked fans and, even while signing autographs, often insulted them in the crudest terms. He got into squabbles, drove recklessly, and smashed up cars. Merlyn was almost decapitated when she was riding with him and he crashed into a telephone pole. Still, the police rarely gave him a ticket. He was Mickey Mantle, after all.

Family

Mantle neglected his wife and four sons to the point of cruelty. Merlyn, who stuck with him from their high-school days in Oklahoma to the end of his life, wrote that he "treated marriage as he did most things, a sort of party with added attractions." He made little effort to hide his numerous affairs from Merlyn and in 1980 walked out on her. He moved into an apartment, then built a house for himself. "I didn't stop loving her," he said. "I just got tired of making excuses, of having to explain myself."

Mantle was no more than a shadowy presence in the early lives of his sons, Mickey, Jr., Danny, David, and Billy. He was somewhere else when each was born. Three times he was missing because of his baseball obligations and once because he was out hunting with his friend Billy Martin.

He didn't become close to his sons until they were old enough to become his drinking buddies. "I didn't even know him until we started drinking together," Danny, the third son, recalled. "For him drinking with us was a way of reliving his days with Billy Martin and Whitey Ford." The entire family became alcoholics.

"I think it's fair to say Mom raised us," Danny said in his part of the family memoir. "There wasn't a whole lot of what passed for family life— we didn't make a big deal out of birthdays. Holidays were usually spent intoxicated."

Mantle's distant relationship with his sons was the opposite of his father's focus on him. When Mickey was 4, Mutt Mantle, an Oklahoma zinc miner, began preparing his son for a baseball career. Mutt had the almost obsessive dream that his son would become a professional ballplayer, and he would pitch to Mickey for hours, training him to become the greatest switch-hitter in the history of the game.

Mantle was devoted to his father and wanted nothing more than to please him, to coax from him a few grudging words of approval. But Mantle had no dreams for his own sons and took no interest in their lives or ambitions. He regretted this indifference late in his life. "Mickey, Jr. could have been a major league baseball player if my dad had been his dad," he wrote in his rehabilitation journal.

By the time of his illness, none of Mantle's sons had started careers of their own. Instead, they joined their father in the business of marketing and exploiting his celebrity. In addition to helping him with his speaking engagements, autograph signings, and restaurant franchise, they took part in the fantasy baseball games that, for $4,000, offered clients the opportunity to play on a team with Mickey Mantle.

Mantle had expected to die young, by 40 at the latest. Hodgkin's disease, a cancer of the lymphatic tissue, had killed his grandfather at that age and his father at 39. But it was his son Billy who fell prey to the disease.

Billy woke up one morning in 1977 with a swollen lymph node in his neck. The node was removed and biopsied the same day. It was found to contain malignant cells, and Billy, who was 19, started chemotherapy immediately.

Treatment drove Billy's cancer into remission, but it returned in 1981. Tests showed it had spread from the lymph nodes to his liver and bone marrow. He entered an experimental protocol in Houston and for six months shuttled between Dallas and Houston with different forms of treatment at each end. He again went into remission, but he had become dependent on Dilaudid, a narcotic painkiller.

Billy's addiction led him into a downward spiral.

Arrested for drunk driving in 1994, he was locked up in the Dallas County jail. After he complained of chest pains during the night, police officers escorted him to Parkland Hospital the next morning. The group was walking down the hall of Parkland when Billy clutched at his chest and collapsed. He was rushed to the emergency room, but it was too late. He was dead of a heart attack.

Mantle turned inward and kept his feelings to himself even more after Billy was diagnosed with Hodgkin's. While he always felt guilty about it, he left taking care of Billy over the years to Merlyn. "I never felt I was there for him when it mattered," Mantle wrote, looking back.

Billy died three months after his father completed the Betty Ford program, but Mantle didn't go back to drinking. He felt he'd turned his life around at last, and, although filled with regrets, he was looking forward to developing a closer relationship with his family. He didn't expect to be teetering on the edge of death while waiting for a donor liver.

The Donor

Late in the evening of Wednesday, June 7, Jeff Place, a Baylor spokesman, released the news that a donor liver might have been found for Mantle. If the liver was examined, tested, and found compatible, the transplant could take place on Thursday.

The anonymous donor had died that afternoon in a small town near Dallas. He was a young man, popular and athletic, somebody still deciding what he wanted to do with his life.

He was also a hero in his own right.

A week before his death, he was water-skiing with friends at a nearby lake when a man trying to swim to a small island started going under, unable to complete the distance. The donor, a trained lifeguard, swam out from shore, got a grip on the sinking man, then towed him back to safety.

The drowning swimmer lived, but his rescuer didn't. About a week later, while he was getting ready to leave for work, a blood vessel in his brain burst. The bleeding from the ruptured aneurysm couldn't be brought under control, and the young man died at a local hospital that same afternoon.

His family decided to donate his organs. "We thought we might as well make something good come out of our tragedy," his mother said. Six people had their lives extended by that generous decision, including a truck driver, a farm manager, a resort operator, and an electrical lineman.

Mickey Mantle was in line to be the sixth.

The donor's liver turned out to be in good condition and a match for both size and blood type. Thus, less than forty-eight hours after Mantle's name was put on the UNOS transplant list, the liver he needed was available.

Favoritism?

Baylor's announcement that Mantle was getting a donor liver triggered a fusillade of criticism. The noise of it still echoes today in public and academic discussions of waiting times and how donor organs ought to be distributed.

The first and loudest complaint was that Mantle's celebrity status had bumped him to the front of the transplant queue. Rather than waiting his turn like an ordinary citizen, he'd been given preferential treatment. He'd hardly been assessed for a liver transplant before he was getting one.

An unusual occurrence, people said. And suspicious.

The phone lines at Southwest Organ Bank in Dallas, the regional agency responsible for procuring and distributing donor organs, were soon jammed with calls protesting favoritism for celebrities. Almost no one who spoke out publicly was inclined to believe Mantle had come by his liver fairly. "It's who you are that counts, not what you need" was the invariant theme of the protests.

The outrage was nationwide, expressed not only in angry phone calls, but in letters to local newspapers and on radio talk shows. "I am a liver transplant patient, but I had to wait over eleven months for mine," a man in Kentucky wrote in a letter to the editor. A caller to Los Angeles's KMPC claimed that as a result of Mantle's special treatment, another person would likely have to pay the price. "Somebody else is probably going to die, . . . because Mickey got the liver because of who he is."

The public was primed to think of favoritism in connection with Mantle because of recent news about other well-known people getting needed organs quickly. Two years earlier, in 1993, Governor Robert Casey of Pennsylvania received a new heart and lungs in less than twenty-four hours, although the median waiting time was 208 days. The next year rock singer David Crosby got a donor liver after only eighteen days, then actor Jim Nabors got one in twenty-four. And now here was Mickey Mantle getting a liver before the news he needed a transplant had quite sunk in.

One critic put the charge against Mantle succinctly in a letter to the *Washington Post*:

> Extremely ill but anonymous children and adults wait many long
> months for a vitally needed organ: many of them die. But a governor,
> a folk singer, a retired baseball player and other "prominents" have
> measured their waiting time in days or weeks.

Reporters unwittingly encouraged the belief that Mantle was getting special treatment merely by mentioning that whereas the national waiting time for a liver transplant was more than four months (130–140 days), Mantle had waited hardly more than a day. How could such a huge discrepancy be fair?

Mantle was stung by the criticism and always turned snappish when journalists asked him if he'd received special treatment. "People think I got that liver because of who I am, but they have rules they go by," he told a writer for the *New York Daily News*.

A Biased Decision?

A second blast of complaint came from transplant professionals and ethicists. They charged Klintmalm, Goldstein, and the other members of the Baylor transplant team with making a bad decision in going forward with Mantle's transplant after discovering he had liver cancer.

People with end-stage liver disease caused by cirrhosis are predisposed to hepatoma (hepatocellular carcinoma), a rapidly spreading and almost invariably fatal form of cancer. About 15 to 20 percent of those with cirrhosis are discovered to have a hepatoma when surgeons remove their livers and biopsy them. When the tumors are too small to be detected until found incidentally by the pathologist after the cirrhotic liver has been removed, those who get transplants do about as well as other recipients.

But some patients like Mantle diagnosed with hepatoma before surgery may have cancer that has already spread microscopically outside the liver. In these cases, it will almost certainly recur, even after the cancerous liver is replaced.

"In the world's experience, the majority of these patients rapidly manifest a recurrence in the new liver or metastases in other sites of the body," said Norman Gitlin, a liver expert at Emory University. "There is minimal advantage to the patient," and given the pressing need for donor livers, "we see no justification for transplanting such a patient."

Some critics suggested Klintmalm and the Baylor team, in considering whether Mantle's cancer had spread, had given him the benefit of the doubt because he was a celebrity. Some said Klintmalm had approved the transplant because he wanted to attract attention to the Baylor program. Transplanting Mantle would be good publicity.

Undeserving?

A third criticism, made forcefully and repeatedly by the public, was that because Mantle was an alcoholic, he didn't *deserve* a liver transplant.

This complaint was directed toward Mantle in a personal way by remarks indicting his character and the free-wheeling, fraternity-party lifestyle he'd lived for decades. He had destroyed his liver by more than forty years of hard drinking. Thus, because he'd caused his own problem, people said, he should have to accept the consequences. He had sown the wind, so he ought to reap the whirlwind.

"It's his fault," a 28-year-old woman told Lauri Goodstein of the *Washington Post*. "He drank himself into oblivion. Everyone knows drinking will kill your liver."

Sports reporters recalled the banter between Mantle and his drinking pal Billy Martin about whose liver would fail first. Mantle had understood where his drinking was likely to lead, but he hadn't stopped. Even when Martin died in an alcohol-related truck accident, Mantle continued to drink. "That Mickey's a bum, man," a caller to a radio talk show said. "He was a drunk."

Some critics pointed out that by giving Mantle a donor liver, somebody else was made to pay for his poor judgment. "He's a loser," a caller to KMPC said. "He shouldn't have gotten that liver. It should've went to someone who really deserved it."

Transplant

Early in the morning of Thursday, June 8, around four o'clock, Mantle was transported to the operating room. Sedated, weak, and almost comatose, as his stretcher was being wheeled down the hall from his suite, he suddenly lifted his head and said, "Good. Let's get it done."

The surgery lasted more than six hours. Several years earlier Mantle had undergone surgery to remove his gall bladder, and as a result, scar tissue had grown over the organs in his abdomen. To get to Mantle's liver and free it from its connections, Dr. Goldstein had to cut carefully and tediously through the tough, fibrous layers of tissue and exercise considerable care to keep from nicking any of the varices or bloated blood vessels found in those with liver disease. Such a misstep and his patient might bleed to death.

Once Mantle's liver was exposed, Goldstein examined it and found it was swollen, rock-hard, and nodular—an appearance entirely consistent with alcoholic cirrhosis.

Goldstein saw nothing to suggest Mantle's cancer had spread to other abdominal organs. Following established procedure, he removed several lymph nodes for biopsy. He then waited while the nodes were flash-frozen, sliced into sections, and examined microscopically by the hospital's pathologists. If they detected malignant cells in the lymph nodes, this would be presumptive evidence the cancer was not limited to the liver and that its cells had already disseminated to other parts of the body.

In case of such an event, Mantle wouldn't get a transplant. He would be sewn up, his old liver untouched, and left to die quickly from his end-stage disease. No further treatment would be useful.

The Baylor transplant team had anticipated the possibility of finding a malignant node. A second patient in the hospital was put on standby status. If metastatic cancer ruled out Mantle as a transplant recipient, the liver would go to her.

But Mantle's lymph nodes turned out to be clean. The pathologist's report on frozen sections showed no evidence of metastatic cancer. The transplant doctors accepted this as confirming that the cancer was confined to his liver.

He was thus good to go for transplant.

More Bad News

Only after Goldstein had removed Mantle's liver did the situation take a turn for the worse. The pathologists examined the liver, and although they found only one cancerous node associated with it, they discovered malignant cells inside the connecting blood vessels and the common bile duct.

"That's when we had our first hint," Klintmalm later said, that Mantle's prospects for recovery weren't optimistic. The discovery suggested critics might be right in believing it was pointless to give a new liver to someone diagnosed with liver cancer before surgery. Yet the malignant cells were found in structures on the underside of the liver, which meant no test could have revealed them until after the liver was removed.

The transplant proceeded as planned.

Quick Fix

The next morning, Friday, June 9, Mantle was wheeled back into the OR. Too much blood was trickling from his abdominal drainage tubes. That, plus his need for four pints of transfused blood and an elevated heart rate, suggested he was bleeding internally. Maybe it was a torn blood vessel or simply a leaky attachment. About one in twenty patients required a second operation to deal with internal bleeding, a hospital representative told the press.

Goldstein discovered that a small clot under the donor liver had broken loose, allowing blood to seep out. He sealed the leak with a single stitch. "It was a very minor problem, more what you would characterize as a nuisance," he said afterward. "The more prominent someone is, the more likely something is to happen."

Postoperative Course

The following day, Saturday, June 10, Mantle was awake and alert enough to watch television reports about his condition. When his breathing tube had been pulled before nine that morning, Goldstein asked him what he thought about the transplant.

"Incredible," Mantle whispered.

The donor liver was working well. Mantle's jaundice began to disappear, and his kidney function returned to normal. The fluid that had accumulated in his abdomen had been drained away, and he was back to his usual size. "The most acute danger seems to have passed," Klintmalm told reporters. Mantle's next challenge would be to cope with the risk that his body would reject the new liver.

Even on Saturday, his first postoperative day, Mantle was able to weave his way from his bed to the bathroom and to sit up in a chair. That afternoon he watched baseball on TV with Mickey, Jr., David, and Danny. His three sons had been taking turns sleeping on the sofa bed in the sitting room of his suite so someone would always be with him.

Mantle was started on a regimen of antirejection drugs to protect his new liver and high-dose chemotherapy to treat his cancer. The combination was considered a bad one. The drugs used to control rejection suppressed his immune response, and this could permit the proliferation of the cancer cells the chemotherapy was supposed to eliminate. Mantle experienced an episode of organ rejection that Klintmalm described as "light." It was quickly ended by treatment with steroids.

Discharge, Readmission

Goldstein discharged Mantle from Baylor Medical Center on June 28, exactly a month after he'd called his son David and asked for help getting to the hospital. He remained an outpatient, however, returning to Baylor regularly for chemotherapy sessions and visits to the transplant surgeons.

Mantle was weak but able to get around and in no pain. He worked to gain his strength back. He drove himself to his country club every day and had a light lunch. This was followed by a few minutes on the treadmill, then a period of recovery in the sauna. He would then drive home and watch TV, too exhausted to do much else for the rest of the day.

He didn't follow a steady course of improvement. The high-dose chemotherapy reduced the production of red blood cells, leading to anemia. His weight dropped from 208 pounds to 170, and he suffered weakness and fatigue. He was treated with a series of seven blood transfusions.

The drug cisplatin was added to his chemotherapy regimen in an effort to prevent any remaining cancer cells from proliferating. The drug made him nauseated, and he checked into Baylor for a second time so he could be treated for the side-effects.

Mantle's physical appearance had undergone a startling change since his first admission. No longer robust and fit, the very image of a professional athlete, he looked pale and shrunken, diminished by his disease. His baseball cap seemed too large for his head, sliding down to the tops of his now more protuberant ears. It was as if over the course of a few weeks he'd aged many years.

Mantle's outgoing, high-spirited manner had altered as well. "He is in a very reflective mood," his lawyer and close friend Roy True told a reporter. "In all the years I've known him, I've never seen him think so hard about life."

He also began to realize that he was alive only because he was lucky enough to have received a donor liver. His transplant raised his awareness of the pressing need for organ donors, and whenever he spoke in public he made a point of encouraging people to sign donor cards. Unsatisfied with such occasional efforts, however, he began to plan some sort of regular recruitment program.

The publicity surrounding Mantle's transplant had dramatic and long-lasting results on donor recruitment. Southwest Organ Bank, the regional procurement organization, reported a rise in requests for donor cards from twelve a week to 700.

"We've sent out thousands of donor cards since Mantle's transplant," Alison Smith, Southwest's director, told the Associated Press. "There is no other event that has occurred that would explain the increased interest."

Worst News

Responding to pressure from the media to provide more information about his condition, Mantle and his doctors held a press conference on July 11. Dr. Goldstein explained why Mantle had been given blood transfusions and how his violent reactions to cisplatin had brought him back to Baylor. The transplant itself, he said, was doing all right, with no signs of rejection.

"Hopefully," Goldstein said, "Mickey can become an example of someone given a second chance."

Mantle had been improving. His nausea and anemia had been brought under control, and he was gaining weight and feeling better. He was eager to play golf again, and he wanted to launch the donor-awareness program he'd come up with. "Mickey's Team," as he planned to call it, would use his slogan "Be a hero, be a donor," and he would tape a series of public service announcements urging people to join the "team."

The day after the press conference, five weeks after Mantle had received his new liver, his three sons and Roy True were in his hospital suite when Goldstein stopped by to deliver some awful news. The CT scans made routinely to monitor Mantle's condition revealed that cancer had spread to his lungs.

"At first Mick looked like he was surprised," True recalled. "And then he said simply, very simply, 'Well, let's just fix it like you did the other things.'"

The doctors tried.

Mantle went back to being an outpatient and continued his chemo-therapy. Then, after a couple of weeks, he began to have severe chest and abdominal pains. He stopped eating. He'd sit at the table and put food in his mouth, then be unable to force himself to swallow. He sustained him-self by drinking cans of liquid diet supplement.

Then on July 28, one month to the day after he was released with a new liver, Mantle again entered Baylor Hospital.

No public announcements were made about his condition, but rumors that he was dying were so persistent he felt the need to address them. Too weak to appear at another press conference, he taped a segment for the ABC program *Good Morning America* that was broadcast on August 1.

"I've been to the hospital for checkups every once in a while," Mantle told the TV audience, "and about two weeks ago, the doctors found a couple of spots of cancer in my lungs."

"Now I'm taking chemotherapy to get rid of the new cancer. I hope to get to feeling as good as when I first left here . . . ." Then he ended with his recruitment pitch. "If you'd like to do something really great, be a donor."

The day of the broadcast, Mantle's doctors, downcast and clearly shaken, confirmed to reporters that Mantle's cancer had spread. While refusing to make any predictions, they admitted a cure was too much to hope for. "For some," Goldstein said, "the chemotherapy has prolonged life two or three years."

Goldstein refused to say how much the recurrence of Mantle's cancer lowered his survival odds. "I never put patients into statistics," he said. "We have a fighting chance."

Despite Goldstein's reluctance to cite figures, reporters quickly uncov-ered them. They learned that nationally 81 percent of the 141 liver trans-plant patients whose cancer returned after treatment died within two years.

Goldstein might call such poor odds a "fighting chance," but physicians not involved in Mantle's care were almost brutally blunt in their assessment. "If he's got cancer in the lung, this is a terminal event, and the whole thing was an exercise in futility," Thomas Starzl, the pioneering liver transplant surgeon, said. "I think it's very sad."

Those who had accused Klintmalm and Goldstein of wasting a donor liver by giving it to someone diagnosed with liver cancer were turning out to be right. But could it have turned out otherwise? Were they right to give Mantle a chance?

Last Inning

Mantle's physicians put him on the most rigorous chemotherapy regimen they thought he could survive. But he was already on a downward spiral they couldn't alter, despite their frantic efforts.

On August 9, Denise Kile, a Baylor representative, announced that the hospital was downgrading Mantle's condition from *stable* to *serious*. Kile added, reminding the public of the attitude that had always characterized Mantle's sports career, "He wants his friends to know he continues to fight."

Outside experts expressed the opinion that now that Mantle's cancer had returned, chemotherapy was pointless. "You can throw some chemotherapy in, but you can't do much," said Gary M. Strauss, a specialist at the Dana-Farber Cancer Institute in Boston. This opinion was echoed by Gregory Curt, an oncologist at the National Cancer Institute. "Treatment at this stage would probably be tried to improve the quality of life, rather than aimed at increasing overall survival," he said.

Mantle's internist, Dr. DeLarios, had already called Mickey, Jr., and Danny and asked them to come to his office. He then showed them their father's x-rays and CT scans. The cancer had spread not only to Mantle's lungs, but to his pancreas and the lining of his heart. The transplanted liver had been ravaged by new tumors.

"What does this mean?" one of the sons asked.

"Ten days, two weeks tops," DeLarios said.

"You have to tell him," Danny said. "I can't do it."

They went to Mantle's hospital suite and DeLarios began to explain to Mantle how the cancer had spread.

"I'm not going to get better, right?" Mantle broke in.

"No," DeLarios said. "And in terms of time—"

"Thank you," Mantle said, cutting him off. "I don't want to know."

Mantle was by now heavily dosed with morphine to control his pain, and he drifted in and out of consciousness. "Why are you making me wait?" he mumbled once. Sometimes he was lucid, and to extend those periods he tried to go as long as possible without drugs. But despite his efforts, the time between doses grew shorter, slipping gradually from four hours to three. If a dose was skipped or delayed, the pain became unbearable.

Mantle kept telling his family he didn't want anybody to see him, that he didn't want sympathy. His once solid body began to waste away. His weight had already dropped from its usual 208 pounds to 170, but now it drifted down to a gaunt 140. His abdomen was bloated, his legs swollen, and his skin and eyes again turned an orangish-yellow. The jaundice had returned, and so had the signs of liver failure.

Mantle's sons began to call his old Yankee teammates to tell them that if they wanted to say goodbye, they would have to come soon. They began flying to Dallas from all over the country. Whitey Ford, Hank Bauer, Bobby Richardson, John Blanchard, and others all spent time with Mantle in his room. During their visits, he somehow found the strength to get out of bed and sit in a chair. He apologized for not being able to speak clearly and easily, but they brushed his apologies aside. "We just wanted to see you and say hi," they told him.

On August 12, Dr. DeLarios cancelled Mantle's chemotherapy session and told him the cancer had reached a point where it was no longer treatable.

"I'm sorry," DeLarios said. "There's nothing else we can do." Mantle again refused to listen to an estimate of how much time he had remaining.

"That was it," Roy True remembered. "He acted like he would live another twenty years."

The next day, half an hour after midnight, Mantle woke up and glanced at his wife Merlyn and his son David. He lifted his hands off the bed, and each took one. The three of them remained that way, holding hands, for the next forty minutes.

Mantle stopped breathing at ten minutes past one. The wavy line on the green EKG monitor flattened out, but no alarm sounded.

Three months after his liver transplant, Mantle was dead.

3

Mickey Mantle's Liver, Part 2

The Issues

It's not necessary to be a baseball fan to be moved by the spectacle of the rapid decline and death of such a vivid and engaging character as Mickey Mantle.

Mantle's story is preeminently a human one, and that he succeeded in staying sober after the death of his son, repented of his past behavior, and looked forward to developing closer relations with his family makes its sudden, sharp ending even more poignant. But touching as Mantle's story may be on the human level, the criticisms of the way Klintmalm and the Baylor group dealt with Mantle as a patient—as an organ transplant recipient—have barbed points.

Summarized, the criticisms raised three crucial questions:

1. Did Mantle get a liver so quickly because he was a celebrity?
2. When Mantle's doctors discovered he had liver cancer, did they show a bias in his favor in going ahead with the transplant?
3. Given that Mantle was an alcoholic, should he have been given a liver transplant at all?

Answering these questions is part of establishing an accurate account of a controversial public debate. But more important, answering them prompts us to examine the issues under dispute and consider what policies about transplantation we're prepared to endorse.

The questions concern Mantle, but I'll view them as personalized versions of ones about how donor livers *ought* to be allocated. While I'll limit the focus to livers, I could as easily focus on allocating hearts, kidneys, or lungs in much the same terms.

Waiting Time

News reports that Mantle was getting a new liver in less than forty-eight hours after being listed with UNOS often contrasted his waiting time with the national average of 130–140 days. This discrepancy, on its face, seemed conclusive evidence of special treatment for Mantle. Judging by the blast of hostility directed toward him, most people accepted it as such. They equated a short wait to celebrity favoritism.

But what the public, including most reporters, failed to realize was that the national average of waiting times (the 130–140 days) was essentially meaningless as an indicator of fairness. While people spoke of Mantle's time on *the* waiting list, in 1995 donor livers weren't allocated on the basis of a single national waiting list. (Nor are they yet.) Sentiment didn't begin to change in favor of such a list until 1999.

Allocation was (as the UNOS statement on Mantle put it) "administered first on a local basis, then regionally, then nationwide." The Baylor transplant surgeons followed UNOS policy in Mantle's case. He was Status 2, and as Joel Newman, UNOS's Assistant Director of Communication, recalled in a statement to me five years later, "A check of the allocation list showed that there were no local Status 1 liver patients, and that Mr. Mantle was the highest-ranked local patient for the organ offer."

While transplant centers were offered organs from the local area first, because of the scarcity of organs they also had to depend on getting ones from the wider geographical region. Thus, the region where a patient was registered was crucial in determining waiting times. With eleven UNOS-defined regions in the United States, this was like having *eleven* waiting lists, instead of one national one.

Some regions had much shorter waiting times than others. Dallas, in Region 4, had some of the shortest waits in the nation for livers. The patient with the most urgent need in Region 4 could expect to wait an average of only 3.3 days. Regions 9 and 2, which included New York and Pittsburgh respectively, had waiting times of several months. Thus, while a national average might be a useful measurement for operations of the transplant system, from the point of view of a particular patient the figure was misleading.

Pittsburgh and New York are in densely populated parts of the country that also have renowned transplant centers. For this reason, not only are there more people from their regions needing transplants, others come from all over the country to become patients. The demand for livers thus outstrips the local and regional supply, so organs must be sought from other regions.

Getting the needed organs was no problem in the early days of liver transplants during the 1970s and 1980s, when there were only a handful of centers nationwide. By 1995, though, there were 119 centers. The new centers wanted to keep the donor livers for their own use, and they were free to do so.

When a liver was donated, local centers, according to UNOS policy, had first call on its use. Organs that previously might have been flown to Pittsburgh were transplanted locally. Waiting times at the major centers became longer, but waiting times at centers in regions with few transplant programs could be very short.

The reason Baylor and Region 4 had such short waiting times was a direct result of the UNOS local-first policy. Also, neither Baylor nor other centers in the area were faced with the sheer number of patients that strained the resources of centers in Regions 2 and 9. Region 4 had a waiting list, but it was never as long as the waiting list for those regions.

The UNOS local-first policy also meant an organ procurement organization (OPO) was free to allocate a liver to a patient in a local transplant center, even when a patient in another region needed it more urgently. OPOs offered livers to other regions only when they had no patients for them. Most livers, by the late 90s, never left the region where they were donated. Often, they never even left the hospital.

By deciding to become a patient at Baylor, instead of going to a larger center, Mantle had unknowingly chosen a region with short waiting times. He then (again unknowingly) benefitted from the UNOS local-first policy. To get a donor liver, he didn't have to be the person with the most urgent need in the nation. He only had to be the person with the most urgent need in North Texas.

Mantle was correct in telling reporters he didn't get the liver because of who he was, because "they have rules they go by." The matching of a donor liver with a recipient was done by a UNOS computer program. It assigned each patient a numerical ranking on the local waiting list on the basis of what had been accepted for years as standard factors: urgency of need, blood type, organ size, and length of wait.

The "urgency of need" status requires a medical judgment about a patient's condition. While making such a judgment isn't as cut-and-dried as determining the other factors, the process isn't arbitrary. Criteria defining urgency are explicitly stated by UNOS, and evidence of their satisfaction must be documented in the patient's chart. Therefore, even if physicians should want to, it's not easy to manipulate the system by representing patients as sicker than they are. "We follow up" to make sure the patient meets the criteria, a representative of UNOS commented on Mantle's case. "This definitely takes place whenever a famous person is involved."

Perhaps the most compelling evidence that Mantle's celebrity status didn't get him a liver is that on the same day he received his transplant, the Southwest Organ Bank offered another, similar liver to New York University Medical Center. This meant no one in Region 4 was a suitable candidate. Thus, Mantle wasn't depriving anyone of a life-saving transplant.

Klintmalm had anticipated charges of favoritism and had wanted to avoid them. He later said that when he'd learned a donor liver was available for Mantle, "My first reaction was unspoken, 'Let's not do him. Let's see if we can do someone else,' to let him wait a few days to let people see that he is waiting like everyone else."

But Klintmalm decided it would be wrong to pass over Mantle. "Mick was extraordinarily sick," he recalled. "He was the only one here in North Texas waiting for a liver who was that sick. The donor liver was the right blood group. You cannot ethically deny a patient what may be the only chance he has, because you do not know if or when you will get another one."

Equating Mantle's short wait with favoritism because of his celebrity status has no discernible basis in fact, so far as I can determine. While Mantle was famous and rich, it was need and luck that got him a new liver so quickly.

Local First: Stacking the Deck

The widely accepted assumption that there was a national waiting list was a stick critics used to thrash Mantle. While this was unfair to Mantle, discussions of his case were useful in calling attention to definite shortcomings of the UNOS local-first policy, particularly with respect to livers.

The idea behind the policy is that charity begins at home, that organs donated locally should be allocated locally. Recruiting donors is easier, policy makers reasoned, when donors can be assured their organs are going to be used to help people in their own community, rather than shipped off to Pittsburgh or some other distant medical center.

Someone might reasonably believe she or a member of her family might benefit directly. If no one in the community needs the organs, then of course no one would object to their being used to help others.

A drawback of the policy is that it favors the wealthy or well-insured. Because they can pay the costs of being evaluated for a transplant at several different centers (at an expense of perhaps $10,000 per evaluation), they can be waitlisted at those centers. This gives them a better chance of getting organs the soonest.

A man needing a liver transplant who lives in New York might become a candidate at Columbia-Presbyterian Hospital, then fly to Dallas and be enrolled at Southwestern Medical Center. He might then move on to St. Louis and be waitlisted by Barnes-Jewish Hospital. These centers are in three separate regions, and the waiting times differ in each. By spending more money, the New Yorker could increase his chances of getting a liver in a shorter time than those listed only at Columbia-Presbyterian.

That multiple listings allow the well-off to stack the deck in their favor (even though the number of cases is small) was a factor fueling the demand to establish (something like) a national listing for liver candidates. Waiting times are particularly crucial for people needing a liver, because at present no machine can take over its functions.

People needing a kidney can rely on dialysis for an indefinite period, and those needing a heart replacement can be sustained by a partially implantable pump (a left-ventricular assist device or LVAD). Liver candidates are simply out of luck when their livers stop working, so reducing the wait may mean the difference between their living or dying.

But Not Sickest First

A second shortcoming of the local-first policy is that donor livers may not go to the people needing them most. Mantle was the patient in the Dallas area in most need of a liver, but was there someone in another region with a more urgent claim? Apparently not. But even if there had been, under the UNOS rules a qualified Status 1 patient in another region wouldn't have gotten the liver that went to Mantle.

It's this anomalous aspect of the local-first policy that disturbs critics the most. A man in New York might be on the edge of death, while the liver in Boston that would save his life goes to a woman who isn't critically ill and could safely wait another six months.

Defenders of the old policy aren't persuaded by such examples, however. Sicker people, they point out, have a higher mortality after transplant than healthier ones. Giving priority to the desperately ill may thus have the consequence of saving fewer lives overall. It fails to make the best use of a scarce commodity.

UNOS, in a recent move prompted by a directive from the Department of Health and Human Services, has changed its liver allocation policy. The new policy requires that when a donor liver becomes available, it go to the patient with the most urgent need, assuming the liver can be transported in acceptable condition. The revised policy (the details of which still haven't been worked out by UNOS) is thus a step toward something like a national waiting list.

Proponents of the new policy say it will save more lives, while critics charge it will mean the greatest number of organs will go to the larger transplant centers, because they have the largest number of patients in urgent need. A number of smaller centers will be forced to close, because they won't be able to get organs for their patients.

Some observers view this result positively, pointing out that not all the nation's current 278 centers do enough transplants to gain the experience needed to offer patients the best outcomes possible. Others see the new policy as nothing but a disguised power grab by the major centers, hoping to eliminate competition and scoop up patients. It's too early to see how this conflict is going to play out and whether the result will benefit patients.

Criteria at Centers

Some ethicists reinforced the public's perception that Mantle got special treatment by observing that his fame and money made it easy for Baylor to accept him as a candidate. "The way he ended up on the list," George Annas said, "was that his name was Mickey Mantle." Or as Arthur Caplan put the point, Mantle's celebrity "got him through the door."

Annas and Caplan weren't saying Mantle got to the top of the transplant list because of his fame and money, but that they prompted Baylor to accept him as a candidate. While this may have been true, nothing about it was (or is) unique. Money talks for people in need of a transplant, and celebrity is an indicator of money.

Most people aren't aware that we have no national policies governing who becomes a transplant *candidate*. Such decisions are usually made according to guidelines adopted by individual transplant centers. The guidelines can't be arbitrary or rely on factors like race, gender, age, sexual preference, or religion that might violate the law. But within these constraints, criteria often vary from center to center.

A center typically employs a committee made up of surgeons, physicians, psychiatrists, nurses, and social workers to employ its criteria in determining whether a patient ought to be accepted as a candidate. Medical need and whether the patient might benefit from the transplant are the primary considerations, but not the only ones.

A committee may also consider whether the patient has some other life-threatening disease not treatable by transplant, is drug- or alcohol-dependent, has a social support network of family and friends to assist during recovery, and shows evidence of being able to adhere to a lifetime regimen of antirejection drugs. The committee will also find out whether the patient has the means to pay for the operation, the subsequent hospitalization, and on-going medication costs.

Large transplant centers often employ a scoring system that involves assigning points to relevant factors. Patients with higher scores are accepted as candidates and given priority rankings. If their medical condition changes, they may be moved up or down in the rankings. Most centers approach the process of candidate selection more informally, but their committees discuss the same sort of factors.

Once a center accepts a patient as a candidate, it supplies information to UNOS. UNOS policies come into play at that point, and the patient is waitlisted and assigned a rank.

The point Annas and Caplan wanted to stress was that not everybody needing a transplant can count on getting one. Because centers operate with their own selection criteria, one center may reject alcoholics while another accepts them. One may reject all patients with cancer, while another may assess them case by case. Patients turned down at one center may not be able to afford to go to another or their insurance may not permit it.

What all centers require, no matter how other selection criteria may differ, is that patients have some way of *paying* for their treatment. The source can be private insurance, Medicaid, Medicare, or personal wealth, but there must be one.

The name Mickey Mantle guaranteed Baylor would get paid. In that respect, Mantle did end up on the list because, as Annas said, "his name was Mickey Mantle." Yet I see nothing to indicate Baylor in any way bent its criteria in selecting Mantle as a candidate. The evidence shows he was selected because he had end-stage liver disease, and his doctors believed he could get long-term benefits from a transplant.

Celebrities in our society are awarded special privileges so often that one need not be cynical to suspect every benefit they receive is unmerited. But it's easy to forget celebrities can also fall sick with life-threatening diseases. When that happens, they're entitled to be treated the same as everyone else.

Sometimes this means going to the top of the waiting list.

Why Not Social Worth?

Not everyone who believed Mantle benefitted from favoritism considered this wrong. Paul Fischer, a Miami resident interviewed in New York at Mantle's franchised restaurant, told a reporter, "I think it's a wonderful thing to get a liver for him and let the legend live on." Also, Fischer added, "special people sometimes deserve special treatment."

That special people deserve special treatment expresses the notion that in deciding how to parcel out scarce resources, it's legitimate to consider what ethicists call the "social worth" of people.

Mantle's critics cited his celebrity to suggest it had given him an unfair advantage, but those like Fischer who endorse social-worth considerations might have mentioned it (or the accomplishment it represented) to *justify* letting Mantle jump the liver queue. Or they might have cited it as grounds for granting him a transplant, while denying one to ordinary ex-alcoholics.

Intuition and Arguments

The strongest appeal favoring social worth as a criterion comes from comparing candidates equally likely to benefit but differing in (apparent) social worth.

The usual contrasts go something like the following: Who deserves a liver more, a mother of two small children or a prostitute who's a crack-cocaine addict? Should a 40-year-old molecular biologist be passed over in favor of a 65-year-old retired gravel truck driver? Should a bartender be preferred over a high-school teacher? Should a prisoner serving a life sentence for murder get a heart that might go instead to a police officer injured in the line of duty?

Most people are likely to feel sure which candidates in these contrasting pairs would be the better choice. But social worth as a criterion need not rest on intuitions. It's also supported by arguments like these three.

1. People making a contribution to society are more deserving of scarce resources than those who aren't. When all candidates are making a contribution, we should choose those whose contributions are proportionately greater. Thus, it's reasonable to prefer the mother, the molecular biologist, the teacher, and the police officer over the prostitute, the truck driver, the bartender, and the criminal.

   Those whose productive life is mostly finished can be rewarded for their past accomplishments. We would thus give a retired social worker priority over an active forklift operator.

2. A variant of this argument is to favor only those whose achievements are outstanding—developing an AIDS vaccine, winning the Nobel Prize, founding a company employing thousands, serving as a state governor. Thus, we could justify letting Mantle jump the liver queue because of his athletic accomplishments and status as a sports hero.

   Mark Siegler, a University of Chicago ethicist, took this view of Mantle explicitly. While Siegler favored ranking alcoholics lower on the transplant list (more about this later), he was willing to make an exception for Mantle, because Mantle was "a real American hero who captures the imagination of a generation through his skill, ability, and personality." In general, Siegler told a reporter, "I think we have to give deference to the rare heroes in American life, and when one comes along, we have to take them with all their warts and failures and treat them differently."

3. The third argument favors giving preference to people in whom society has invested substantial resources in the expectation of receiving future dividends.

   Everyone has benefitted to an extent from the investment of social capital, but some have benefitted significantly. A pediatric oncologist, for example, has received an education subsidized by federal, state, and private funds. Hence, if a liver she needs goes to a cable installer, society will suffer a net loss equaling the difference between its investments in the two. Prospectively, it will also get less of value out of the work of the installer.

Inherent Worth

These arguments defend allocation principles that reward service and merit or promote the general good, and they could be employed to shape a "meritocratic" world. We have no trouble imagining a society in which a "hero of the state" is accorded special treatment and people making even modest contributions are given precedence over those who are a drain on resources.

But our society isn't like that. None of the allocation principles is compatible with our fundamental commitment to the democratic principle that each person has an inherent worth that is equivalent to the inherent worth of anyone else.

The democratic principle instructs us to overlook all differences among people, whether personal traits like talent, race, age, intelligence, and gender or acquired ones like wealth, social position, or artistic or scientific achievement. Equally irrelevant is whether one is the mother of six, the only child of a widower, or the President of the United States.

Each person is equal as a person; everybody counts as one and nobody for more than one. The incompatibility of social-worth principles with our commitment to a democratic society is thus a decisive reason for rejecting them.

Liver Cancer

The discovery that Mantle had liver cancer put his doctors in a difficult position. If the cancer had spread beyond his liver, a transplant would be useless. What's more, a liver that could have saved the life of someone else would have been wasted.

It "was a hard decision" Klintmalm later said. Yet he decided to list Mantle with UNOS, because the Baylor doctors saw no evidence Mantle's cancer had spread.

"I wonder how carefully they looked?" George Annas asked after the recurrence of the cancer that led to Mantle's death. "That's the question when dealing with celebrity medicine, how carefully you screen for contra-indications for a procedure you'd like to do."

Klintmalm's response to such criticisms was that they had screened very carefully. The scans hadn't revealed cancer outside the liver, and although Mantle's alphafetoprotein measurement was high, the test wasn't specific for cancer. Why, critics asked, hadn't the Baylor team used a test under development at the University of Pittsburgh to detect the presence of abnormal liver cells in the blood? Klintmalm explained that the test was still experimental and its accuracy and reliability hadn't been established in clinical trials.

Klintmalm also scorned the suggestion that Baylor had been eager to transplant a celebrity to raise the profile of its program. He and his team, he pointed out, had been forced to spend hours giving interviews and holding press conferences to supply information to help prevent misunderstandings among people waiting for transplants. The whole episode had distracted them from their work. "Anyone who has had experience with the press would be insane to do a case like this for the sake of receiving notoriety," Klintmalm said.

Liver Cancer and Transplantation

Baylor in 1995 was only one of a handful of centers willing to transplant hepatoma patients. Klintmalm was doing research on the effectiveness of transplants as a treatment for liver cancer, and Mantle appeared to fit his research criteria. Thus, Mantle was initially considered as only another patient in a series.

Although centers were routinely turning down all hepatoma patients, thanks to the work of Klintmalm and others, people with non-metastatic liver cancer are now routinely accepted as candidates. Those who get transplants have decent prospects for surviving at least three years.

In a recent study involving 404 patients with hepatocellular carcinoma and cirrhosis, a diagnosis like Mantle's, the survival rate after transplant was 87 percent for one year and 76 percent for three. By contrast, 369 transplant patients without cancer had a survival rate of 77 percent for one year and 72 percent for three.

Other studies have produced similar statistics, but not everyone with liver cancer, even if it hasn't spread, is likely to benefit from a transplant. People with tumors larger than ten centimeters (about four inches) in diameter, for example, tend not to do well. Thus, even centers that accept hepatoma patients may turn down those with large tumors.

While it may seem unfair not to give everyone an opportunity, donor livers are so scarce they must go to people who have a reasonable chance of surviving. Mantle's CT scan showed he had three or four tumors "between pea and marble size" and two smaller ones. None of the tumors approached the ten-centimeter limit. Klintmalm's group, in accepting Mantle as a candidate, thus had good reason to believe he could benefit from a transplant.

Benefit of the Doubt

John Banja, an ethicist at Emory University, suggested, like Annas, that Mantle's celebrity might have biased Baylor's decision to give him a new liver after he was diagnosed with cancer. "Mantle's doctors might be more willing to give a person like him the benefit of the doubt in terms of the probability of the success of the operation," Banja told a reporter. "They were more willing to take a chance with someone like him than they would be with the average Joe."

Annas's and Banja's suggestions that Klintmalm's group either conveniently overlooked Mantle's cancer or gave him the benefit of the doubt in deciding to accept him for transplant are undercut by decisions the group made in other cases two years before Mantle even became their patient.

Scott McCartney, in *Defying the Gods*, his 1994 book about Klintmalm and the Baylor program, recounts two cases resembling Mantle's, those of Charles Palmer and Kristan Reading. Both involved ordinary people, not celebrities, who were accepted for a transplant by Baylor, although diagnosed with liver cancer. Chuck Palmer's case shows how similar the issues were and how similarly hard the decision.

Palmer was a 23-year-old Seattle resident, a cook in the National Guard, who came to Baylor already diagnosed with a liver tumor. Palmer's Seattle doctor, to confirm his diagnosis, had biopsied Palmer's liver by slicing out a wedge of tissue. This technique produces bleeding, and when cancer cells are present, they are disseminated throughout the abdomen.

The Baylor doctors believed this increased the probability that Palmer's cancer had spread (a view no longer accepted). This seemed confirmed by a sonogram and a CT scan showing a mass of tissue in his abdomen, but the oncologist changed his mind when further tests showed the mass was only a blood clot. Even so, there were still the presumed effects of the wedge biopsy to consider.

Klintmalm had a strong motive to deny Palmer a transplant. His research protocol for treating liver-cancer patients excluded those whose cancer had spread, and he had already demonstrated a four-year survival rate of greater than 50 percent in following his protocol. Palmer, if he died from cancer, might make these results look worse. More was also involved than Klintmalm's personal disappointment, because the worse results might discourage the adoption of his protocol and thus deny a potentially effective treatment to a large number of patients.

As if this were not pressure enough on Klintmalm's group, fifty-three patients were already on the Baylor waiting list. Any one of them might have a better chance of survival than Palmer.

The transplant committee, after much discussion, decided to accept Palmer as a candidate. But almost at once a new test showed cancer in his hepatic artery. The cancer had definitely spread, and this automatically made him ineligible for a transplant under Klintmalm's protocol. Yet Daniel DeMarco, who would later become Mantle's gastroenterologist, pressed the transplant surgeons to break the rules and give a 23-year-old kid his only real chance to live.

DeMarco and the surgeon reached a compromise. A surgeon would open up Palmer and explore his abdomen. If no cancerous changes were found, he would remain on the transplant list.

Palmer stayed on the list. Ultimately, however, he didn't get a transplant. A month passed before a suitable liver became available, and when a surgeon opened him up for the second time, he discovered the cancer had spread widely. A transplant would be pointless, so the donor liver intended for Palmer went to the backup patient. Palmer was sent home to die.

While the Palmer case lacks a happy ending, it shows that Klintmalm and his group were prepared all along the line to give the benefit of the doubt to a patient coming as close to Banja's "average Joe" as can be imagined. Palmer wasn't rich, well-connected, or famous. He wasn't even particularly well-educated or accomplished. He was simply a young man with bad luck.

I see nothing to suggest the Baylor group treated Mantle any differently than they did any other patient. To their credit, they apparently did everything possible to help their average-Joe liver-cancer patients. But outsiders weren't watching then. Thus, when Klintmalm and his colleagues decided to transplant Mantle despite his cancer, some observers got the impression Mantle's celebrity was influencing their decisions.

Apparently it wasn't.

Alcoholics

Perhaps the sharpest of the critical barbs hurled at Mantle was that he didn't deserve a donor liver because he'd destroyed his own by years of two-fisted drinking. He'd made his own bed, the criticism went, so he ought to lie in it.

This way of thinking about alcoholics remains widespread. Polls show most people don't think alcoholics should qualify for liver transplants, and some ethicists argue they should be given a lower priority ranking. Several centers won't accept alcoholics as transplant candidates, while others penalize them with longer waits. Oregon's priority listing of diseases the state will pay to treat reflects the national attitude; liver transplants for alcoholics ranks above only hemorrhoids and terminal AIDS.

Perhaps the most influential judgments about alcoholics are by primary-care physicians who simply fail to refer them to transplant centers for evaluation. No one has studied what criteria (if any) these physicians use or how many patients are affected by their decisions.

Damage

Most people seem aware that the heavy consumption of alcohol is associated with liver damage. (Witness Mantle's running joke with Billy Martin about whose liver was going to go first.) What happens is that alcohol eventually damages liver cells and produces internal scar tissue. The surviving cells multiply and form "regeneration nodules," but the scar tissue keeps blood from reaching them. The liver then ceases to be effective in removing toxic substances from the blood. When the toxins reach a critical level, the brain is affected, and confusion and coma may result.

The blockage of the liver also produces high blood pressure in the veins leading into it, because the heart isn't able to force blood through the scarred tissue. As the blood backs up and the heart keeps pumping, the thin veins in the esophagus may rupture. An untreated person may bleed to death.

While the ultimate outcome of cirrhosis is liver failure and death, the disease begins insidiously. Mantle, like many, was free of symptoms until a routine physical revealed an abnormality. But by then he'd been an alcoholic for almost forty years. Alcoholic cirrhosis (not all cirrhosis is caused by alcohol) is a serious public health concern, because it's the primary cause of end-stage liver disease in the western world. Approximately 5 to 10 percent of the population in the United States are chronic alcohol abusers.

About 15 percent of this group will develop cirrhosis over a ten to twenty year period, which means at any time 500,000 to a million Americans suffer from alcoholic cirrhosis. Every year, 10,000 to 20,000 Americans die of chronic alcoholic liver disease.

The medical evidence shows that liver failure caused by alcoholic cirrhosis can be successfully treated by a liver transplant. A transplant, indeed, is the *only* effective treatment. Alcoholics dying of liver failure thus might be expected to take their place in line to wait for a donor liver, but the objections to Mantle's getting a transplant reflect the widespread public and professional view that alcoholics, even after a long period of sobriety, shouldn't have equal access to transplants.

The Medical Argument

A common justification for this bias is what's usually called the "medical argument." It makes sense to deny alcoholics livers, according to this argument, because the organs would be wasted. Either alcoholics will have a lower rate of survival or they will ruin their transplanted liver by going back to abusing alcohol and becoming unable to adhere to their regimen of anti-rejection drugs; therefore, donor livers could be better used where they could be counted on to extend people's lives.

This argument was persuasive in the 1970s and 1980s when it rested either on speculation or research involving relatively few patients. But over the last decade more than a dozen studies tracking the progress of liver transplant patients have repeatedly shown alcoholics do as well as or better than non-alcoholics. One recent study found the one-year survival rate for alcoholics was 75 percent; the five-year rate was 62 percent. The figures for non-alcoholics were 83 and 61 percent respectively. The causes of death were also similar for the two groups.

And what about alcoholics who start drinking again? Strangely, those who lapsed (defined strictly as consuming any alcohol) after getting a transplant did as well or better than those who didn't. Their one- and five-year survival figures were 80 and 55 percent.

Nor did alcoholics fail to stick to their regimen of antirejection drugs and lose their new livers prematurely. Alcoholics had a 5.6 percent rate of (chronic) rejection, while others had a 6.2 percent. Alcoholics who lapsed into drinking had the best rate of rejection of any group—zero percent. Those who remained abstinent had a rate of 9 percent.

The medical argument rests on empirical evidence about the relative success of alcoholics and non-alcoholics after getting transplants. Whatever early data showed, current data fail to mark any meaningful differences between the two groups. So the medical argument can no longer be used to justify treating alcoholics differently.

The Moral Argument

The belief that alcoholics shouldn't be entitled to equal access to transplants must now be supported, if at all, on moral grounds. Those who argue for the view consider it rooted in the notion of individual responsibility.

Alcoholic cirrhosis is thought of by those taking this position as a lifestyle disease, one resulting from a pattern of personal decision-making. In contrast to a disease like breast cancer, alcoholism can be prevented. Individuals need only restrict or eliminate their consumption of alcohol. Hence (the argument goes), somebody like Mantle who persists in years of hard drinking is responsible for causing his disease.

People who caused their disease shouldn't be entitled to a claim on scarce resources equal to that of those who played no role in their becoming ill. (Who should get the remaining ice cream cone, the kid who tossed his away or the one whose cone was stolen?) Donor livers are scarce and the costs of transplants considerable, so people who didn't cause their diseases should be given priority.

Commenting on the Mantle case, Caplan put the point succinctly: "Spending $300,000 for a liver transplant for somebody who brought harm upon himself is not a prudent use of scarce money and scarce livers." Restricting the allocation of livers to alcoholics is thus a way of holding people responsible for their choices. If they choose to live as drunks, they must risk dying as drunks.

This argument has a strong appeal. If asked, "Who do you think should get a liver, a 63-year-old alcoholic like Mantle or a bus driver the same age whose liver was destroyed by a raging viral infection?" most of us would tend to favor the bus driver. Mantle destroyed his liver by his behavior, while the bus driver simply had bad luck. An alcoholic competing for a liver against an innocent victim of an accidental infection is almost sure to lose the popular vote.

But should he?

Predisposition

The basic principle underlying moral judgments is that (as philosophers say) "ought implies can." If you *ought* to do something, you must first be *able* to do it. For example, we don't hold people accountable for earthquakes, because there's nothing they can do to cause or prevent them.

Ought implies can.

Alcoholics need transplants because they destroy their livers by drinking. To the extent people are responsible for becoming or remaining alcoholics, they are responsible for destroying their livers. But to what extent is that?

For those inclined to deny donor livers to alcoholics on moral grounds, this is the crucial question. It is, unfortunately, a vexed and murky one without an established answer.

Once alcoholism was attributed to a weak will and alcoholics held wholly accountable for their behavior. They were alcoholics because they were morally flabby, spineless weaklings surrendering to temptation time and again. If they didn't stop drinking, it was because they didn't want to and so repeatedly made bad choices.

The recent conception of alcoholism as a disease casts doubts on this traditional view, replacing the moral account with a medical one. "Alcoholism," according to a typical definition (this one by Nicola DeMaria), "is a primary, chronic disease due to a variable combination of genetic, psychological, and social factors that affects the psycho-physical integrity of the individual and often proves to be progressive and fatal."

No one believes alcoholism is a hard-wired, genetically determined disease like muscular dystrophy or cystic fibrosis. Evidence suggests it involves, rather, a genetic *predisposition* to becoming dependent on alcohol. Thus, in the way someone with fair skin who never ventured outside couldn't get sunburned, someone predisposed to alcoholism who never took a drink couldn't become an alcoholic.

If alcoholism develops from a predisposition, we could hold people responsible, under the right conditions, for becoming alcoholics. Maybe once they become alcoholics their power to make choices is restricted, but they could decide not to take those first few drinks. The genetic program predisposing them to continue drinking would then never have a chance to kick in and activate the biochemical changes in their brains that erode their power to control their behavior.

This was the position taken by Mary Dufour, Deputy Director of NIH's National Institute on Alcohol Abuse and Addiction, in commenting on Mantle. "Although taking the first drink is a willful behavior," she said, "once the person is addicted, it's beyond their control." So by choosing to take that first drink, we might say, the predisposed person becomes responsible for becoming an alcoholic. Because of the consequences of being an alcoholic, he also becomes responsible for developing cirrhosis and needing a donor liver.

But the catch in this argument is its assumption that people either know or ought to know they're predisposed to alcoholism before they decide whether to take their first drink. Yet how could they know? While some family patterns have been identified suggesting alcoholism has a hereditary component, despite various attempts no scientist has succeeded in identifying a genetic marker or a gene for alcoholism.

We have, in short, no way of diagnosing a predisposition for alcoholism. Thus, in the absence of a definitive test, we can't hold people responsible for acting in ways that may lead to alcoholism. We can't say somebody "ought to have known" he was predisposed, because *no one* can know that, either about himself or about anyone else. Maybe someday, but not now.

Everyone knows it's *possible* to become an alcoholic, and maybe the most prudent people might choose not to drink. But it would be unfair to deny livers to alcoholics alone on the grounds they weren't as prudent as they could have been. To be fair, we would also have to deny them to people who acquired virulent infections during foreign travel and those who had accidents while rock climbing. We would end up choosing only people who had lived very narrow, if unlucky, lives.

Not Getting Treatment

Alvin Moss and Mark Siegler are among those who believe alcoholics needing liver transplants should be ranked lower than others. While acknowledging that, granted alcoholism is a disease, people might have no control over becoming alcoholics, they consider alcoholics responsible for *remaining* alcoholics.

In particular, Moss and Siegler say, "alcoholics should be held responsible for seeking and obtaining treatment that could prevent the development of late-stage complications" like cirrhosis. By making alcoholics accountable for the damage to themselves leading to the need for a liver transplant, we are simply "holding people responsible for their personal effort." Their failure to seek treatment is thus legitimately reflected by assigning them an allocation ranking lower than others of the same medical status.

This proposal is too flawed to bear the serious weight Moss and Siegler load onto it. First, not everyone has equal access to treatment. Mickey Mantle and his family could afford to go to the Betty Ford Clinic, but many people, particularly those who are poor or live in rural areas, either can't afford private treatment or lack access to alcohol rehabilitation programs.

Second, to satisfy Moss and Siegler, alcoholics must seek treatment early enough "to prevent late-stage complications." But this assumes people are sufficiently able and medically informed to anticipate the consequence of their drinking to act at an appropriate time. This seems to be asking too much of any but a small segment of the population.

Third, alcoholics often live disorganized lives, ones marked by poverty and practical difficulties. Even those who want to get treated may have too many barriers to overcome. Perhaps they can't take off from work, have no access to transportation, or need to care for family members.

Fourth, what about those who seek treatment and fail? Moss and Siegler quote statistics indicating that "more than two-thirds of alcoholics who accept therapy will improve," but they have nothing to say about the one-third who don't. If those in this group develop cirrhosis, are they entitled to compete equally for a liver? Is trying to quit drinking sufficient or is success also required?

Finally, Moss and Siegler's views about alcoholism seem too simplistic. People seek treatment for most diseases because they are prompted by pain or some dramatic symptom like bleeding. But the symptoms of alcoholism aren't obvious and may not be noticed by the alcoholic until irreversible damage is done. It does seem unfair to penalize someone for not seeking treatment for a disease he doesn't realize he has.

Alcoholism also clouds judgment, and as Peter Ubel, a critic of Moss and Siegler, observes, one of its symptoms is denial. People often don't believe they have a drinking problem, even when it's pointed out to them. (Mantle dismissed Dr. DeLarios's several warnings that drinking was ruining his liver.) They see no need to seek medical attention, and by the time they're treated, they already have severe liver damage. But it's plainly unfair to withhold transplants from people whose disease may have caused them to delay getting medical help.

The notion that it's legitimate to discriminate against alcoholics who don't seek treatment is so unpersuasive it's tempting to view it as an effort to harmonize the old moral account of alcoholism with the new medical account so as to keep alcoholics answerable for their behavior. That we simply don't know how responsible alcoholics are for their actions, that we are ignorant of the basic facts about alcoholism, tends to undercut this whole approach.

Why Alcoholics?

Alcoholic cirrhosis isn't the only "lifestyle" disease treated by organ transplants. People who smoke, for example, tend to develop chronic obstructive airway disorder (including emphysema) and may require a lung transplant. But perhaps heart disease offers a closer parallel to alcoholic cirrhosis. Evidence indicates some forms have a genetic basis, but specific genes predisposing individuals to it haven't been identified.

Most heart disease seems to involve an interplay between hereditary factors that cannot be altered and behavioral ones (exercising, eating properly) that can. While no single factor can be connected with heart disease, patterns of behavior can be linked to it. To this extent, we know how to prevent it (that is, reduce its probability). Because individuals can exert some control over heart disease, they thus bear some responsibility for it.

Should we, then, adopt the position that people needing heart transplants are responsible for their own problem and deny them a donor heart? Or should we (à la Moss and Siegler) put lower on the list those who haven't taken steps to prevent heart disease by abandoning their couch-potato, high-fat lifestyle?

Either would be a mistake. What we know about heart disease is statistical. Although we can identify "risk factors" like family history, high cholesterol, obesity, and sedentary lifestyle, we can't say in a particular case what caused someone's heart disease—whether her heart disease could have been prevented. It's unreasonable, then, to hold her responsible for her disease. She might not have been able to prevent it, even if she'd lived according to currently accepted prevention guidelines.

All people who develop alcoholic cirrhosis do so because of drinking alcohol. When the disease occurs, we know its cause. But an alcoholic, from his viewpoint, doesn't know his drinking is going to result in liver disease, anymore than a heart patient knows her fondness for hamburgers is going to result in a heart-damaging infarct. Not every alcoholic develops cirrhosis and not every Big Mac maven ends up with a damaged heart. We can generalize statistically about groups, but people can't know whether those generalizations apply to them as individuals.

We have, to put the point bluntly, no more reason to hold alcoholics responsible for needing a liver than we have for holding heart patients responsible for needing a heart. Both have problems requiring medical care, not moral censure.

Where Do We Stop?

Those wanting to set the bar for liver transplants higher for alcoholics appear not to realize that, if generalized, their line of reasoning would skew society in the direction of favoring health and medical concerns over most others.

We pride ourselves on protecting and promoting individual freedom, and this means allowing people to shape their futures according to their concept of the good life. Freedom has to operate within restrictions, of course, but do we want to pressure people to regulate their lives by standards they must meet to qualify for an organ transplant should they ever happen to need one?

It appears reasonable, at first sight, to discriminate against alcoholics, because their problem is "their own fault." But where should we stop? What about somebody who knows little about fungi and eats the liver-destroying Death Cap mushroom he finds in the woods? Do we want to deny him a liver on the basis of his hubris?

And what about the mountain-bike racer who wipes out topping a hill and shreds her liver? Should we deny her a new one on the basis of her reck-lessness? Or should we outlaw mountain-bike racing? Then what do we do about the attempted suicide who gets drunk and swallows all the tablets in a bottle of Tylenol? Should we put him low down on the list because his need results from self-inflicted damage?

If we begin penalizing people on the grounds that they are responsible for putting themselves in need of a transplant, we may end up with a small pool of "blameless" candidates. But to prepare people to qualify for the pool we would have to encourage them to avoid a variety of activities and life-styles and to shape their lives along the lines of a medically approved model.

We would need to discourage, as a society, diversity and spontaneity of action to foster prudence and uniformity. Rather than our current commit-ment to promoting individual autonomy, we would end up promoting social conformity. We would, in effect, reward the medically virtuous and punish the medically wicked.

This is too high a price to pay. Let's give people the organs they need because they need them, not as a way of rewarding them for having lived some medically correct idea of the virtuous life. The traditional aim of medicine is to comfort and care for sick people and try to make them better. How they came to need help has never been the concern of medicine.

I suggest that's the way it should remain.

Legacy

Mickey Mantle has already started fading from the public's consciousness. He's on the way to being forgotten as a living presence and recalled only as a column of statistics and a handful of anecdotes.

Yet Mantle's legacy extends beyond baseball and isn't the result of anything he attempted to achieve. That he was a celebrity, an ex-alcoholic, and a patient with end-stage liver disease put him at the center of the debate over the rules for distributing donor livers. His fame and his problems attracted the public's attention to the crucial issues involved and forced us to rethink and defend our solutions.

This is a legacy that won't appear in the record books.

4

That Others May Live

The Dead-Donor Rule and Anencephalic Infants

Community Hospital: Monday, June 1, 9:00 A.M.

"That's where it should be," the radiologist said, tapping the green and yellow image on the screen. "But there's a complete blank there. Zip, zero, nada."

The light in the radiology suite of Community Hospital was grey and watery, but the rows of stacked monitors glowed with an almost painful brightness.

"Damn it all, I'm sorry to be right," Dr. Carl Greer said, running a hand through his frizzy gray hair. He turned to face Dr. Chen, the senior resident. "Okay, Tom, she's your patient, so you're going to have to explain the situation."

"The dad's in the waiting area, and I'll talk to him first." Dr. Chen hesitated. "Could we get the surgeons to look at these images? I'd like to mention some options to the parents."

"Sure, sure," Dr. Greer agreed, nodding. "I can tell you what the surgeons are going to say, but let's explore all the possibilities." He took a deep breath and expelled it in a long whoosh. "Otherwise, the baby's a real keeper. What a shame."

MARK HERTZLER sat up straight in his chair in the waiting room. He stared at the swinging doors, rhythmically tapping his fingers on the wooden arm rest.

He sighed and glanced at his watch. It had been a long time since they'd wheeled Lola into the delivery room. Almost two hours. Maybe something wasn't going right. Or maybe the baby was just taking a long time.

They'd told him he could stay with Lola if he wanted to, but medical stuff always made him feel sick. But he wouldn't mind having a baby. The doc at the clinic said it'd be a boy, that he could tell from the pictures they'd made of Lola's belly. Mark liked the idea of having a kid to show off to his friends. He could take him fishing, go to ball games.

But he and Lola ought to get married. A kid needed a family. He was only 23, and he'd planned on being single for a few more years. But life didn't always ask you what your plans were. Things just happened.

He could do worse than marry Lola. She was pretty and smart, and she'd make him do things he ought to do anyway. Like get some of the guys on the job to teach him welding so he could make some real money. He'd been a helper for eight months, and it shouldn't take him long to break out. Strike an arc, then keep the puddle moving—that's about all there was to it. They'd need money with a kid, and Lola's job at Don's Market barely paid the rent.

Mark patted his shirt pocket and wondered if he had enough time to take the elevator down and go outside for another smoke. Probably. He wouldn't be gone ten minutes. As he stood up and took a few steps toward the hall, Dr. Chen pushed through the swinging doors. Mark was the only one in the waiting room, but Dr. Chen's eyes swept around, checking for other people.

Mark liked Dr. Chen, even through they had talked only a few minutes before Lola was taken away. Dr. Chen, with his smooth face and clipped black hair, looked so young he wasn't as scary as the other doctors, but also he spoke in plain English without using fancy medical terms.

Dr. Chen's smile had been white enough for a toothpaste commercial, but now he wasn't smiling. Something about the way he kept his head down and avoided meeting Mark's eyes suggested things weren't all right.

"Is something wrong with Lola?" Mark hadn't personally known of anybody dying in childbirth, but women on the soaps his mom used to watch did it all the time. Dr. Chen slipped out of focus for a moment as Mark imagined never hearing Lola's loud, brassy laugh again.

"Lola's fine," Dr. Chen said. "But come over here and sit down so I can explain something to you."

Mark sat in the same upholstered grey chair with the varnished wooden arms, and Dr. Chen took the one beside him. He turned around so he could face Mark.

"Has the baby come yet?" Mark asked.

"The baby was born half an hour ago," Dr. Chen said. "It's a boy, just what you were expecting."

Thank God Lola was all right. So he had a son. He'd need some time to adjust to the idea. "We're going to call him Mike, after Lola's dad."

"That's a nice name," Dr. Chen said. But he didn't smile at all, and he shifted around in his chair, looking uncomfortable. "Look, Mark, Mike's got a serious problem."

"A problem?" Something about the way Dr. Chen pronounced the word made him feel cold all over. He said it the way people said cancer. "What's wrong?"

"It's his heart." Dr. Chen put a hand up to his chest. "Something's wrong with the left side, the side where the blood comes back from the lungs and gets pumped to the body."

"Yeah?" He didn't understand. "So what's wrong exactly?"

"Mike's missing nearly all the left side of his heart." Dr. Chen frowned. "His heart didn't develop properly, and apparently that didn't show up on the early ultrasound."

"But he's alive?" The world seemed to spin around him.

"He's got some left side function." Dr. Chen nodded. "But very little. The technical name for his problem is hypoplastic left heart syndrome. We can use a machine to help his heart circulate the blood, but he can't stay on it for long."

"How about an operation?" Mark for the first time understood what the doctor was telling him. Mike's heart was like a pump with half the pieces missing. "Can you fix it?"

"The surgeons don't advise trying." Dr. Chen shook his head. "Too much of the heart is gone, and we'd be putting him through heavy-duty surgery without any hope of long-term success."

"So he's going to die?" Mark said the words flatly, but even as he spoke them, his own heart ached.

"Unless we can get him a new heart."

"What do you mean, a new heart?"

"A transplant."

"I don't know if Medicaid will stand for that," Mark said. "My insurance won't pay a dime for Lola or Mike, because we're not married." He shrugged. "We don't have the money for anything like that."

"Medicaid will pay," Dr. Chen said gently. "But are you and Lola going to stay together? You think you'll be able to care for a kid who's got to have medicine on a regular schedule for the rest of his life?"

"I don't know if I could," Mark said. "But I know Lola and me both could, particularly if he's going to die if we don't." He hesitated. "I need to talk to Lola."

Midwest Medical Center: Monday, 9:30 A.M.

Dr. Susan Stein felt her stomach clench into a tight knot. Despite fifteen years as a neonatologist, she had to stifle a gasp as she caught sight of the baby's head crowning at the vaginal opening.

Maybe I'm wrong, she thought. Dear God, let me be wrong.

Harold Vitner, the obstetrics resident presiding at the delivery, cradled the baby's head in one hand, while with the other, he turned the shoulders slightly to ease their passage through the birth canal. Behind the plastic shield covering his face, his eyes were hard and his lips tightly compressed.

The delivery was going smoothly, as smoothly as any could. But the outcome was wrong. Terribly wrong.

Dr. Stein stepped toward the end of the delivery table, moving closer for a better view. Perhaps the blood and the lights and the angle had made her eyes play tricks on her.

But now she could tell they hadn't. Harold was completing his extraction, and she could see the baby was a girl. Good weight and well developed—except for the head.

The vault of the skull was completely missing from the eyebrows upward, making the head look strangely collapsed. It reminded her of the peculiar shape of the mantle of a squid, except the face was so strikingly human.

Dr. Stein bit at her lower lip as she surveyed the scene. The cerebral hemispheres were almost certainly missing, along with the skin and bone normally covering them. Only the brain stem seemed present, covered with a fibrous membrane looking like soft grey parchment. It was the most basic and primitive of the brain's components, differing little in its function from that of a crocodile. It would govern the child's breathing, trigger her sucking response, and regulate her crying and sleeping.

But the brain stem couldn't sustain life. Eventually, in a few hours or a few days, it would begin to lose its functioning. The baby would sporadically stop breathing, then gasp for oxygen and breathe again. Eventually, mercifully, the brain stem would cease functioning, and there would come a time when breathing stopped and there wasn't a gasp to start it again.

Dr. Stein looked away from the baby as Ellen Howard, the baby's mother, groaned sharply and writhed beneath the green surgical drape covering the upper part of her body. She had been given an epidural for the pain and was also lightly sedated. Dr. Stein decided Ellen shouldn't see her baby until she was back in her room and had recovered from the effects of the sedation.

"Just hold on, Mom," Harold called out, his voice strained. "We're almost done here. Then you can get some rest."

Ellen Howard had arrived at Midwest Medical Center already in labor, and Dr. Stein had talked to her only briefly before they moved to the delivery room. But she had read Ellen's chart carefully, looking for clues that the baby might be in trouble. She hadn't seen any, but she hadn't had much to go on either.

Ellen was a 27-year-old law librarian, a primigravid sailing through her first pregnancy. She'd been seen by her family practitioner, who had confirmed her pregnancy, and once by an obstetrician. Ellen had failed to act on the obstetrician's recommendation that she have an ultrasound around the end of the first trimester. She'd also never returned to have her blood drawn for an alphafetoprotein test, which might have predicted the present trouble.

Dr. Stein had asked Ellen why she hadn't followed any of the medical recommendations, or at least sought regular prenatal care. She was an educated person who should have known the importance of being monitored during pregnancy.

"Yeah, but I'm young and in excellent health." Ellen had smiled as she relaxed between one of her contractions. "I didn't see any reason to turn something as natural as pregnancy into a high-tech production. I eat right, don't drink, smoke, or do drugs. I swim ten laps every day. I didn't feel like I needed anybody to tell me what to do."

But there was something else too, Dr. Stein had learned from Ellen Howard's chart. Ellen's younger sister, who had died in her tenth year, had been profoundly retarded from Down syndrome. Ellen had loved her sister, and abortion wasn't an option for her. So she probably hadn't wanted to find out how the fetus was developing. If it was abnormal, but she didn't know it, she wouldn't be tempted to have an abortion.

Don Howard, Ellen's husband, was a tall, thin man with a quick smile. He had stood beside Ellen's bed and gripped her hand during the contractions. "I'm a lawyer, but I'm a tax lawyer," he told Susan when she introduced herself. "I'm more likely to help doctors get rich than to sue them." He smiled.

Harold clamped off the umbilical cord with two yellow plastic clips, then cut between them with scissors. The nurse holding the baby walked toward the bright lights of the warming table. Susan Stein followed. The baby would now be her responsibility. Her medical responsibility, she corrected herself. Ellen and Don Howard would have the real responsibility.

The baby lay on the table under the lights moving her arms and legs feebly as the nurse suctioned out mucous from the nose and mouth. As Dr. Stein looked down at the child's distorted head and thought of having to tell the Howards their baby was anencephalic, she felt a leaden gloom settle over her.

Community Hospital: Monday, 1:00 P.M.

Lola Slade pulled a tissue out of the box on the nightstand, wiped her eyes, then blew her nose.

"What do you think we ought to do about Mike?" Mark asked.

He was sitting stiffly in the chair opposite the end of her bed, and in his dingy jeans, scuffed work boots, and red plaid shirt, he seemed out of place in the hospital. He was too rough to fit in with all these smooth people.

A wave of pity washed over Lola as she noticed the expression on his face. He looked stunned and confused, as if he'd been hit on the head at his job and was still dazed. He was a good person, warm-hearted and hard working, but he wasn't good at handling responsibility.

"What do you want to do?" Mark asked again.

"Get him a new heart, if we can." Lola's voice was rough from crying. "We're going to stay together, and we're going to take care of him." She turned and looked at Dr. Chen, who was standing by the chest of drawers, leaning on it with one elbow. "When can you do it?"

"I won't be doing it myself." Dr. Chen stood up straight. "Dr. Morgan would do the actual surgery. But the big problem is going to be finding a heart."

"What do you mean?" Lola asked.

"Transplant organs for infants are in short supply." Dr. Chen paused. "Also, Mike needs a heart in a hurry. We can't count on keeping him stabilized for more than a few days."

"Oh, Jesus." Mark spoke softly, the words almost a prayer.

"I'll get Mike's name on the waiting list, if you both agree about wanting a transplant," Dr. Chen said. "He'll have top priority, because of his condition. But I want you to know before we get into this that it may be a long haul, and there's no guarantee Mike's going to get a heart in time."

"It depends on somebody else's child dying, doesn't it?" Lola said.

"We've got to hope another baby dies so Mike can live." She shook her head. "That's horrible."

"The other baby will die anyway," Dr. Chen said quietly. "That you want a heart for Mike won't have anything to do with it. The worst thing is having a baby die and not getting the heart for Mike or somebody else."

"I see what you mean." Lola clenched her teeth to stifle the sob she felt rising in her throat. "Is there something we could do to speed up the process?"

Dr. Chen pursed his lips. "I guess we could go public," he said after a moment. "Encourage the parents of a sick newborn to donate the heart to help Mike, if their baby dies."

"That's like begging," Mark said. "I don't know about that."

"We'll do it," Lola said fiercely. "If it's begging, I'll beg. And you will too." She turned toward Dr. Chen. "Just tell us how to go about it."

"I'll introduce you to Hal Burton," Dr. Chen said. "He's the Channel 3 medical reporter."

Midwest Medical Center: Monday, 3:00 P.M.

Ellen Howard leaned back against the cranked-up hospital bed and focused her attention on Dr. Stein, who was perched on the edge of the mattress. She'd slept for more than an hour, but she was still tired, as if she had just completed a twenty-mile run. She was also sore, but not as much as she'd expected.

Dr. Stein's face was lined and serious, framed by greying black hair tied back. Ellen swiveled her head to the right and glanced at Don. His face was stricken, his skin blanched white, his jaw clamped tight. His brown eyes were as blank and hard as marbles. She probably looked even worse, she reflected, after what she'd gone through.

And now this.

It surprised her she wasn't hysterical. But she didn't feel much of anything, really. She dreaded what would happen later, when her feelings started sneaking out from behind the wall her mind had erected. But right now she needed the wall to get her through whatever she needed to get through.

Sounds of muted talking came from the television. The maternity ward was overcrowded, and the woman in the room's other bed had the set on with the volume turned low. A flimsy beige curtain hanging from an aluminum track separated them, but the TV was suspended from a metal arm and was visible from both sides.

Her neighbor was watching the Sandy Stone Show, a tabloid talk program, and three large women were explaining to Sandy how they had lost the men in their lives because they refused to go on diets. They sounded both absurd and pitiful.

"She's not going to get any treatment at all?" Don asked. He wanted to make sure he had the facts straight, as if knowing the facts would somehow make it possible for him to change them.

"Claire," Ellen said. "Her name is Claire. Not she or it."

"Claire," Don said, not meeting her eyes.

"There is no treatment," Dr. Stein said. "We'll keep Claire warm and comfortable. Give her fluids, including a sugar solution to satisfy any hunger." Her face clouded. "Then we'll wait for nature to take its course."

"How long?" Ellen had a sudden image of her baby lying all alone, crying for her. Tears stung the corners of her eyes, and she swallowed hard to push down the lump in her throat.

She hadn't seen Claire yet. Dr. Stein promised a nurse would bring around a wheelchair and take her down to the neonatal intensive care nursery. She wouldn't be able to hold her baby, but she could at least touch her and make sure she was being taken care of. That she wasn't in pain.

"Maybe only a few hours." Dr. Stein gave a small shrug. "A few days at most."

"We don't want anything done to increase her—Claire's—suffering." Don sounded stern, and Ellen knew he was doing his best not to burst into tears. "We don't want extraordinary steps taken to make her live longer."

If anything, Don had wanted a child even more than she had. Maybe because he was ten years older. They'd been married for five years, and after the first year, she'd gone off the pill. They hadn't talked about doing anything to help matters along, but as soon as she was pregnant, they had become as excited as two kids waiting for Christmas.

Don had moved his study into the basement so the room across from their bedroom could be a nursery. They had spent weekends going to baby stores and shopping for furniture, equipment, linens . . . everything there was for babies.

"We won't do anything to extend Claire's life," Dr. Stein said. "I understand how you feel about that."

Ellen was about to say she was ready to see the baby, when something Sandy Stone was talking about on the TV caught her attention.

"Little Mike Hertzler needs a new heart," Sandy Stone said. "According to doctors at Community Hospital where he was born this morning, the infant has only days to live unless a heart can be found to replace his defective one."

A picture of a baby in a plastic-sided hospital isolette appeared on the screen. The small body, with its dark hair and pale wrinkled skin, was surrounded by a tangle of plastic tubes. The child was completely inert, and only the slight motion of the chest under the blue hospital blanket showed he was breathing.

"Mark Hertzler, Mike's father, is going to tell us about the situation," Sandy Stone said. She turned toward a very young blonde man in jeans and a red plaid shirt.

He looks scared, Ellen thought. But who wouldn't be? His son is dying, but what can he do? He can't buy a heart. Then, in an instant, without any reflection, she knew what she wanted.

"Dr. Stein," Ellen said. "Could Claire's heart be donated?"

"So you heard that?" Dr. Stein waved her hand toward the TV.

"That's what we should do," Don said, nodding vigorously. "Claire wouldn't have lived in vain, because some good would have come of her death. The way it is. . . ." His voice trailed off.

"Well?" Ellen looked at Dr. Stein.

"It's not an easy situation," Dr. Stein said, sighing. "Her organs are usable now, but even though she has only brain-stem function, she's not brain dead." Dr. Stein looked uncomfortable, and her eyes fell away from Ellen's. "By the time she is, her organs will be damaged from lack of oxygen and won't be suitable for transplant."

"Isn't there some way they could be kept usable?" Don swiveled around and turned his gaze onto Dr. Stein. "We've suffered a terrible tragedy, but it looks like we might be able to keep something similar from happening to another family."

"Well," Dr. Stein took a deep breath and sighed again. "If you're serious, there's a protocol established in Canada we can follow to keep Claire's organs in good shape." She paused, looking worried and unhappy. "I have to warn you, though, all this will make it harder on you."

"Will Claire suffer any pain?" Don asked.

"We don't think infants like Claire can feel pain," Dr. Stein said. "But we always treat them as if they could." She shook her head. "No, Claire won't experience any pain."

"Can you donate her heart to the baby at Community Hospital?" Ellen asked.

"It's unusual," Dr. Stein said, "but yes, I can get in touch with the doctors there."

"Then that's what we want to do," Ellen said. Her voice was steady. "We want to give Claire's heart to the little boy who'll die without it." She felt the tears welling up in her eyes, and she reached out and gripped Don's hand, squeezing it so hard she made the joints in her fingers pop. "Mike," she said, her words thick and blurred. "The baby's name is Mike."

Midwest Medical Center: Monday, 4:45 P.M.

Dr. Susan Stein stopped at the nursing station outside the glassed-in NICU and waited while Carl Woodrow, the Nursing Supervisor, finished typing something into the computer.

"Hi, Susan," Carl said, a smile lighting up his broad mahogany-colored face. "Sorry for the wait."

"No problem," she said. "How's the Howard baby doing?"

"Still stable," Carl said, his smile disappearing. "Good pulse, but the breathing is a little irregular."

"When she shows signs of serious ventilatory distress, I want her put on a ventilator."

"Put an anencephalic kid on a vent?" Carl's face took on a puzzled expression.

"Right," Dr. Stein said. "Her parents want her to become an organ donor, and we're going to follow the Ontario protocol. We're also adding antibiotics along with her glucose drip."

"That won't do her any good," Carl said.

"Look," Dr. Stein said, keeping her voice level, "there's no chance for this baby—none. But maybe her heart can save the life of another child."

"But that's a dangerous way to go," Carl said, his voice rising and taking on an edge. "You can't tell when an anencephalic baby's dead. Not really."

"We're going to follow a testing protocol."

"Testing?" Carl said, shaking his large head. "No test works on a kid like that. You start saying babies without a brain are dead and treat them like a spare-parts warehouse, what's to keep you from treating ones born retarded or deformed the same way?"

"There's a big difference, Carl," Dr. Stein said. "But if you don't see it, I can't convince you now. Getting back to the protocol, after the baby is on the ventilator, I want it turned off every six hours. If she doesn't start breathing on her own within three minutes, start the machine again and page me."

Dr. Stein noticed that Carl was glaring at her, his jaw clenched tightly, but she ignored him. "When I hear from you, I'll confirm death, then call the transplant surgeons at Community, and they'll send over a team for the heart. I've notified the other transplant centers the kidneys and liver might be available, but I haven't heard from any of them yet."

"You'll have to write those orders in the chart," Carl said. He turned and removed a red folder from an aluminum rack, then dropped the folder in front of Dr. Stein.

"I'm not asking you to agree with me," Dr. Stein said, opening the chart.

"I don't," Carl said curtly. "I think it's wrong. I'll see if one of the nurses will carry out the orders."

"I'm thinking about a baby named Mike," Dr. Stein said, without looking up. "He's missing half his heart. We can do something about that, but we can't help Baby Claire."

She lifted her head and found herself staring into Carl's stony eyes. She looked back down and resumed her writing. She knew she was right, but even so, her hand shook, turning the lettering into shaky scribbles.

She couldn't deny there was a problem about establishing death, but she'd get somebody experienced to back her up. Also, there was something creepy about keeping the body of a anencephalic baby functioning so the organs would be in good condition for transplant. But creepy wasn't wrong.

Community Hospital: Monday, 5:15 P.M.

Lola snapped awake as she heard Dr. Chen's voice. She sat up in bed and rubbed her eyes.

"I have a little good news," Dr. Chen said, closing the door behind him. "A doctor at Midwest Medical Center called me, and she says they've got a potential donor for Mike."

"Sounds real good," Mark said. He got up from his chair and stood beside Dr. Chen at the foot of Lola's bed. "Did they say when we can we get the heart?"

"We don't know for sure." Dr. Chen sounded almost embarrassed.

"He means we've got to wait for a baby to die," Lola said. "But maybe Mike will die first. It's possible, isn't it?"

"Or maybe another heart will become available first," Dr. Chen said. "The parents saw you on TV and wanted to help Mike." "That's so wonderful," Mark said, his voice breaking. "I can't believe people would do that for complete strangers."

"Who are they?" Lola asked. She felt a tide of warmth rise up in her, an almost overwhelming mixture of gratitude and joy.

"They didn't want their names revealed," Dr. Chen said.

"Whoever they are, I can't thank them enough," Mark said. "It's like winning the biggest lottery in the world."

"Now the waiting's really going to get hard," Dr. Chen said.

"But there's more hope," Lola said. "Mike's got a real chance now." Her voice dropped. "I only wish we weren't waiting for somebody else's baby to die. Hoping it will happen soon. That almost makes me feel evil."

Midwest Medical Center: Tuesday, June 2, 4:45 A.M.

The nurse awakened Ellen to say they were going to take Claire off the ventilator at five o'clock. Ellen wanted to walk down the hall to the NICU by herself, but the nurse made her sit in the wheelchair. That was hospital policy for new mothers.

The nurse parked her a few feet from the isolette, but as soon as she left, Ellen maneuvered the chair forward until she was beside the clear-sided plastic box holding her baby.

Electrical leads ran from the heart monitor attached to Claire's chest, and brownish-orange splotches on her arms and hands marked the places where IV needles had been inserted. A thin plastic tube was threaded through a nostril, and a larger blue-tinted tube was stuck down her throat and taped into place. The machine that breathed for her produced a whispery, sighing sound, like a wind blowing gently though tree branches.

Claire was lying on her back, covered only by a diaper that was much too large for her tiny body. Her arms and legs twitched slightly from time to time, but otherwise she was still. Despite the machines attached to her body, her face was tranquil, and she showed no signs of pain or distress.

You're a beautiful baby, Ellen thought. I wish I could take you home with me so you could grow up and go to school and I could love you forever.

Dr. Stein had stopped by her room around 10:30 to say that Claire was starting to have trouble getting enough oxygen and they were going to have to hook her up to the breathing machine.

"We'll take her off in six hours," Dr. Stein said. "If she can't breathe on her own . . . well, that will be the end." She gave Ellen a questioning look. "I'm telling you this, so you can decide if you want to be there."

"I do," Ellen said.

Don had kept quiet, and later, when she had encouraged him to go home to rest, he had made only a token objection. "Don't you want me to come with you?" he'd asked.

She told him she would be all right, and she had rather see him take care of himself. She had meant it, too. With his shoulders slumped, his eyes teary, and his voice slurred as if he'd been drinking, Don had seemed at the limit of his endurance. Ellen felt a hand on her shoulder, and she looked behind her to see Dr. Stein. A young, balding man in a floppy green scrub suit was standing at her side. Ellen thought Dr. Stein looked almost as tired as Don. Her complexion was pale, and a few wisps of hair had come loose and were dangling over her forehead.

"This is Dr. Tishman," Dr. Stein told her. "He's a pediatric neurologist, and he's with me to assess Claire."

Dr. Tishman nodded gravely at Claire. He then turned away to pick up the long strip of paper that had scrolled out of one of the machines hooked up to Claire.

"I know this is hard," Dr. Stein said gently. "If you've changed your mind, somebody can take you back to your room."

"No," Ellen said, not daring to try to say more.

Dr. Stein nodded, then walked to the other side of the isolette. Ellen reached over the edge and wrapped her fingers around Claire's tiny wrist. The skin was exquisitely smooth and supple. And warm. That's what surprised Ellen. The warmth. If only the rest of you was so perfect. No, she caught herself, you wouldn't have to be perfect. If only you had a club foot or a cleft lip or something that could be fixed.

Dr. Stein inserted the earpieces of the stethoscope and held the diaphragm against Claire's chest. The doctor looked up at green numerals of the digital clock on the wall at the end of the nursery. After listening a moment, she glanced at Dr. Tishman.

Dr. Tishman did something to the breathing machine at the end of the isolette, and the soft, sighing sound abruptly ceased. The silence was noticeable. Like the wind dying down, Ellen thought. Dr. Stein again put her stethoscope against Claire's chest, and for a moment her face froze in concentration. Dr. Tishman watched but did nothing.

Ellen stroked her baby's arm, then her cheek, avoiding the plastic tube. Her skin was smooth, soft, and unblemished. She's beautiful, Ellen thought.

Dr. Stein moved the stethoscope, checking one part of the chest, then another. The chest didn't move. The tiny movements that had occurred while the breathing machine was running had stopped completely. Dr. Stein looked up at the clock, then pulled the ends of the stethoscope out of her ears. She glanced at Dr. Tishman. "That's three minutes," she said.

"I can't detect any sign of spontaneous respiration," Dr. Tishman said. "The EEG is compatible with that."

Dr. Stein nodded then walked around the isolette to Ellen. "Claire's gone now," she said in a soft voice. "Let me take you back to your room."

Ellen squeezed the small arm gently, noticing it was still warm, then pulled her hand away. Goodbye, she thought. I wish we could have known one another better.

As Dr. Stein wheeled Ellen from the room, she heard the whispery, sighing sound of the breathing machine start again. Then, for the first time, a torrent of hot tears streamed down her face, and her shoulders heaved with uncontrollable sobs.

Community Hospital: Tuesday, 11:15 A.M.

Lola was sitting in a chair beside her bed watching a young Frank Sinatra and a group of his buddies planning a big robbery on the high seas. At least that's what she thought they were doing. She couldn't keep her mind on the story, and every few minutes, she glanced away from the TV toward the door, expecting to see Dr. Chen or Dr. Morgan, the transplant surgeon.

The volume was turned low, and she could hear Mark's heavy, regular breathing. He hadn't wanted to lie in her bed, but she had insisted. She had slept most of the night, until one of the nurses woke her up to say they'd sent for the heart and the transplant team would be starting the operation in about an hour.

Lola had called Mark at home, waking him out of a dead sleep, and he had started for the hospital. Then he'd had a flat tire on his pickup. His spare turned out not to have any air, so he'd had to hitch a ride to a service station, and finding one open so early hadn't been easy. By the time he arrived, Mike had already been put to sleep for the surgery.

Dr. Morgan had told her the operation might last six or eight hours, but even so, she hadn't been able to settle down. She stared at the TV, because she couldn't sleep.

"Ms. Slade?" she heard somebody say. She jerked her head up and opened her eyes. She must have been napping.

Dr. Morgan was standing in front of her. Still dressed in his baggy blue operating outfit, with his hair held back under a flat blue cap, he looked tired, but he was smiling slightly, and she took comfort in that.

"Mark," she called sharply, reaching over and shaking his leg. "Wake up. Dr. Morgan is here."

Lola got up from her chair and stared at the surgeon with her eyes opened wide. Questions swarmed through her mind, but she suddenly seemed unable to speak.

"How is he?" Mark asked. He slid off the bed and stood beside her. He put his arm around her, and she leaned against him. Together they faced the surgeon.

"He's doing okay." Dr. Morgan said, raising a hand as if giving a blessing. "The operation went fine, and we didn't encounter any problems we hadn't anticipated."

"Thank God, thank God." Mark pulled her tight against him.

"He's not out of the woods yet." Dr. Morgan held up an index finger, cautioning them. "Anesthesia is hard on babies, but he's got good lung function, so I'm not worried. Also, we'll have to cope with his body's rejection of the new heart, but we're pretty good at controlling that with drugs."

"How was the heart?" Lola asked. "Was it a good one?"

"As perfect as could be," Dr. Morgan said. "I've never seen a better heart."

Lola felt the tension drain out of her, and she bit her lip to keep back the tears. I'm going to write the parents, she resolved. I'm going to thank them for saving my baby, for making him whole.

"I'll take you to the recovery room, and you can see Mike for yourselves," Dr. Morgan said.

Following him down the hall, she and Mark walked so close together they bumped into one another. It happened so much they found it funny. By the time they reached the recovery room, both of them were laughing and crying.

Mike's skin was no longer a pale bluish-white. It was a vibrant pink, almost red. He looked wonderful.

LIKE ELLEN AND KEN HOWARD, some parents faced with the devastating news their child is anencephalic find the courage needed to act unselfishly. Despite anguish and heartache, they offer their child's organs to save the lives of other children.

Every year, about 500 babies like Mike are born with hearts so defective they need a new one simply to go on living. Yet you won't find any medical center in the United States eager (and not many even willing) to transplant the heart from an anencephalic infant like Claire into a baby like Mike.

Not that such surgery is illegal. Rather, the atmosphere surrounding it so crackles with the electricity of ethical controversy that hospitals and transplanters alike prefer to steer clear of it. Public disputes are divisive, time-consuming, and potentially bad for the reputation of both institutions and individuals.

I used to be contemptuous of such wary attitudes when I read about the parents of an anencephalic child having a hard time finding a hospital willing to transplant their child's organs. Sure, I thought, it might be a bit controversial, but the lives saved ought to make a little bad PR worthwhile.

I still believe this, but after a couple of years of thinking about the ethics of organ transplantation and reading more widely in the medical and philosophical literature, I've softened my hasty condemnation of the hospitals as spineless bureaucracies. The issues are more tangled and intractable than, in my innocence, I had imagined.

Even so, I've also learned that when we take the trouble to untangle the skein and clear up some confusions, it's possible to demonstrate how using organs from anencephalic infants to save the lives of other babies is both morally acceptable and compatible with good public policy.

Anencephaly

To grasp the issues and understand why they're so hard to resolve to the satisfaction of even reasonable people, it's necessary to start with anencephaly itself. Most of the facts about it aren't in dispute, but what to make of them is a source of sharp disagreement.

Anencephaly is a developmental neurological abnormality, a defect so profound it's without parallel in the sad index of birth impairments. In addition to being born missing the dome and back of the skull, anencephalic infants also lack both hemispheres of the brain. Without the cerebral cortex, the layer of grey matter lining the hemispheres, anencephalic infants permanently lack consciousness. Hence, they are incapable of having even the most rudimentary thoughts, emotions, wishes, or intentions. An anencephalic baby will never be able to recognize her mother's face, smile and squeal in anticipation of some delight, or reach out to grasp a bright new toy.

The brain stem, however, is present in anencephalic infants, and it initiates and directs the body's basic housekeeping activities. These are the ones performed automatically, like breathing and circulating the blood. The sucking instinct is likely to be present, as well as the gag reflex and blink response. The babies may cry, squirm, or kick their feet, and while it's not likely they can feel pain, lacking the necessary neural equipment, some may respond to a needle stick by jerking away. Apparently this is only a reflex.

Anencephalic infants aren't blobs of protoplasm so much as complex biological systems governed by a primitive program of information. They're reminiscent of one of those alien cities of John W. Campbell's science fiction in which complicated machines go on working to supply the needs of a long vanished population. The city stands vacant, unoccupied but full of sound and motion. With anencephalic infants, it's as if their functioning bodies are waiting for personalities that will never arrive. Their bodies, like the vacant cities, are hauntingly empty, and the whir and clank of the machinery underscores that fact.

Only about 25 percent of anencephalic infants are born alive, and just 40 percent of these survive for a full day. A third of these survivors live as long as three days, and a mere 5 percent live a week. Although some anencephalic infants have been known to survive for months on life support, this is a rare event. The infants, as a rule, flutter through life quickly, leaving behind mostly sorrow and wistful parental dreams of what might have been.

Parental Wishes

Like Ellen and Ken Howard, the parents of anencephalic babies, grappling with news that can crush the spirit, sometimes decide the best way to give meaning to their child's brief life is by donating the organs to help others. This notably occurred more than a decade ago when an anonymous couple in London, Ontario, learned that their daughter, referred to as Baby Gabrielle by her doctors, was anencephalic. (I used their experiences as the basis of the story about the Howards and Claire.) After consulting with specialists at the medical center, the parents decided they wished to donate her organs.

"The parents insisted they wanted their infant's organs used," Dr. Tim Frewen, the head of pediatrics at Children's Hospital told a reporter. "They wanted to see that their baby would touch others and contribute to life in some way."

As soon as Baby Gabrielle, who had been put on a ventilator, failed to breathe on her own, transplant coordinators in Canada and the United States got busy and located a recipient for her heart. Still on a ventilator, she was flown to California and transported by ambulance sixty-three miles east of Los Angeles to Loma Linda University Medical Center.

On a Friday morning, two days after Baby Gabrielle had been declared dead, her heart was removed and transplanted into the chest of a baby delivered by caesarean section earlier that same day. His name was Paul Holc, and he became the youngest heart recipient in the world. (Paul's surgeon was Dr. Leonard Bailey, who had earlier caused controversy by transplanting a chimpanzee heart into the infant known as Baby Fae. She was also born with hypoplastic left heart syndrome. See Chapter 7, "Kurosawa in California.")

Even before the Holc transplant put Loma Linda Medical Center in the spotlight, it had received almost 200 calls from parents asking about the possibility of their anencephalic newborns becoming organ donors. In response, the hospital had established a program for maintaining anencephalic infants on life support to preserve their organs for transplants. The program had strong advocates, people who saw it as a means of increasing the supply of transplant organs, but it also had severe critics.

Shortage

Loma Linda initiated its program not primarily to help parents, but because of the shortage of transplant organs. Organs for people of all ages are scarce commodities, but the weight of the shortage presses especially hard on babies, because they need small organs. A heart from a 10-year-old is useless to a 10-day-old; it won't even fit into the chest cavity.

Organs for infants are particularly difficult to come by. Comparatively few babies die in the catastrophic ways that render them brain dead while leaving their vital organs unscathed.

Gunshot wounds, motorcycle accidents, primary brain tumors, and strokes are calamities befalling mostly teenagers or adults. Infants are more typically carried off by slower acting diseases like leukemia or viral and bacterial infections, and if the disease doesn't damage their organs, the treatments usually do.

Hooked up to a ventilator, an infant may be kept alive for an indefinite time, but when she is removed and allowed to die, her organs will deteriorate as a result of oxygen starvation. When, in transplant jargon, "tissue perfusion" is poor, the cells making up the tissues of the organs don't get enough oxygen and begin to die (become "ischemic"). Thus, the organs of an infant unable to breathe spontaneously who doesn't die while on a ventilator probably won't be in good enough condition to justify transplantation.

A few statistics show how devastating the organ shortage is for infants. Each year about 500 children need heart transplants; about the same number need a liver, and 400 to 500 need a kidney. Between 40 and 70 percent of these children die while on the transplant waiting list. Thirty to 50 percent of children under the age of 2 needing a transplant die before getting one. Probably many more die than this figure represents, because those born with severe defects (like Baby Mike's missing half his heart) don't live long enough to reach the waiting list.

No Consensus

If organs from anencephalic infants were donated by their parents and surgeons agreed to transplant them, the lives of many children who otherwise would die could be saved. Exactly how many is uncertain. Some in the transplant community think several hundred organs might be available every year, while others claim the number is a hundred or fewer. While the numbers are in dispute, no one doubts lives would be saved and that over time hundreds of babies could be rescued from certain death.

So what's to keep grieving but beneficent parents like Ellen and Ken

Howard from insisting they want their anencephalic child to become an organ donor? And what's to keep transplant surgeons from using the organs to save the lives of other children?

Nothing in principle stands in the way of the whole process playing out with the smoothness of a Masterpiece Theater production. Yet before transplant surgeons become easy about removing organs from anencephalic infants, the surgeons must feel confident that every step involved, in addition to being legal, is also morally legitimate. It's not surprising that a consensus is lacking about some of the steps.

The absence of agreement among ethicists, neonatologists, transplant surgeons, legislators, and others isn't because anyone believes the use of anencephalic organs is inherently wrong. Rather, knotty moral and conceptual problems connected with removing the organs of anencephalic infants stand in the way of consensus. The problems mostly originate with a rule of medical ethics that has evolved to protect potential donors—the Dead-Donor Rule.

The Dead-Donor Rule

The Dead-Donor Rule is simple and direct: before vital organs are removed, the donor must be dead. While people may consent to surrendering a patch of skin or a single kidney, they aren't allowed to consent to the removal of any organ required to sustain their life. Transplant surgeons, for their part, are constrained not to cause a donor's death by removing an organ necessary for life, even if the purpose is to save the life of someone else.

In the early days of heart and liver transplants during the late 60s, to follow the rule surgeons often had to keep a death watch over a donor, hovering outside his hospital door until he was declared dead, then rushing the body into an adjacent operating room to whip out the organs before they were damaged by the loss of circulation.

The organs might turn out to be useless anyway, if a donor took a long time to die. His weakened heart or slowed respiration could fail to deliver an adequate supply of oxygenated blood throughout the body and cause ischemia. In a desperate situation, the surgeon might go ahead and transplant the organ, but the recipient almost always died.

To eliminate these sad and frustrating episodes and increase the availability of usable donor organs, under the influence of the federal Uniform Determination of Death Act, states during the 1970s enacted laws introducing the concept of brain death and criteria for determining when it occurs. The Act's definition of brain death followed the formulation by a

Presidential Commission set up to study the issue, and its definition was modeled on the one in the 1968 report of the Harvard Medical School's Ad Hoc Committee to Examine the Definition of Brain Death.

The Committee was explicit about its aim and why a new definition was called for. "Our primary purpose," the report stated, "is to define irreversible coma as a new criterion for death," because "obsolete criteria for the definition of death can lead to controversy in obtaining organs for transplantation."

The "obsolete" criteria are the traditional cardiopulmonary or heart-lung criteria, according to which a person is dead when her heart has stopped and she's no longer breathing. Despite the Committee's label, these criteria haven't been displaced by brain death as a definition of death. Rather, we now operate with two sets of criteria. (See Chapter 8, "But Are They Really Dead?," for a discussion of the confusion this can cause.)

The question of whether someone is brain dead arises mostly in circumstances in which a patient's respiration or heartbeat is maintained by life-support devices and drugs. The great majority of people who die are declared dead in accordance with the same criteria King Lear appeals to when, cradling the pulseless body of Cordelia in his arms and holding a mirror to her lips, he says, "If that her breath will mist or stain the stone, why, then she lives."

The criteria for brain death presented in the Determination of Death Act and enshrined now in state laws are for whole-brain death. Death is defined as the irreversible cessation of all brain function. This means, essentially, there can be no electrical activity in the brain. Not even the brain stem can be producing signals.

In determining death, physicians may use, along with other measurements, EEG (electroencephalographic) data, and the "flat line" on an ER monitor has become as familiar in TV dramas as "He's stopped breathing, Doctor" was in the days of radio. Such data, however, serve only as evidence that brain function has permanently ceased, and by themselves they don't define death.

Physicians are enjoined by the criteria to consider a comatose patient's medical history and diagnose the cause of his loss of consciousness. These requirements are precautions to prevent someone unconscious as a result of taking drugs or (particularly in the case of a child) being submerged in icy water from being declared dead without further investigation. Ultimately, the determination of death, including brain death, is a physician's clinical judgment, a decision based on physical examination, tests and measurements, and a body of information.

Legally Dead

Anencephalic infants are not legally dead, whether judged by the old cardio-pulmonary criteria or the new brain-death criteria. An anencephalic infant's brain stem functions, and as a result his heart beats and his ventilatory muscles move his chest muscles to fill his lungs and then to expel the air. This is only the autonomic nervous system blindly doing its job, yet so long as the brain stem keeps issuing its instructions, the whole brain isn't dead. Thus, an anencephalic infant's organs can't be removed without violating the Dead-Donor Rule.

This is the conclusion the physicians at Children's Hospital came to when they faced the question of how they were going to treat Baby Gabrielle. "We felt we should stick with the classic definition of brain death," the head of the transplant unit said. Yet if Baby Gabrielle's organs were going to be worth transplanting, they would have to be kept perfused with oxygen-rich blood. This wasn't a problem at first, because for twelve hours she breathed on her own. But then her breathing slowed, and so with her parents' permission, she was put on a ventilator.

In an interpretation later disputed by some critics, Baby Gabrielle's physicians decided her failure to breathe regularly was an indication that her brain stem was deteriorating—that she was on the way to becoming brain dead. With the aim of detecting when her brain activity ceased entirely, the Ontario physicians adopted a procedure (a protocol) to check on her brain stem's activity.

After she had been attached to the ventilator, they tested her breathing reflex (like Dr. Stein's monitoring of Claire in the scenario) by turning off the ventilator for three minutes to see if she could breathe on her own. If she couldn't breathe spontaneously, that would be evidence her brain stem had failed. She would then be dead by the whole-brain criteria, and her organs could be removed without violating the Dead-Donor Rule.

Forty-eight hours after her birth, Baby Gabrielle was removed from the ventilator. When she didn't start breathing reflexively, she was pronounced dead. Her body was reconnected to the ventilator, then flown to California.

Loma Linda Medical Center, known already as the only hospital in the country willing to accept anencephalic infants as organ donors, had its own protocol for assessing their status. Anencephalic infants were allowed to remain on a ventilator for one week, and if during the week, they met the criteria for brain death, their organs would be used for transplantation. If brain death didn't occur by the end of the week, the infant would be taken off the ventilator and given only what hospitals call "comfort care" until he died. The protocol didn't extend to Baby Gabrielle, because she had already been declared dead.

Problems

Physicians at both Ontario's Children's Hospital and the Loma Linda Medical Center were committed to honoring the Dead-Donor Rule. Because the rule requires establishing brain death, they formulated procedures for testing for brain activity. While different, the approach taken by each group seems reasonable, yet critics were quick to object that no test for determining brain death can be assumed reliable for infants a few hours or even a few days old.

Imaging techniques, such as MRIs, CT- and PET-scans, easily detect the lack of such large brain structures as the cerebral hemispheres, but brain death isn't the sort of condition images can reveal. The electrical tracings of an EEG might seem a more promising method, but techniques for using the equipment were developed for adults and children with cerebral hemispheres, and there's no accepted way of measuring electrical activity in the brain stem alone. Further, EEGs must be interpreted, and experts don't consider their meanings clear for very young infants, anencephalic or not. Machines, in sum, provide relevant data, but they can't determine brain death.

The Ontario protocol relied on the failure of an anencephalic infant to breathe spontaneously, but critics charged that this isn't necessarily proof of brain death. If an infant's breathing falters and he's put on a ventilator, the brain stem is likely to remain as functional as the heart or liver. No evidence shows that, as time passes, it's likely to deteriorate in some inevitable programmed fashion.

Also, such clinical signs of death as a patient's eyes being fixed and the pupils dilated aren't reliable indicators in anencephalic infants, because they often are born with anomalies such as malformed retinas or nonfunctioning optic nerves. Similar reasons also rule out as unreliable the use of reactions to loud sounds or painful stimuli like sharp pinches.

In the matter of determining death, critics of the Ontario and Loma Linda protocols are generally acknowledged as correct. Scientific medicine, despite all its machinery and technical expertise, isn't able to guarantee a correct diagnosis of brain death in anencephalic infants. Hence, even when physicians do their best to abide by the Dead-Donor Rule, they have no way of being sure they aren't violating it.

It's this uncertainty more than any other factor that's led transplant surgeons to abandon the use of organs from anencephalic infants. Neither the surgeons nor their hospitals want to be charged with killing babies for their organs.

Revising Death

In trying to circle around this impasse, proponents of transplanting organs from anencephalic infants have explored several avenues. The most obvious solution is to revise the Uniform Determination of Death Act (and relevant state laws) and count anencephalic infants as brain dead without requiring them to meet the usual criteria.

Another solution is to drop the whole-brain concept of brain death and revise the criteria to define brain death as permanent and irreversible loss of cortical function. The cerebral cortex, the grey matter forming the outer layer of the brain's hemispheres, is necessary for intelligence, imagination, language, memory, and everything else referred to as higher brain function. Cortical function is permanently missing in anencephalic infants. Hence, they would be brain dead.

A difficulty with modifying the Universal Determination of Death Act criteria to define anencephalic infants as brain dead (and thus as dead) is that the infants are obviously not dead in any ordinary sense. Granted their mental status is nonexistent, they still breathe, suck, excrete, move their eyes, and flail their arms. They aren't corpses ready for burial, and we would consider it pathological for their parents or anyone else to treat them as if they were.

A second difficulty is that merely declaring anencephalic infants brain dead has an arbitrariness suggesting we're free to treat other groups the same way whenever we find it convenient. If the category "brain dead" is no more than a social construction, babies born blind, brain-injured, or with blue eyes might also be classified as brain dead. This is why advocates for the disabled usually oppose proposals to transplant organs from anencephalic infants. They see all disabled people threatened.

Another danger of playing fast and loose with the definition of brain death is that the part of society already skeptical about the current concept is likely to believe brain death is nothing more than a gimmick doctors use to get their hands on transplant organs. Enough suspicion already exists to make increasing organ donations an uphill struggle.

More appealing than declaring anencephalic infants brain dead is the redefinition of brain death as absence of cortical function. Death as the permanent loss of the capacity for thinking, feeling, and imagining captures our sense that anyone so unfortunate as to be deprived of these abilities is no more than the shell of a person.

But the net cast by this definition may catch too many fish. If manifesting cortical activity is the standard, then along with anencephalic infants, people in persistent vegetative states would be classified as brain dead.

Broadening the definition like this may not be unreasonable in an abstract way. Karen Quinlin's ten years of lying comatose in an extended care facility, ten years of blank days that for her could have been ten minutes or a thousand years, is for most of us a nightmare. How much better, we think, if we were given an anesthetic (to prevent the possibility of pain) and our organs were removed and distributed to people able to make better use of them.

But whatever we may think of such a proposal for ourselves, extending the category of the legally dead to include people in chronic vegetative states is too big a step to take to justify removing transplant organs from anencephalic infants. The proposal, at the least, would force us to face the range of problems associated with active euthanasia and eugenics and demand a radical restructuring of our social practices and institutions.

Setting Aside the Rule

Rather than engaging in a variety of philosophical contortions to permit us to use anencephalic transplant organs without violating the Dead-Donor rule, why not simply set aside the rule? More accurately, why not recognize anencephalic infants are an exception to the rule and allow their organs to be removed without their being dead?

This position was taken by the American Medical Association's Council on Ethical and Judicial Affairs in its 1995 report "The Use of Anencephalic Neonates as Organ Donors." The Council is explicit: "It is ethically permissible to consider the anencephalic neonate as a potential organ donor, although still alive under the current definition of death. . . ."

The reason the Council cites for making anencephalic infants an exception to the Dead-Donor Rule is that "the infant has never experienced, and never will experience, consciousness." In taking this as the crucial factor, the Council reflects a view common among those of us who think seriously about the status of anencephalic infants—namely, there is something very different about them, something that distinguishes them radically from other infants, even ones born with serious neurological defects. They are, biologically, human babies, but they lack something distinctively human.

No analogies seem helpful in understanding anencephalic infants. Although they've been compared to snails and fish, creatures we don't believe capable of consciousness, they don't resemble either, because animals have their own complicated ways of life and fit perfectly into ecological niches. Anencephalic infants have no niche, no natural place in this world.

Another group of physicians and ethicists, the Ethics Committee of the Transplantation Policy Center in Ann Arbor, Michigan, refused to take a stand on the question of whether an anencephalic infant should be thought of as alive or dead, preferring to sidestep the issue entirely.

Yet the Ann Arbor group in effect made taking organs from anencephalic infants an exception to the Dead-Donor Rule on the ground that they aren't like other infants. Rather, they "should be viewed as a class that is entirely sui generis, and one for which special rules and laws should apply." Or perhaps more to the point, certain rules and laws should not apply—in particular, the Dead-Donor Rule and laws defining death.

The AMA Council expresses the hope its report will help build a consensus favoring "removing organs from anencephalic neonates before the neonates die" and lead to a change in the law. The hope is based on the way the report of the Harvard Committee influenced the society in coming to accept the concept of brain death so quickly.

Two Questions

The AMA Council's 1995 opinion was a sharp departure from its earlier one. In 1988 the Council held that while using organs from anencephalic infants was ethically acceptable, the infants had to be dead before their organs were taken. Thus, the earlier opinion required following the Dead-Donor Rule.

However, in December of 1995 the Council was asked by the AMA House of Delegates (the organization's governing body) to reconsider its ethical position, leading the council to "suspend its opinion deeming use of anencephalic organs prior to legal death ethically permissible." The Council then reiterated its support for the Dead-Donor Rule.

Should we think of the Council's retreat from its bold position as a matter of a group forced to truckle to superior power? Perhaps that's what happened, but even if so, it doesn't establish the Council's original 1995 opinion as superior. I think the opinion manages to blur, if not confuse, two distinct questions best dealt with separately:

1. Is it ethically permissible to remove transplant organs from living anencephalic infants?
2. If it is, should this become public policy?

I suggest the correct answer to the first question is the one given by the Council—yes—but the answer to the second question is no. Setting aside the Dead-Donor Rule shouldn't become public policy, but even so, the uncertainties of correctly determining death in anencephalic infants shouldn't stand in the way of our using their organs for transplantation.

Let me explain.

The Best Interest Rule

The Council's claim that it's ethically acceptable to ignore the Dead-Donor Rule when transplanting organs from anencephalic infants seems correct. Anencephalic infants, as ethicists say, don't have an interest that would be violated by having their organs removed, even though it means the end of their lives.

The Best Interest Rule is a standard medical ethicists appeal to when deliberating about whether the treatment of a patient is morally justified. Is it, for example, in the best interest of Baby Sue, born nine-and-a-half weeks prematurely, to be treated aggressively? Extremely premature babies, because they haven't finished their growth in the uterus, aren't likely to survive, and if they do, usually have severe physical and mental impairments. Perhaps Baby Sue's interest would best be served by making her comfortable and allowing her die without becoming the object of painful, expensive, and probably futile efforts.

This case and hundreds like it are hard to deal with because our ignorance of the future makes any answer uncertain. The extremely premature baby may escape the statistical predictions and grow up to be a person with no deficits and an outstanding talent for mathematics. Or the child may lead a brief life, characterized chiefly by pointless agony. Still, the question about her best interest makes sense because we must make decisions on the basis of projecting a future for her.

With anencephalic infants, a question of best interest isn't so much difficult as inappropriate. It produces a mental cramp, because no answer can be either right or wrong. It's not a matter of waiting to see how things turn out and thinking maybe we should have decided some other way, because for anencephalic infants, things always turn out the same—the infant dies without ever having become conscious.

It doesn't even make sense to ask whether it's in the best interest of an anencephalic infant to live or die. When we talk of best interest it's always in a context in which people can be imagined to have a future or at least a past. We can reason it's in the best interest of a badly burned teenage boy to be kept alive, even though he begs to be allowed to die. We believe once he's made a recovery, he can live a satisfying life. He's got a future ahead of him that we can imagine for him.

Or we can say it's in the best interest of our unconscious Great Aunt Meg to be taken off a ventilator and allowed to die, because we remember "Meg never wanted to be kept alive by machines." She's got a past, one we can consult in making a decision.

The expectations of the future or the reality of the past guide us in our deliberations in making best-interest decisions. But anencephalic infants have neither past nor future in any meaningful sense. Their lack of even the possibility of consciousness and everything that implies (thinking, feeling, imagining, or remembering) translates into a lack of interest so complete that whether they live or die is, taking their point of view, a matter of indifference. There is no good for them in this world, though there is also no bad. There's only a void.

While it seems neurologically impossible for anencephalic infants to experience pain, they may react to what for others would be painful treatment. Because our knowledge of the brain is imperfect, the ethically safe course is to assume the reactions may be expressions of pain. In which case, the only possible interest anencephalic infants can have is to be protected from unnecessary pain.

But this concern that they not suffer is more a mark of our caution than the recognition that they are like other infants. Anencephalic infants are, as the Ann Arbor group holds, sui generis. They are human offspring, and by virtue of that and out of consideration for their parents and the practices of our society, they deserve to be treated with dignity.

Having no interest, anencephalic infants can't be treated in a way that will be against their interest. Granting this premise, the argument that organs from even live anencephalic infants can be used for transplantation can be put in a nutshell: (a) Lacking any interest, anencephalic infants can't be said to have a need for their organs, even though the organs keep them alive. (b) But dying children, who have a best interest and whose lives could be saved by a transplant, do have a need for the organs. (c) Also, the parents of some anencephalic infants might achieve some measure of solace by donating their child's organs to save the life of other children. Thus, we have powerful reasons to use (with parental consent) the organs of anencephalic infants and no reason not to.

On the view that anencephalic infants have no interest, the Council's opinion that it's morally acceptable to ignore the Dead-Donor Rule in removing organs from them is justified.

Making Public Policy

But would the Council's opinion make for good public policy? Put bluntly, would it be a good idea to change the law and allow a particular group of infants to be killed for their organs?

I suspect it was thinking about the matter in the broader social context, and not as an abstract ethical question, that persuaded the House of Delegates to encourage the Council to suspend its opinion and go back to the drawing board.

Turned into law, the Council's recommendation for even a limited suspension of the Dead-Donor Rule threatens to erode the prohibition against killing one person to save the life of another. In transplant medicine, this is an important stricture, for were it set aside, then on purely utilitarian grounds we could justify sacrificing the life of any single donor to acquire organs to save the lives of five or six other people.

While it might be natural to respond by arguing that an anencephalic infant isn't really a person and so it would be all right to kill one to get transplant organs, this would put us in the position of having to develop criteria to determine who is and who isn't a person. This is a rock that has sunk many philosophical ships. Despite all efforts to frame reasonable and adequate criteria, the results have been about as successful as gaining acceptance for a world language.

In the unlikely event that ethicists, physicians, and jurists could settle on criteria for identifying persons, it's doubtful society at large would be willing to accept the subtle distinctions they would inevitably involve. Also, criteria stringent enough to classify anencephalic infants as non-persons would most likely put fetuses into the same category. Thus, the abortion question would become hopelessly intertwined with debates about taking organs from anencephalic infants. Going down this road leads only to unnecessary frustration and confusion.

If we start killing human infants for their organs, we're also establishing a precedent dangerous to the society. "The slippery slope is real," Dr. Joyce Peabody, head of the Loma Linda program observed in a Los Angeles Times interview. Because of the prominence of her program, Dr. Peabody received referrals of infants as potential organ donors who were "born with an abnormal amount of fluid around the brain or those born without kidneys but with a normal brain." What's more, the referring physicians, she reported, "couldn't understand the difference between such newborns and anencephalics."

If such essentially normal infants are on the other side of the barrier against killing, setting aside the Dead-Donor Rule would leave them too vulnerable. The widening circle of donor "eligibility" can too easily spread from anencephalic infants to impaired newborns, then to impaired adults. Not that this would happen, but it could happen. And that's too big a risk.

But if we can avoid violating the Dead-Donor Rule while achieving the same positive results, we've won the game.

Winning the Game

At the center of the whirlwind of argument is a single problem: uncertainty over determining the death of anencephalic infants. It's this problem that prompted efforts to alter criteria for brain death and led the AMA Council to avoid the issue by recommending a suspension of the Dead-Donor Rule.

If anencephalic infants came equipped with plastic strips on their foreheads that changed from green to red when they died, the tangled issues about transplanting their organs would become irrelevant. But we're never going to get such an unambiguous indicator; we don't have it even for adults. The Council, in the course of suspending its 1995 opinion, calls for more research on ways of establishing death in anencephalic infants.

While additional research is likely to produce scientific findings useful to determining the cessation of brain stem activity, suspending the use of transplant organs from anencephalic infants while waiting for those findings is unnecessary. If it's unnecessary, it's also unconscionable, because while we're waiting for the research to be carried out—and how many years will that be?—children are dying who could be saved by receiving an organ from an anencephalic infant.

Now let me say why it's unnecessary.

The determination of death is ultimately a clinical judgment. It's a decision by a knowledgeable physician using relevant available information. The possibility of error is always present in making any kind of medical judgment, including one about death. When the cardiopulmonary criteria are applied to adults, death is sometimes misdiagnosed, and the same is so when brain-death criteria are employed. Experts say determining brain death in very young infants is especially difficult and the judgments aren't as reliable as they are in adults. For anencephalic infants, the judgments may be even less reliable.

This makes it hard for a physician to know whether she's following the Dead-Donor Rule when she says an anencephalic infant is dead and the organs may be removed for transplant. Has she misdiagnosed death? Is the infant really still alive?

The possibility is always there—but a mistake of this kind has no important consequence for anencephalic infants. Because they have no best interest, it's morally acceptable to remove their transplantable organs before they are dead. The important consideration, rather, is that following the Dead-Donor Rule makes for better social policy than setting it aside. Hence, physicians knowledgeable about anencephalic infants should use their best clinical judgement to determine that an infant is dead before approving the removal of the organs for transplantation.

Yet if a physician should make a mistake and wrongly diagnose death, no moral wrong will be done. An anencephalic infant may die earlier than otherwise, but this is neither good nor bad. Having no past, having no future, without even the possibility of consciousness, the infant has no best interest, no good to be promoted.

Protocol

Most people when they hear about the parents of anencephalic infants wanting to donate their child's organs for transplantation imagine the process must be quite simple. It should be, and I believe the following three conditions (call them a protocol) are sufficient for protecting everybody's interest, while also making organs available for saving lives.

1. The diagnosis of anencephaly should be made independently by two physicians with relevant expertise (e.g., a neonatologist or pediatric neurologist) who aren't members of the transplant team. Because anencephalic infants have no best interest, a correct diagnosis is crucial.
2. The parents of an anencephalic infant should be given an opportunity to consent to donate their child's organs. The parents may initiate the process or a hospital staff member may mention the option to them. Parents can't be assumed to be sufficiently knowledgeable and self-possessed to think of the option themselves.
3. Once parental consent is given, the anencephalic infant must be declared dead by two physicians with relevant expertise before the organs are removed. The physicians cannot be members of the transplant team.

THE LOMA LINDA PROGRAM was closed down after only eight months. Generally regarded as a failure, the program's closing more than a dozen years ago marked the end of any on-going effort to make use of transplant organs from anencephalic infants.

During the eight months the program operated, twelve anencephalic babies were placed on ventilators, but none became an organ donor. Only one ever met the brain-death criteria, and no recipient could be found for his organs. The other eleven were disconnected from their ventilators when the week specified by the protocol was up. All were given only comfort care and eventually died.

The flaw in the Loma Linda program was in its protocol of keeping infants on ventilators until they died. We have no moral duty to keep anyone on a ventilator who has no possibility of recovering, and anencephalic infants lack the potential for any condition resembling recovery.

We have no moral obligation to sustain their lives, and if we put them on ventilators to preserve their organs, we can remove the ventilators to check their status. If their hearts stop or they stop breathing or evidence indicates their brain stem is no longer functioning, they can be declared dead. They can then be reattached to the ventilator to protect the organs.

This was the procedure physicians at Ontario's Children's Hospital followed in dealing with Baby Gabrielle. And they saved the life of Paul Holc, who's now a teenager.

That should be recommendation enough for anybody.

5

Kidney for Sale

Is it Ever Right to Sell Your Kidney?

Cleveland Medical Center: September, 2000

ALICE CUSHMAN

"I need to see Dr. Hauser," Alice said in a wheezy voice. She was breathing hard, her heart thumping. She'd run from her car. "It's about my daughter, Karen Cushman."

"I'll page him," the nurse said. She pointed past the door to the stairs. "You can wait over there."

As Alice turned, she caught sight of a short, balding man sitting in one of the upholstered chairs. Tom Weaver, the manager at Rendezvous Stables. He got up and hurried over to her.

"I'm so sorry, Ms. Cushman," Weaver said. His brown eyes were so large they made her think of the horses he managed. "I saw it happening, but I was helpless."

"What did you see?"

"It had nothing to do with horses." Weaver was so emphatic she was sure he was worried she'd sue. "Karen and the others stabled their horses and hung up their tack. Jill said she and Karen went up into the hayloft, and Karen decided to crawl out on the hoist arm. She wanted to reach the big sycamore that grows beside the stable."

"Did she fall?" Alice wanted the story to be over.

"I saw her swing up onto a limb," Weaver said. "Then she lost her grip. When she fell, she hit the end of the hoist." His face took on a pained expression. "I heard a sharp crack, like a stick breaking. Then she was on the ground."

"Thank you." Alice stiffened. She noticed a tall, dark-haired man in green scrubs at the nursing station. "I've got to talk to the doctor now," she told Weaver. "You don't have to stay."

Alice approached the man in the green scrubs. "Dr. Hauser?"

"Karen is doing fine, Ms. Cushman." He shook her hand. "But we need to talk about her treatment. We've run into a situation that's a bit unusual."

"Could I see her first, . . . please?" She needed to study Karen's face. Touch her. She needed to know the worst.

"We had to perform emergency surgery to stop the bleeding from her damaged kidney, so she's still recovering from the anesthesia." Dr. Hauser's voice was so soft she had to strain to hear. "She came through well, and we're moving her to the surgical ICU."

Alice walked with Dr. Hauser into a narrow room that was hardly more than an alcove. A nurse in a flowered jacket was bending over the bed adjusting a wire leading to a monitor. She stepped to the side, giving Alice a clear view of Karen.

Her heart froze. Tears welled up. Karen's face was swollen, and her black hair was matted and stringy. The area around her eyes was greasy. The pale-blue plastic tube in her mouth was held in place by a crisscross of white tape. A smaller tube ran down one nostril, and what seemed like a dozen wires and leads were attached to her body. Behind her bed, a blue computer screen displayed an array of numbers in yellow characters. Somewhere another machine was producing a soft whooshing.

Everything blinked out of focus a moment. Alice reached out and put her hand on top of Karen's. Karen's silky skin was warm, and Alice stroked it with her index finger.

"Is she going to be okay?" Her voice was husky, and so small she wondered if she'd spoken aloud.

"She's doing fine," Dr. Hauser said. "She'll look better when we pull the tubes and she wakes up."

"But will she be okay?" Alice persisted. "And what's the strange situation?"

"Come into my office," Dr. Hauser said. "Karen's being well taken care of."

BETTY BURKE

Betty Burke rapped on her son's door, then stepped into the room. Chris lay stretched out on his bed watching the small TV she'd bought him for his fifteenth birthday.

"How come you're not at soccer practice?" She glared at him. "This is the second time. Coach Bronfman is gonna drop you from the team."

"I'm trembling." Chris shrugged. "So I'll have more time to study." His eyes drifted back to the screen.

"Or watch TV," Betty snapped. "How come you didn't go?"

"I'm too beat." Chris didn't look at her.

"Do you feel sick?"

She had noticed around the time of Chris's birthday his skin had the pale translucent look of porcelain, but she'd put it down to the fading of his summer tan. Like her, Chris had straw-colored hair, pale blue eyes, and fair skin. But she could also see her ex-husband reflected in the line of his jaw. Chris would be a good-looking man, but he was going to be her little boy for a few more years.

"I just feel tired," Chris said. "And I've been going to bed early, too. It's not fair."

Betty wondered if Chris wasn't depressed. She'd gone through a bout of depression eleven years earlier, when Tom had divorced her and moved to Seattle with his 20-year-old girlfriend. Betty had been 28 when she'd found herself completely responsible for a 4-year-old child and no real job skills.

Tom hadn't asked for custody, but he hadn't paid child-support either. She'd worked as a waitress, then as a cashier at Lottsa Pasta for four years before passing the test for a real estate license. It took another three years before she started earning enough to give up work as a fill-in cashier.

Two weeks after that evening, Chris met her at the door when she returned from work. He was on the verge of tears.

"Look at this, Mom," he pulled up a leg of his jeans. His right shin and calf were marked by a scattering of liver-covered spots. Some were the size of a quarter, but others were no larger than a pencil point.

"The other leg is like that too." His voice was panicky. "Those look like bruises." Betty fought back her own panic. She ran a finger over Chris's skin, touching the spots. "Did you get kicked a lot at soccer?"

"No," Chris said. "My stomach hurt, and Coach Bronfman said I didn't have to play."

"I'm going to call the doctor. Probably it's only an allergy." She tried to sound normal, but her voice trembled.

ALICE CUSHMAN

Dr. Hauser's office was small and spartan, furnished with little more than a metal desk and a tall bookcase. Alice sat in the armchair and waited while Dr. Hauser fetched coffee.

He handed her a paper cup, then slid into in his swivel chair. She took a sip of the coffee, welcoming its warmth and bitterness. Now that she'd seen Karen, some of the raw fear she'd felt had subsided.

"Your daughter's left kidney was crushed in her fall. She also broke two ribs and has a lot of bruising. But the kidney is the main problem."

"The surgery didn't fix it?"

"When she was brought to the trauma unit, we suspected hemorrhaging." Dr. Hauser ignored her question. "To combat shock, we started giving her fluids IV and hurried her down for a CT scan. We could see her kidney was badly damaged and bleeding to beat the band, so we knew we had to operate. But it was what we didn't see that worried us more."

"What do you mean?" Her shoulder muscles tightened.

"We couldn't see her right kidney. Sometimes scans don't show you everything, and it was possible it was in some unusual location."

"Is that common?" She put the coffee on the edge of the desk. The sip she'd taken had made her stomach sour.

"It happens." Dr. Hauser shrugged. "We injected her with a contrast dye, then scanned her again." He checked her expression, and she nodded. "We weren't able to locate a right kidney."

"What does that mean?"

"Karen was apparently born with only one kidney. That's not as unusual as you might think. By some estimates, as many as one out of every 11,000 people have a single kidney."

"But wouldn't a doctor have found out before now?" She thought of the many times she'd taken Karen to her pediatrician for checkups.

"Not necessarily." Dr. Hauser shook his head. "A single kidney is enough to do the job, and unless somebody gets an infection or has an accident like Karen's, they can live a normal life and never learn they have only one kidney."

"But what about Karen?" Alice fought to keep her voice at a normal level. "She *did* have an accident."

"We didn't take out her kidney. We tried to repair it, but it's so damaged, I can't hold out much hope we can save it."

"But you said she was stable." She made the statement an accusation. "I thought that meant she wasn't in danger."

"She's not in immediate danger." Dr. Hauser snatched a drink of coffee. "The kidney is still bleeding a little, and if it doesn't stop, we'll have to remove it. It's also likely to get infected, because there's been so much tissue damage."

"But what can you do?" She felt the darkness closing in. She'd thought Karen was safe. But she still might die.

"She'll have to start dialysis. In fact we're putting her on the machine immediately, because her kidney is no longer functioning." He paused "Of course I'd like to get her off dialysis as quickly as possible, because kids on dialysis don't always grow normally. There can be other problems too."

Alice thought of having to take Karen to be hooked up to a machine for several hours three or four times a week. Her great aunt had been on dialysis for almost a year and had found it so difficult that eventually she'd finally refused to go and had died a week later. How could she subject Karen to that?

"Oh, God." Alice put both hands over her face. "Poor Karen."

"Don't let the idea of dialysis get you down too much," Dr. Hauser said. "If Karen loses her kidney, she's an excellent candidate for a transplant."

"That's better than dialysis?" Her voice was bitter.

"Night and day," Dr. Hauser said. "With a transplanted kidney, her growth will be normal, and she'll feel better. She'll have to take antirejection drugs, but she can live almost like any other teenager."

"Then you'll give her a transplant?" Alice asked. "If she needs one."

"If a donor kidney is available. We can put her on the UNOS list, but I'm warning you now, it's a long one."

"How long?"

"She's probably looking at two, two and a half years."

"Years! That's impossible."

"If Karen can get a kidney from a living donor, the transplant becomes elective surgery. The results are also better, in terms of rejection and long-term survival."

"Then I'll be the donor," Alice said. "My husband was killed in a plane crash when Karen was ten, and my closest relative is a cousin in the Virgin Islands. Somebody I've never met."

"We're not going to let you be a donor until we make sure *you* have two kidneys that are both in working order."

"How soon can you test me?"

Alice picked up her coffee and took a long swallow. She almost felt happy. Karen had a way back to health, and her mother was going to provide it.

BETTY BURKE

Dr. Harvey Langhorn, the pediatrician Chris went to for sports exams, was uncharacteristically glum after he had examined Chris, paying particular attention to the spots on his legs. Leaving Chris to get dressed, Dr. Langhorn asked Betty into his office for a private talk. He'd never done that before.

"I want you to take Chris to see Dr. Brenda Fox at the Cleveland Medical Center," Dr. Langhorn said. "I'm sending her blood samples, and my office will make an appointment for you."

"What's wrong with him?" Betty asked. She was reluctant to leave without finding out something.

"He might have a blood disorder," Dr. Langhorn said. "But he'll need some tests I'm not able to perform. Dr. Fox is a pediatric hematologist, and she can give you some answers."

Dr. Brenda Fox was a small brisk woman with a quick smile and an easy manner. She shook hands with Betty and Chris as she escorted them into her tiny, cluttered office.

She chatted with Chris for a moment, then got down to business. "Dr. Langhorn was right," she said, looking at Betty. "Chris's symptoms point to a blood disorder, and the tests show he has an abnormal number of immature white cells." Dr. Fox paused. "But to confirm what we suspect, we need to take a sample of Chris's bone marrow."

"Will it hurt?" Chris asked.

"A little bit," Dr. Fox admitted.

A week later Betty was back in Dr. Fox's cluttered office. Chris sat outside, watching *Bingo* on the waiting-room TV.

"The tests on the bone marrow confirmed what we suspected," Dr. Fox said. "Chris's marrow is filled with a high percentage of immature cells called myeloblasts."

"What is the disorder exactly?" Betty was getting frustrated with the vague way everybody talked. "Does it have a name?"

"Acute myeloid leukemia," Dr. Fox said gently. "Or AML."

"Blood cancer." She felt too stunned to think. Dr. Fox's voice seemed to be reaching her from a distant place. It was worse than she had imagined. She'd thought Chris would have to take drugs or vitamins to build up his blood. But leukemia?

"More accurately, AML is bone-marrow cancer. That's where the bad cells originate. They're related to white blood cells called granulocytes."

Betty no longer understood anything Dr. Fox was saying. She wanted to snatch up Chris and run away someplace where the sky was a bright blue and it was sunny and children didn't have to think about cancer or death. Death. Chris? It happened to other people's children, so it could happen to him.

"I gave you the worst news," Dr. Fox was saying. "But the good news is AML is treatable. Even better, treatment can lead to a complete cure."

"What's the treatment?"

"It has two possible phases," Dr. Fox said. "We begin with chemotherapy to try for a remission. We test that by checking for a normal number of blast cells in the marrow. If the number is normal, that's the end of treatment."

"But if it isn't?"

"We go to the second phase and use a high-dose course of chemotherapy to wipe out the bone marrow," Dr. Fox said. "We then re-seed it with cells from normal marrow. If they divide and establish themselves, we begin to think we've got a cure." She looked directly at Betty. "Close relatives make the best marrow donors, because they're more likely to be a match. We'll need to test Chris's relatives."

"You're looking at pretty much all he's got," Betty said. "His dad lives in Seattle. Or at least he did. I don't even know how to find him." She shrugged. "He hasn't got any brothers or sisters, and his grandparents on both sides are all dead."

"We can go the National Marrow Donor Program, but that's a long shot."

"I'll be tested whenever you want," Betty said. If she could take Chris's disease away and make it her own, she would.

"Let's not get ahead of the game," Dr. Fox said. "It may never come to that. Right now I want you to take Chris to a surgeon to get a shunt put in. He can then have the chemo drugs injected directly into a blood vessel, and we won't have to stick him with needles all the time."

ALICE CUSHMAN

In the three days after the accident, Alice followed the path of her ordinary life like a robot going through programmed motions. She wished she had someone to share her worries with. She missed Peter more than ever. When he was killed, their daughter and the business they'd started together became the twin poles around which her life revolved.

She and Karen lived well, but more important, she could provide Karen with whatever she needed. She hoped to leave her a trust fund large enough to allow her to decide what she wanted to do in life without worrying about money. If she wanted to be an actress or an artist, she could. But now Karen's accident cast a shadow over her whole future.

On Thursday, two days after Alice had submitted herself to a battery of tests, when she returned to Cleveland General she received two pieces of bad news.

"Karen's kidney is going to have to come out," Dr. Hauser told her. "It's so badly damaged it's pulpy, and we can't get it to stop bleeding. Also, as

I was afraid might happen, it's infected. We're treating the infection, but the best thing would be to get rid of the kidney, which isn't doing any good, before the infection spreads and becomes life-threatening."

"Then do it." Alice had been prepared for the news and wasn't shocked to hear it. "But how long do we have to wait before you give her my kidney?"

"I'm sorry." Dr. Hauser glanced away. "You're doing okay with your kidneys, but both of them are seriously scarred."

"How could that be?" Alice stood up. "I've never had a kidney problem in my life."

"You could have had one without knowing it. It might have been a urinary tract infection that spread and damaged your kidneys before it was brought under control."

"Are you telling me I can't be a donor?" She barely registered what Dr. Hauser was saying about her. It was Karen she was thinking about.

"It would be too dangerous for her. We don't want to subject her to the risks of surgery and infection to give her a kidney that might not work." Dr. Hauser spread out his hands. "Also, you're doing fine with your kidneys, but if we took one, you might start having trouble. You might need a transplant yourself, then you couldn't help Karen as much."

"I understand your point." Her voice was dull.

"Karen will do okay on dialysis. And remember, she's already on the UNOS waiting list."

Two years. Or more. Will Karen stop growing? She won't be the same lively, funny kid. She'll become a sad child, forced to be brave, always in and out of the hospital.

"Do people ever die while waiting?"

"I . . . I'm afraid they do," Dr. Hauser said. "But there's no need to think about that now."

Alice suddenly had trouble getting her breath. Tears welled up behind her eyelids. She tried to blink them away, but they spilled over and ran down her cheeks. Ignoring Dr. Hauser, she put her face in her hands and sobbed.

BETTY BURKE

Chris tolerated the chemotherapy surprisingly well. Starting on the day after each treatment, he began to throw up. But the drugs prescribed by the pediatric oncologist brought the nausea under control.

Chris spend four weeks in the hospital. Because his immune system was suppressed, he was at risk for accidental infections and had to be isolated in his room. Betty, gowned and gloved and wearing a sterile mask, stayed with him as much as she could, but most of the time, Chris was bored. He worked at his school assignments in a half-hearted way and watched too much television. He was allowed to walk around the halls wearing a gauze mask, but he felt so weak he spent most time in his room. One of the boys he made friends with died a week after they met.

The doctors were always drawing blood from him, yet it was puncturing his hip to take out marrow that Betty hated the most. Chris learned to tolerate it, but each time it happened, she left the session with tears in her eyes.

Three weeks after Chris completed the last round of chemotherapy and was allowed to go home, Betty got a call to see Dr. Fox. "Bad news, I'm afraid," Dr. Fox said. "Chris has about 30-percent blast cells in his marrow, and that's not good." Betty nodded, feeling numb. "But we've still got the bone marrow transplant to fall back on, and it's very successful in treating Chris's disease." She gave Betty a sympathetic look, then dropped her gaze. "But there's one problem."

"I told you I'll be the donor."

"That's not it," Dr. Fox said. "A bone marrow transplant, with hospital stay, tests, and everything, costs about $300,000."

"I've got insurance," Betty said. "It covers Chris too."

"I've been on the phone with your carrier myself," Dr. Fox said. "They'll okay the BMT, but they pay only 70 percent. So you need to come up with 60,000." She gave Betty an embarrassed look. "Can you do that?"

"Sixty-thousand?" Betty shook her head. "If I sold my car and everything I own, I might be able to come up with three." She squeezed her hands into fists. "Isn't there some way I could owe the hospital? Or maybe get on welfare?"

"The hospital won't admit Chris without proof of ability to pay," Dr. Fox said. "Even if Chris could qualify for Medicaid, which he probably can't, it wouldn't help you. The state funds budgeted for cases like his have already been spent for this fiscal year. Next year the funding starts again."

"But that's crazy," Betty said, her voice rising in anger. "He needs the treatment now, not next year."

"I wish I could suggest something," Dr. Fox said.

CHANCE MEETING

The waiting area of the cashier's office at Cleveland General was crowded, and Alice felt fortunate to find a seat. As she squeezed into the chair next to the wall, a woman with short blonde hair shifted her purse to give her more room.

"Thanks." Alice smiled. "They don't make it easy, do they? If I knew they wouldn't kick my daughter out, I'd make them wait for their money."

"My son's here." The woman turned her head, and Alice noticed her eyes were red-rimmed and her makeup blotchy. "They're kicking him out, because I can't pay for his treatment." Her voice was low, but tight with anger.

"My God," Alice said. "I didn't know that was legal. Is he very sick?"

"Leukemia. He needs a bone-marrow transplant, and I don't have $60,000 to pay my part." She tightened her lips. "What's the matter with . . . ?"

"She needs a kidney transplant," Alice said. "But we may have to wait two or three years. They won't use one of my kidneys, because they're shot to hell." Alice felt tears stinging her eyes. "My husband is dead, and I don't have any relatives to ask."

"Sounds like me. Only, my ex-husband just disappeared, and even if he hadn't, I doubt he'd have any money." She looked at Alice for a moment. "I wish I could help you."

"That's a nice thought." She held out her hand. "I'm Alice Cushman."

"Betty Burke." Alice noticed the woman's short nails were torn and ragged.

"Maybe I should surf the net, and see if I can find somebody with a spare kidney." Alice gave a snorting laugh.

"Are you serious?" Betty sat up in her chair, suddenly alert. "How much would you pay?"

"I was just spouting off. I hadn't thought about it really." Then she caught on. "You mean you'd give up a kidney?"

"For sixty-thousand dollars?" Betty nodded vigorously. "In a heartbeat."

"But the blood and tissues have to match." Alice's mind was racing ahead, imagining what would have to be done. What could go wrong. "I know that much."

"I'm willing to be tested." Betty's voice had an edge of excitement. "Today. Right now."

"Even if you didn't match, I know they do kidney exchanges," Alice said, half to herself. "Probably we could swap the right kind of kidney for yours." Then she stopped. "But they won't accept you as a donor here, unless you're a relative."

"So who's to say we're not? Maybe I'm a half-sister or an aunt or a cousin—anything." Betty leaned closer. "You do have sixty-thousand? You could pay me in cash?"

"Not a problem," Alice said. "I've got enough in the bank."

Betty smiled, then began to cry. Alice felt tears spring into her own eyes. Each held out her arms for the other, then coming together, they clutched each other tightly.

KAREN

Betty was a crossmatch for blood and tissue compatibility. Alice was ready with a cooked-up story about how she and her cousin Betty had been out of touch since they were teenagers. But only Margo James, the transplant social worker, asked her about her Betty, and Margo seemed satisfied with the story.

Alice paid Betty half the promised money, and Betty gave it to the hospital as a deposit. Betty donated bone marrow for Chris, and the hospital authorized his doctors to proceed with the bone-marrow transplant.

Karen was up and walking the day after her surgery, and her new kidney started producing urine immediately. Her blood pressure, which had been abnormally high, returned to normal, and the fluid making her feet and legs puffy was eliminated by her new kidney.

"I never thought I'd be this happy again," Alice told her daughter as they drove home from the hospital. She kissed her fingertips and pressed them against Karen's cheek.

Betty didn't regain her strength until a month after surgery. Her abdomen remained sore, and she still tired easily. Even so, she was strong enough to see Chris through the bone marrow transplant.

CHRIS

Chris had a harder time than Karen. Over a course of four days he was given high doses of chemicals to destroy his bone marrow. He vomited uncontrollably, and chill and fevers racked his body. Drugs helped very little.

For a month he was unable to tolerate food, even the thinnest of broths, and he was fed intravenously. Sores broke out in his mouth, and yeast colonized his mouth and throat. The antifungal drug caused severe headaches and a constant tingling in his arms and hands. But he improved. Thirty-one days after his first dose of chemotherapy, he was allowed to return home.

"His blood count is essentially normal," Dr. Fox told Betty. "About 80 percent of the time, when marrow comes from a close relative, we get a good outcome." She smiled at Betty. "I'd say you can consider Chris cured."

Betty glanced at Chris huddled against the door of the car. His face was thin and pale, but his blue eyes were huge. They were looking everywhere, taking in the world. Winter had passed, and it was May. The air was cool, but the sun reflected from Lake Erie made the day spectacularly bright.

ALICE CUSHMAN had the money to buy the kidney Karen needed, and Betty Burke was willing to donate a kidney for the money needed to pay for Chris's treatment. In a society committed to a market economy, a partial solution to the problem of the shortage of kidneys for transplants seems simple—those needing a kidney can purchase it from those having one to spare.

When a willing buyer meets a willing seller, as the economists say, a kidney could be exchanged at a price acceptable to both parties. Those with a spare kidney turn out to be virtually every healthy person, because kidneys, like eyes and ears, are paired organs, and we can get along about as well with one kidney as with two.

International Kidney Exchange, Inc.

This solution was appreciated as long ago as 1983 by H. Barry Jacobs, a Virginia physician who lost his license as the result of a 1977 mail-fraud conviction. Jacobs possessed a keen appreciation of advances in the field of transplant medicine. Kidney transplantation had steadily improved during the 70s, and by the early 80s, it was rocking and rolling. Because of the federal End-Stage Renal Disease Act, dialysis was guaranteed to everyone needing it, regardless of the ability to pay, and many who would have died a decade earlier were kept alive by kidney machines. The act also paid for transplantation, so as dialysis extended the lives of an increasing number of people, the need for transplants also increased.

But where were the kidneys to come from? Enter Dr. Jacobs with a plan. Not coincidentally, the plan also constituted a business opportunity for Dr. Jacobs.

Jacobs founded the International Kidney Exchange, in September 1983, to broker kidneys from living donors. Jacobs planned to advertise for healthy people willing to surrender a kidney for financial gain. The potential donor would set the price, and Jacobs would undertake to match up a donor with a recipient. For the services involved in bringing them together, he would collect a brokerage fee ranging from $2,000 to $5,000.

The recipient-buyer would ordinarily be expected to pay this fee. If, however, the recipient were covered by Medicaid or some other government-funded medical program, the program would pick up the fee. It would become a part of the overall medical bill for a transplant, like the surgeon's fee or the cost of the hospital stay.

Jacobs was aware that in an affluent nation like the United States he might not be able, despite extensive advertising, to attract enough people willing to sell a kidney. His company wasn't called the *International* Kidney Exchange for no reason, and his plans included recruiting donors from third-world countries. People conscripted from abroad would be transported to the United States for surgery, then returned home with money in their pockets.

Jacobs even anticipated the problem of securing informed consent from donors who might be illiterate. They would be warned of the dangers and complications of having a kidney removed, then, if they were still willing, they would express their consent by means of a conversation with a physician. If needed, an interpreter would be supplied. The conversation would be tape-recorded to form a permanent record.

Jacobs's brokerage plan was roundly condemned by all who took notice of it. A distinguished bioethicist characterized the scheme as involving "profiteering," because it took advantage of those who are desperately poor, as well as those desperately in need of a kidney. The public and professional organizations involved in kidney transplants—the National Kidney Foundation, the American Society of Transplant Surgeons, the American Society of Transplant Physicians, and the Association of Independent Organ Procurement Organizations—issued statements condemning Jacobs's brokerage plan. The National Kidney Foundation denounced the sale of kidneys as "immoral and unethical."

Freelancers

While Jacobs was the only medical entrepreneur proposing to broker live kidneys, a number of potential donors saw an opportunity to freelance their own kidneys. The following ad appeared on Christmas Day, 1983, in the Burlington County edition of the *New Jersey Times*:

> **Kidney for Sale**
> From 32-yr.-old Caucasian female
> in excellent health.
> Write to P.O. Box 654 . . .

In Georgia, a man offered to sell a kidney for $25,000 so he could buy a McDonalds' franchise. A woman later undercut this price by offering one for a mere 5,000. California seemed to have more freelancers than other states, but the prices asked ranged as high as a 160,000.

Such ads triggered at least one best-selling novel. Robin Cook claimed that *Coma*, with a plot hinging on supplying transplant organs for a large-scale blackmarket, was inspired by an unsigned ad in a California newspaper offering to sell any organ the reader wanted to buy.

Laws

The freelancers apparently never got any takers, and Jacobs's brokerage operation never got off the ground. Without the cooperation of the surgeons and physicians in the professional organizations, Jacobs's scheme could never have worked, but even so, the state of Virginia delivered a *coup de gras* to the International Kidney Exchange by passing legislation specifically prohibiting the sale of human organs. Within a few months, California, Maryland, and New York passed similar laws, and several other states were soon lined up to follow.

The need for additional state laws ended in 1984 with the passage of the National Organ Transplantation Act (Public Law No. 98–507). The OTA holds, among numerous other provisions, that:

> It shall be unlawful for any person to knowingly acquire, receive,
> or otherwise transfer any human organs for valuable consideration
> for use in human transplantation if the transfer affects interstate
> commerce.

Lawyers still speculate about whether this wording will stand up to scrutiny in a court of law. Does "transfer" for "valuable consideration" outlaw awarding an honorarium as an expression of gratitude? Is paying a donor for enduring pain and suffering illegal? The transplant community, even so, sees its meaning as clear: no organ sales under any description.

During the Congressional hearings preceding the passage of the OTA, Jacobs testified that while he preferred to see the government handling the procurement of organs, if it failed to do so, he was prepared to step into the breech. He regarded his brokerage plan, he admitted, as the foundation of a "very lucrative potential business."

Albert Gore, then a Senator from Tennessee, joined his colleagues in denouncing Jacobs's plan. Summoning a familiar image, Gore declared, "People should not be regarded as things to be bought and sold like parts of an automobile."

Britain

Despite numerous newspaper ads soliciting buyers for live kidneys, no evidence shows that anyone in the United States actually succeeded in becoming a paid kidney donor. Britain, by contrast, had at least one case and perhaps several.

In 1988, Colin Benton, a British citizen, died of renal disease after a kidney transplant failed. Benton's widow later revealed that the kidney had been obtained from a Turkish citizen who had traveled to London to have it removed at a private hospital. He was said to have been paid 2,500 pounds (about $4,400). When reporters asked the donor why he'd agreed to sell his kidney, he explained that he was a poor man and his daughter required surgery. Selling a kidney was his only way of raising the money needed to pay for it.

Prime Minister Margaret Thatcher, reacting to the Benton case and to newspaper reports that other Turkish citizens had also been brought to Britain to become paid donors, denounced the "sale of kidneys or any other organ of the body" as "morally repugnant." While Mrs. Thatcher's commitment to a free market remained strong, it was obviously not absolute, and her government rushed emergency legislation through Parliament to outlaw all organ sales.

Condemned as Illegal and Immoral, but . . .

By the end of the 1980s, virtually every country in Europe and North America had passed legislation forbidding commerce in kidneys from live donors. Yet the Jacobs and Benton cases continue to be discussed, and whenever they are, the use of paid living donors is typically denounced.

Often those censuring the practice mention as a justification only its apparent seaminess and the disgust it evokes. Over the years, however, a number of ethicists, lawyers, and members of the transplant community have produced a veritable Chinese menu of objections to paying live kidney donors.

The more prominent and recurrent include: a paid donor loses the psychological benefits that reward a voluntary donor; the practice reduces altruism in the society; the quality of donated kidneys will decline; the donor may suffer harm and become a burden to society; selling a kidney involves putting a price on the priceless; organ selling treats the human body as a commodity and thus reduces our respect for people.

While these complaints are serious, they are overshadowed in importance by the protest that the practice exploits the poor and thus is rightly outlawed. While I'm prepared to endorse the exploitation aspect of this complaint, I think if we take the world as we find it, as a place where basic needs aren't always met, in some situations paying a kidney donor isn't morally objectionable. I want to argue this point and suggest the OTA be amended to permit paying living donors in special circumstances. The issues emerge, however, only against the background of a few facts about dialysis and transplantation using donor kidneys.

Dialysis

Faced with people who were sick and dying because their kidneys had been choked up by disease or crushed by injury, physicians at the turn of the twentieth century desperately began searching for a means to assist them. The two methods attempted are the ones still used—kidney transplants and dialysis—even though it took fifty years of experimentation before either produced anything resembling satisfactory results.

Dialysis, thanks to the steady commitment of the Dutch-American researcher Wilhelm Kolff, became a practical reality in the 1950s. It did much to make the development of transplant surgery possible by keeping patients alive while a donor kidney could be located. It also gave surgeons a backup in case of organ rejection. Transplant surgery was already enough like high-wire walking not to have to be done without a net.

Dialysis is nothing more than using a machine to take over the kidney's filtration function. A patient's blood is slowly drained from her body and after traveling through a dialyzer, is returned to the system. The blood in the dialyzer passes through layers of membranes surrounded by a specially formulated fluid. As the blood travels, urea, potassium, and other waste materials pass through the membranes and into the surrounding fluid. The cleansing process takes from two to six hours.

Dialysis is cheaper than ever, but still expensive. The cost of each treatment session is $115–120, and some people require two or three sessions a week. When the expense of the equipment and its operation, hospital facilities, and the time of nurses, physicians, and technicians are taken into account, the real cost of dialysis may be as much as $100,000 a year for a single person. Some 200,000 people in the United States undergo the process for a yearly total of about eight billion dollars. Expenses are paid for all patients under the federal End-Stage Renal Disease Act.

Dialysis saves lives, but it's a miserable experience. People who are chronically ill may have to endure being hooked up to a machine for four- or five-hour sessions three days a week and must carefully regulate their diet and fluid intake. Despite the name "artificial kidney," dialysis machines perform only the filtration function, and the regulatory hormones produced by a normal kidney aren't supplied. Children on dialysis, despite drug therapy, often fail to develop properly, and prolonged treatment can lead to anemia, generalized infections, neurological damage, gastrointestinal bleeding, recurring headaches, and bone disease.

Psychological and physical stress also exact a heavy toll. Depression is common. Five percent of dialysis patients take their own lives, and another 7 percent commit "passive suicide" by dropping out of treatment programs or refusing to stick to their diets. Failing to adhere to the rigid requirements governing successful dialysis is the third most common cause of death among older patients. Dialysis is so hard to endure that only the prospect of certain death keeps most people tethered to the machines, and for some even that prospect eventually becomes preferable to prolonged suffering.

Transplants

Kidney transplantation is far superior to dialysis for most people with chronic kidney disease. Living with a transplant is no picnic, but what a real kidney does is more and better than what an artificial one does. A transplant can dramatically restore the health of someone weakened by disease and weeks of dialysis and thus allow her to live an almost normal life.

Not only is a transplant better for people than dialysis, it's cheaper. The surgery may cost $40,000 or $50,000, and the check-ups and drug therapies needed to monitor and prevent organ rejection may run 10,000 to 15,000 a year. Yet such sums are peanuts compared to the hundred-thousand a year required by someone needing frequent and continuing dialysis. Many people getting a new kidney can even go back to work, improving both their incomes and their psychological health.

So why don't people in need skip dialysis and get a transplant? Because, as with other transplant organs, not enough kidneys are available. Most kidneys come from people who have recently died. During a typical year, 8,000 cadaver kidneys are transplanted, but at the end of the year, *six times* that number of people remain on the waiting list.

The people left lingering aren't necessarily those who started the year. The waiting time for a kidney averages almost two-and-a-half years (824 days), and people needing a kidney aren't in good health. While waiting, they must cope with the ravages of their disease and suffer the rigors and hazards of dialysis. They then deteriorate even further. Every year more than 22,000 people die while they and their families cling to the hope a new kidney will soon become available to save their lives. The shortage of kidneys is growing worse. Each month two new people are listed for each transplant performed. A few years ago the United Network for Organ

Sharing loosened the criteria for determining when a cadaver kidney is acceptable for transplant. Without the change and the inclusion of organs of marginal worth, the gap between kidneys needed and ones available would have widened even further.

Roger Evans's study of the efficiency of retrieving cadaver organs suggests that even if we all agreed to be organ donors and hospitals improved their retrievals, the demand for kidneys might still not be met. Thus, the goal of getting enough cadaver kidneys is likely to remain as elusive as finding the path to Shangri La.

Living Donors

Living donors offer the only immediate hope of closing the gap. More people would die each year and the waiting list would be considerably longer if live donors didn't contribute some 4,000 kidneys. The yearly total of transplants is 12,000, and so about a third of the kidneys used come from living people.

Considering that as late as the 1950s and early 1960s, little or nothing could be done to save the lives of people with end-stage kidney disease, the success of transplants shines bright against a dark sky. Those receiving a cadaver kidney (according to UNOS data) have a 94 percent chance of being alive after a year, and an 85 percent chance after four years. Some are still doing well who received a cadaver kidney in the 1960s.

While these figures are impressive, those for people transplanted with a kidney from a live donor are truly stunning. Nearly 95 percent can expect to be alive at the end of the first year, and 93 percent at the end of the fourth. Judged on the basis of the probability of staying alive longer, someone needing a transplant is significantly better off receiving a kidney from a live donor.

That kidneys from living donors work better is connected with the fact that cadaver organs are always, to some extent, damaged. During the process of death, blood flow is often reduced for an extended period and small emboli may block circulation. Prevented from getting oxygen, tissues start to die. Blood clots may form in the kidneys, and enzymes released by dying cells begin eating at the tissues.

Cadaver kidneys also typically have to be preserved and transported to the hospital where they will be used, and this extra time without a blood supply produces yet more tissue damage. The damage may be subtle, but it's real.

Taking Stock

Here, then, is the situation with kidneys: a kidney transplant is both cheaper and better than dialysis; kidneys from living donors are preferable to kidneys from cadavers; the need for kidneys far outstrips the supply (and perhaps always will); thousands die while waiting for a transplant; even more would die, if living donors didn't contribute their kidneys.

These facts lead to the obvious conclusion that (all things being equal) to reduce human misery and save lives, we should try to increase the number of living kidney donors.

Many transplant centers, following this same train of reasoning, have swelled the number of living donors by loosening their requirements. Once most centers demanded a donor be a spouse or blood relative, but now the majority ask only that the donor be "emotionally close" to the recipient, opening the way for friends and lovers to step forward.

Some in the transplant community have gone further and argued for establishing a registry of people willing to donate a kidney to anyone medically appropriate, even a complete stranger. While no registry has yet been set up, a few generous people have given a kidney to strangers. The event is still rare enough, though, to receive national news coverage when it occurs.

We're now back to the point where we started—the kidney shortage could be ameliorated, if not solved, by allowing people needing a transplant to pay a healthy and willing donor to supply a kidney.

Of course if paying a donor is morally wrong, this solution can't be accepted. We couldn't endorse it any more than we could approve of someone's murdering his aunt so he could inherit the money needed to pay for his son's transplant. Both cases violate the rule that it is generally wrong to use wrongful means to achieve an end, even if the end is praiseworthy.

But is it wrong to pay a kidney donor?

Exploitation?

The major objection to paying living donors is that it involves financial coercion and thus exploits the poor. Selling a kidney is (in George Annas's words) "an act of such desperation that *voluntary* consent is impossible." Were we to permit it, we would be faced with the unedifying spectacle of the rich literally plundering the bodies of the poor to save or improve their own lives.

Annas's phrasing of this objection is a bit over-the-top. It suggests that live donors like Betty Burke have no choice at all, but this isn't strictly true.

Not every parent would want to make such a sacrifice for her child, so Betty is in a coercive situation partly because of what she values and wishes to achieve. Her desperation is, similarly, a function of her objective. She isn't pressured into becoming a kidney donor by overt threats, but by her commitment to helping her son.

The objection is substantially correct, however, and in a just world (or even one where adequate medical coverage is guaranteed), people wouldn't have to sell a kidney to meet the basic needs of their children. We don't live in such a world, however, and the relevant question is whether, in the society we inhabit right now, we should condemn paying living donors as unethical and prohibit the practice.

I suggest the coercion-exploitation objection doesn't carry the day and that, given our commitment to allowing individuals to be self determining, we should, in some circumstances, permit paying living donors.

Exploitation and Options

The key idea behind the exploitation objection is that the poor are inherently vulnerable, because they can so easily find themselves in coercive situations. Betty Burke was faced with the problem of finding the means to pay for Chris's bone-marrow transplant. Some parents might have given up, but she was determined to do her best for Chris. She took the only option open to her in the circumstances and sold her kidney.

A rich person in the same situation could have paid for her son's treatment without a thought. Someone short of cash but owning substantial property or having well-off relatives could have considered a mortgage or a loan. For none of these people would selling a kidney be the only solution to the problem. Chances are it would be among the last possibilities to occur to any of them.

Annas may be right that selling a kidney is an act of such desperation no one would choose the option, if another were available. (Crime is not an acceptable alternative.) In our society's version of the market economy, our financial status does much (if not most) to determine the range of options available to us. Where we live, how we live, the car we drive or whether we even have a car can be a function of the financial resources at our command.

To be poor is to have fewer of the options money provides. Our society has shown itself generally willing to tolerate disparities in income and the disparities in the range of options that roughly parallel them. Most people can't afford to drive a BMW. If they want to and can't, we don't have much sympathy for them, because they could buy a cheaper car or find some other means of transportation. Most people can't afford to have a house on the beach, but they can afford to live somewhere.

We aren't completely tolerant of the lack of options in all aspects of life. We have introduced a variety of social programs to provide the poor with education, food, clothing, housing, and various degrees of legal assistance and medical care. We have, in effect, given the poor options where previously they had few or none. Yet even in the area of undisputed basic needs, the society has left gaps.

Bridging the Gap

We've made sure anyone needing dialysis can get it, regardless of ability to pay, but we haven't made sure anyone qualifying for a liver transplant can get one. Nor have we made it possible for anyone needing any other potentially life-saving therapy to receive it. (That dialysis and kidney transplants are paid for is a triumph of the kidney lobby.)

Bone-marrow transplantation has been shown to be effective in the treatment of childhood leukemia. Yet someone like Chris Burke may be unable to get treated, because he doesn't qualify for Medicaid, his mother's insurance doesn't pay an adequate amount (or doesn't cover him), the state has run out of Medicaid funds, or his family lacks the money to bear the cost. How can the gap be bridged?

The United States and other Western countries made paid donors illegal primarily on the ground that donors are exploited by the arrangement. But the result of the prohibition is to slam shut the only door leading out of the dilemma people like Betty Burke and the Turkish father find themselves in. They are protected from exploitation only at the cost of not being able to achieve their aim of helping their children.

Society has failed to help the poor by providing such options as guaranteeing life-saving treatments for children or offering long-term family medical loans, yet it takes away the only option open to them. The notion of protecting the poor by outlawing paid donors begins to look like the smug moralism of those repelled by the idea of selling organs, yet not willing to remove the motive behind such a desperate action.

If our society isn't going to meet the needs of a child, it seems reasonable that a parent ought to be left free to do so. Laws against paying kidney donors squeeze people like Betty Burke between the jaws of a vice—society refuses to help their child, then refuses to let them help in the only way they can.

People in such situations (not just parents, either) must be allowed to demonstrate their love, commitment, and courage by doing what society doesn't do. Because of their lack of alternatives, they are being exploited, but even so we should at least leave them free to choose self-sacrifice.

Our society's commitment to the principle that people ought to be free to shape their own lives, including controlling what is done to their bodies, supports the notion that paying kidney donors is not morally wrong.

This opens the question of whether we should permit paying donors as a matter of public policy. While a strong case can be made for adopting such a policy, I'm not going to try to make it here. I'm committed only to the more modest goal of showing that we should at least permit paying a kidney donor in special cases.

Autonomy

The self-sacrifice of a kidney donor like Betty Burke is real, not merely symbolic. Removing a kidney is a major surgical procedure that can take as long as three hours. The donor may die from anesthesia or an uncontrollable hemorrhage, suffer a stroke or heart attack from a blood clot, experience organ or nerve damage due to a slip of the knife.

Postsurgical pain is considerable (more than for the transplant recipient, ironically), and the risk of infection is inescapable. Most donors can return to their usual activities within a month or two, but the muscles of their abdomen may never recover their strength and elasticity.

Given the safety risks and personal costs associated with being a kidney donor, we might ask whether we should leave people like Betty Burke free to make the decision. Our society sometimes regulates people's behavior to protect them from their own actions. We require motorcycle riders to wear helmets and car passengers to belt up. We require prescriptions for a variety of drugs and don't allow passengers to stand in front of the white line when riding on a public bus.

While society does restrict some actions, we recognize a prior presumption in favor of autonomy. We believe rational individuals should be permitted to be self-determining—that their actions should be the result of their choices and decisions.

We endorse the notion that, by virtue of their rational nature, people are uniquely qualified to decide what is in their own best interest. To use Kant's terms, we consider people ends in themselves, not means to some other end. Thus, people have an inherent worth, and others have a duty to respect this and avoid treating them as if they were parts of the ordinary world and subject to manipulation—even when the manipulation is "for their own good."

Autonomy is not an absolute value, but we as a society demand compelling reasons to justify limiting the power of individuals to make their own choices. We generally restrict actions only when they may cause harm to others or violate a rule intended to benefit society as a whole. We thus outlaw assault and require people to pay their taxes.

The grounds for restriction becomes shakier when the behavior at issue is (as ethical theorists say) self-regarding and not other-regarding. How can we justify such overtly paternalistic practices as motorcycle-helmet and seat-belt laws? One answer is that such laws are only to protect people from their carelessness or ignorance. Either they aren't making a reasoned decision about fastening a seat belt or maybe they don't know the risk they are taking. The ignorance of patients could similarly be offered to justify requiring prescriptions for potentially harmful drugs.

Justifying a prohibition against becoming a paid kidney donor along such lines doesn't seem possible. The prior presumption favoring autonomy, of allowing people to be self-determining, also favors allowing people to sell a kidney. We can, of course, make sure would-be donors are adequately informed and not coerced in making their decisions. Ultimately, however, the decision is theirs to make.

Risks

If a donor were very likely to be killed or grievously injured by giving up a kidney, we might decide to outlaw the procedure as so dangerous that, overall, little good could come of it. We admire courageous actions, but we don't support social policies that place the life of one individual at serious risk in the hope of extending the life of another. (Some might regard rejecting such policies as unwarranted paternalism, however.)

This is not an issue with living donors, because the actual risk to a kidney donor is quite low. The operative mortality is three deaths per 10,000 cases. (Statistically, about one donor every four years dies from surgery.) University of Minnesota researchers found serious complications in only 2.8 percent of the thousand cases they examined. They found no deaths.

Living with only one kidney also seems to have no serious long-term consequences. University of Alabama researchers were "unable to demonstrate any adverse long-term effects." Some studies show donors have a lower clearance of creatine (a byproduct of protein metabolism), but this apparently has no health consequences. Donors seem to have no greater incidence of high blood pressure than the population as a whole, and all available information suggests that the average life span of donors remains unchanged. Insurance companies don't even charge donors higher rates for health and life insurance.

No case can be made in terms of high risks for forbidding the use of living donors. Thus, paid donors can't be forbidden on the basis that they are coerced by economic necessity into taking extraordinary chances.

Lifestyle Risks

That some risk is involved in being a living donor isn't enough to rebut the presumption favoring autonomy. Our society permits people to engage in activities that are much more risky than donating a kidney and living with the outcome. Motorcycle racing (1 per 50), mountaineering (4 per 10,000), smoking (36 per 10,000), and even traveling by air (30 per 10,000) have greater rates of mortality than kidney donation.

Because we value autonomy, we allow people to take calculated risks. We may sometimes regulate their actions to increase the safety margin, but we don't forbid them. The presumption favoring permitting someone to decide to become a living donor is at least as strong as that favoring the highly dangerous sport of rock climbing.

Control Over the Body, Unpaid Donors

Justice Cardoza's famous statement that "Every human being of adult years and sound mind has a right to determine what shall be done with his own body" captures an emerging consensus in our society. Although Cardoza's ruling and dozens of other judicial judgments are usually cited in support of a patient's decision to refuse or terminate medical treatment, the principle behind them supports the notion that, guided by our own values and judgment, we are free to take risks with our safety.

That we acknowledge the right of individuals to take such risks is illustrated by the honor we accord to those who donate a kidney to someone in need. The honor goes with their personal sacrifice, but the legitimacy of their action is based on our recognizing that people have a right to control their bodies, even to the extent of giving away one of their organs.

Yet the same principle that makes it legitimate to give away an organ also makes it legitimate to sell one. Suppose a man donates a kidney to his son, but the tissue matching is poor, so the hospital trades with another hospital for a more suitable kidney. The second kidney comes from a woman who has donated it to her daughter.

No one could object to the transaction, because the consent, the risks,

and the motivation are all the same in the trading situation as in the donation. (Kidney exchanges of this sort aren't hypothetical but already take
place routinely at major transplant centers.)

Now suppose Betty Burke sells her kidney to Alice Cushman. Betty uses
the money to pay for Chris's chemotherapy, and Alice's daughter Karen gets
the kidney. Except that money changes hands, the consent, risks, and motivation in this transaction are the same as in the trading and in the donation.

If nothing is wrong with donating a kidney, I suggest nothing is wrong
with selling a kidney to achieve the same purpose of extending or improving someone's life.

An Exception to the Law

We recognize people's autonomy by permitting them to make their decisions
and take their risks. We acknowledge their right to decide what is done to
their bodies. Hence, so long as their choice is free and informed, we consider their decision to *donate* a kidney morally legitimate, even praiseworthy. The same considerations that support allowing people to donate a
kidney also support allowing them to sell one.

The coercion objection is supposed to demonstrate that no one who sells
a kidney can be making a free choice. But, as I said, this is only half right.
While the poor can make free choices, their options are limited. I suggest
that our endorsement of autonomy commits us to allowing the poor at least
to choose among the options open to them. We don't promote the
autonomy of the disadvantaged by narrowing still further the range of
their options.

These considerations support amending the 1984 National Organ
Transplantation Act to permit paying living kidney donors in at least some
situations. When healthy and competent adults need money to meet the
basic medical needs of a member of their family or themselves, they should
be allowed to receive (in the language of the Act) "valuable consideration"
for donating a kidney.

Building such an exception into the law is no more complicated than
framing laws governing capital gains, gifts, or retirement accounts. Also,
paying donors need not be done in a private transaction or an open market.
The exchange of a kidney for money could be orchestrated by an organization like UNOS and the fee set by a panel of experts. Once we accept that
it is morally legitimate to pay a donor in some circumstances, our society
has the administrative skills to make the exchange work.

The Poor

I've talked about "the poor" who want to sell a kidney and "the rich" who want to buy one. That's the language that those objecting to paying donors use, but it's not quite accurate. It's true that if selling a kidney were permitted, we wouldn't see Bill Gates or Donald Trump signing up for donor surgery, but many more people might need to consider the option than those teetering on the economic edge, on welfare.

Most people in the economic middle are able to meet daily needs, but many lack the savings or other resources required to cope with extraordinary expenses. If a crisis arises, they, like Betty Burke, have no way of meeting a sudden demand for money. Thus, more people are potentially in Betty's position than discussions of "the poor" suggest.

How Far to Go?

I took on the modest task of demonstrating that in cases like that of Betty Burke we should modify the law forbidding the sale of organs. Yet the arguments from autonomy favoring such an exception may be strong enough to support the conclusion that it is morally acceptable to allow paid donors in general.

If so, we need to ask whether we are prepared to accept this as a social policy. Do we want a society in which people are willing to sell a kidney to get the money for a new car or a Caribbean cruise? To pay for an Ivy League education for their kids or a more comfortable retirement?

Faced with such a prospect, opponents of organ sales begin talking about the loss of altruism in society, the poor quality of purchased kidneys, the "commodification" of humans and the consequent lost of respect for persons. They talk about bidding wars for organs, high-pressure tactics to recruit poor donors, post-donation regrets, and the repellent aspects of an organ market. We're back, that is, to Dr. Jacobs and the International Kidney Exchange.

I'd have to offer additional arguments to answer such objections and support a broad policy change. I'm not going to go so far here, but I believe these objections can be answered. Bidding wars and open markets can be avoided (as I mentioned) by turning over buying and distributing kidneys to an organization like UNOS. We already have procedures to protect voluntary living donors that would also protect paid donors. The negative aspects of commodification and the decline of altruism, furthermore, must be balanced against the gain of saving thousands of lives.

We need to keep in mind, with respect to this last point, that "the rich" don't want to buy the kidneys of "the poor" to display them on the mantle in glass jars. Those needing kidneys include people on Medicaid as well as ones who drive BMWs. Someone who buys a kidney from a living donor benefits, but in leaving the waiting list, also makes available a cadaver kidney that can then go to someone else.

Some may deplore, as Al Gore once did, thinking about kidneys as spare parts and living people as potential suppliers. They may be repelled by the idea that some people would give up a kidney, not because they want to help a fellow human being but because they want money to start a laundry or pay for their kid's education or merely to finance a trip to Paris.

But what the critics tend to overlook is that such people would be pursuing their dreams and deciding to take a risk to make them possible. Critics also tend to overlook that what repels them may result in saving or prolonging the life of a sister, a mother . . . a child.

Or perhaps even their own.

6

Donors of Last Resort

Protecting Vulnerable People

Boston, 1954

In the fall of 1954, Dr. Daniel Miller, a United States Public Health Service physician, called Dr. John Merrill, the head of the renal disease unit at Harvard's Peter Bent Brigham Hospital, to tell him about a startling opportunity.

Dr. Miller had a patient on the verge of kidney failure. This wasn't unusual for Miller, because he was a specialist in kidney diseases. What was unusual was that the patient had a twin brother—an identical twin. Dr. Miller was thus offering Merrill the possibility of performing a kidney transplant that, for the first time in medical history, had a chance of complete success.

The Brigham (now Brigham and Women's Hospital) was one of the world's leading research centers for kidney disease, and Merrill was participating in the development of the Kolff-Brigham artificial kidney. He and his colleagues David Hume, Joseph Murray, J.H. Harrison, and Francis Moore were already known internationally as transplant pioneers.

During the years 1951–1953, the Brigham group had performed fifteen kidney transplants. But all their patients died. Their failures repeated the experiences of researchers in England and France and forced them to accept the conclusion the others had reached—successful kidney transplants were impossible.

Murray and his group realized the problem couldn't be solved merely by developing better surgical techniques. The surgery had already been more or less perfected. What stood in the way of success, rather, was the inability to prevent the recipient's body from rejecting foreign tissue.

A donor kidney might be tolerated for a few days, perhaps a week, but eventually the recipient's immune system would destroy it. Attacked by antibodies and white blood cells, the kidney would become inflamed and swollen. Clots would form inside, choking off the blood supply, and the organ would stop functioning. The patient would die of kidney failure.

Yet recognizing it was the immune system's response to a foreign organ that produced rejection pointed to a possibility surgeons had never tried. If a donor could be found who was the twin of the recipient—an *identical* twin—a kidney transplant ought to work.

The donor kidney, immunologically speaking, wouldn't be alien to the recipient and thus shouldn't trigger an immune response. For decades physicians had known patches of skin moved from one place to another on the body of same person would always "take." Thus, a kidney from an identical twin should also take.

Richard and Ronald Herrick

Richard and Ronald Herrick grew up as farm boys in Northboro, Massachusetts. When Richard was five, he fell ill with scarlet fever. Although very sick, he made a good recovery, and as both twins grew into adulthood they stayed healthy. Richard joined the army, while Ronald entered college to become a teacher. With sturdy builds, dark hair, dark eyes, and ski-slope noses, the two young men were obviously twins.

Richard's first medical problems surfaced in 1952, when he was 21. His legs and feet swelled so much he couldn't walk, and his blood pressure soared. Lab tests detected red blood cells and protein in his urine and an elevated level of urea in his blood.

The doctors at the army hospital decided he was suffering from chronic kidney failure, probably as a result of kidney damage from his childhood bout with scarlet fever. They gave him a diagnosis of glomerulonephritis.

Richard was treated with diet and drugs over the course of the next two years, but the treatments did little good. He became progressively sicker. His lungs filled with fluid and his heart increased in size as it struggled to push blood through his scarred kidneys. He was approaching complete kidney failure.

It was then that Dr. Miller called John Merrill.

Identical?

Richard was admitted to the Kidney Study Unit of the Brigham. He immediately underwent dialysis with the Kolff-Brigham artificial kidney, an improved version of Wilhelm Kolff's original machine. With the urea cleared from his blood, Richard's condition stabilized.

Merrill and his colleagues were decidedly interested in Richard. A contemporary photograph shows Murray, Merrill, and Harrison standing behind Richard and Ronald, the doctors in their long white lab coats. Merrill has a square-jawed, determined look, like a boxer about to go into the ring, while Harrison, taller than the others, stares into the camera, his face fixed in a serious expression. Murray, his glasses sparkling and his balding head reflecting the light, is smiling with what might be construed as suppressed excitement.

The researchers were prepared to offer Richard a kidney transplant, if Ronald would consent to be a donor. But first they needed to be certain the brothers were identical twins. Their close resemblance seemed to make it obvious. One was slightly shorter than the other, but both had the same tiny birthmark on their right ears. Also, the obstetrician who had delivered them reported they'd shared a single placenta. When their blood was typed, the samples not only fell into the same ABO category, the antigens matched in more detailed respects.

But the researchers needed irrefutable biological evidence. Another transplant using a kidney from a genetically distinct donor was certain to end in another failure. Also, unless they knew the brothers were identical, they wouldn't be able to test the theory that a kidney from a genetically identical donor would be tolerated by the recipient's body.

The only definitive test for genetic identity then available was a skin graft. The Brigham doctors cut postage-stamp sized patches of skin from Richard and Ronald, then exchanged them, sewing the skin from one onto the arm of the other. The researchers monitored the patches for several weeks, then biopsied them. Under a microscope, tissues from both brothers looked completely normal and showed no signs of rejection.

Richard and Ronald were definitely identical twins.

Doubts

With the genetic identity of the twins established, no medical or scientific barrier stood in the way of proceeding with the transplant. Yet a moral question made the surgeons hesitate. Richard Herrick was in the final stages of his life. Dialysis could stave off death for a while, but eventually he would die from uremic poisoning or infection. A transplant offered him the only possibility for extending his life. Indeed, he was the first person in history for whom that possibility was more than speculative.

But what about making Ronald Herrick a kidney donor? Ronald was perfectly healthy and wouldn't be helped by having a kidney removed. Indeed, he would be put at risk of infection and death from the surgery. Medicine's primary rule, one honored in more than two millennia of medical practice, is "First, do no harm." Wouldn't the surgeons be violating this rule?

Ronald could get along without two kidneys. One in 11,000 people is born with only one, and most never find this out. Some learn it when they get sick and require imaging studies or have an accident that damages their kidney, but such cases are rare. Ronald would know he had only one kidney, and he would be advised not to take part in activities like tackle football that might damage it.

Another question also troubled the surgeons. Was Ronald at risk from the same kidney disease threatening Richard's life? Epidemiological studies suggested it was unlikely Ronald would develop glomerulonephritis, even though he had been exposed to scarlet fever, but the possibility couldn't be ruled out. If he did, his brother would be unable to help him with a transplant. Ronald would then follow the same path to death as other end-stage kidney disease patients.

The Brigham group explained to Ronald the risks he'd be taking in becoming a donor. He made it clear he was willing to do whatever he could to help his brother. The two young men, still hardly more than boys, shared a deep emotional bond. Ronald consented to the surgery enthusiastically, pleased by the prospect of contributing something to save Richard's life.

But the surgeons had one more doubt. Could Ronald's consent really be free, knowing his brother's life depended on his decision? The group debated the question, sometimes heatedly. They eventually decided it would be morally justifiable for them to go ahead with the transplant.

Surgery

The surgery took place in 1954, two days before Christmas. J.H. Harrison removed Ronald's left kidney, and Francis Moore rushed it into the adjacent operating room. Joseph Murray, the man with the eager smile, was preparing Richard to receive the graft by dissecting out the blood vessels of his left kidney.

Although the surgeons worked rapidly, an hour and a half elapsed between the time Ronald's kidney was removed and then sewn into Richard's abdomen. The kidney wasn't cooled during the wait, although this would later become a standard practice to slow deterioration.

Ten seconds after the new kidney was hooked up, urine poured out of the ureter, splashing onto the operative field. "So much ran onto the floor,"

Murray recalled years later, "we had to get the nurses to mop it up." Once the ureter was sewn to the bladder, the urine flowed into it in an entirely normal way.

"How does it feel to have three kidneys?" a journalist asked Richard at a press conference several weeks later. The reporters had been told that leaving Richard's own kidneys in place was the most conservative course to follow. If they were removed and the transplant failed, he'd have no kidney function at all.

"Just fine." Richard smiled broadly.

"How does it feel to have only one?" Ronald was asked.

"I can't tell the difference." Ronald smiled as broadly as his brother. "I feel just like anybody else."

With Richard's new kidney working overtime, the signs of his disease began to disappear. The fluid bogging his lungs drained away, his enlarged heart shrunk to normal size, and the puffiness in his ankles and feet disappeared. The urea in his blood dropped back to normal. He recovered his appetite and vigor.

Richard's blood pressure remained high, however. Hoping to bring it down, the surgeons decided to remove his diseased kidneys. Six months after this second round of surgery, he'd recovered enough to return to ordinary life. He married one of the nurses who had taken care of him during his hospitalization, and the couple soon started a family.

That Richard was living such a normal life settled a question that had worried researchers. Would a recipient from a living donor be so troubled by a mixture of guilt and gratitude as to be psychologically disabled? No previous recipient had lived long enough to suggest an answer. While Richard was grateful to his brother, he showed no sign of allowing Ronald's sacrifice to ruin his life.

More Cases

Richard Herrick's kidney transplant was the world's first successful organ transplant. It proved what the Brigham group had suspected—that when the tissues of the donor and recipient are perfectly matched, the recipient's body tolerates the graft.

The proof of this concept triggered a spate of transplants between identical twins. By 1958, four years after Richard's surgery, the Brigham team had done six twin transplants, and researchers in Paris, Montreal, and Oregon had performed several more. The number rose to thirty by 1963, and ten years later it had increased to fifty.

Joseph Murray received the Nobel Prize for Medicine in 1990, in recognition of the advancements in transplantation he and his colleagues had made. Their success with twins demonstrated the importance of tissue compatibility, and researchers began working out methods for matching donors with recipients. This, along with the development of new drugs and drug combinations to control the immune response, opened up a new era in kidney transplantation.

But the new powers of transplant surgery also began to produce new ethical problems. Like sparks flying from an anvil, they glowed brightly, started several fires, and even now continue to smolder and flare.

New Territory

The Brigham group was concerned about the moral legitimacy of risking the life of a well person to help a sick person. This isn't a problem that has gone away, but their decision was made easier by the fact that Ronald Herrick was 23 years old, intelligent, and well-enough educated to understand his risks. He was also manifestly eager to do what he could to extend his brother's life.

But several of the twin cases following Richard Herrick's presented the surgeons with an even thornier ethical issue. A number of twins with end-stage kidney disease were small children. Thus, although they needed a kidney from their siblings to extend their lives, those siblings weren't capable of consenting to becoming donors.

Legitimate consent requires people to possess the capacity to grasp what it means to become a donor. They must understand they will undergo surgery and thus risk dying and experience pain. They must also understand that living with a single kidney may limit their activities or cause permanent damage. But a young child can't be presumed capable of reckoning such risks.

But (the surgeons asked) if a child isn't qualified to give consent to becoming a donor, who should decide? Parents seemed the most obvious decision makers, because they've always been the ones to consent to medical treatment on behalf of their children. A long tradition of legal rulings recognizes the power of parents to make such decisions, even in cases in which a therapy may threaten a child's life.

The problem with kidney transplants was different, though. Parental decisions had always concerned treatments intended to *benefit* a sick child. But never before had it been necessary to risk the life of a healthy child for the sake of a sick one. The Brigham group had faced the problem of risking the life of an *adult* with his consent, but what about risking the life of a child incapable of consenting?

This was new ethical territory.

Sophie's Choice

The problem became more widespread as the crossmatching of tissues was introduced and surgeons extended the success of kidney transplants beyond identical twins and began accepting family members who were good tissue matches as donors.

This put tremendous pressure on families. What were parents to do when a younger child was a match with an older child needing a transplant? More and more parents were suddenly forced to deal with questions that earlier had been faced only by the parents of a relatively few identical twins.

The problems of decision making were ramified by special considerations for a number of unfortunate parents. What if the child who was a potential donor was mentally retarded? Or what if he was an adult, yet suffered from a debilitating mental illness like schizophrenia?

Parents of children needing a transplant were thrust into a position similar to Sophie Zawistowska's in William Styron's *Sophie's Choice*. Just as Sophie was coerced into deciding which of her children would be condemned to the risk of death in a Nazi concentration camp, parents of children who were minors, mentally impaired, or mentally ill were asked to decide whether to risk the life of one child to save the life of the other.

Still a Problem

Kidneys remain in short supply, and transplants from living donors are more successful than ones from cadavers. Families continue to be pressured by circumstances to make wrenching decisions about risking the health and safety of one child to benefit another.

The scope of the problem may also be increasing once more. No machine can take over the functions of the liver, even to the extent an artificial kidney can take the place of a real one. Every year 14,000 people need liver transplants, but only 5,000 get them. Donor livers are in short supply, and 1,200 people a year die while waiting for one.

To cope with this desperate situation, a new technique has been developed. Surgeons remove a segment (or the left lobe) of a donor's liver and transplant it into a recipient. Because the liver, unique among organs, has the capacity to regenerate, both the donor's liver and the transplanted segment will eventually grow to normal size.

Only adults are currently accepted as donors. But when the procedure becomes better established and is demonstrated to be reasonably safe (which seems likely), children and other legal incompetents may become regarded as potential donors.

It's easy to imagine circumstances in which a child might be the only available liver-segment donor for a sibling. The surviving parent of a couple, for example, might not have a blood type compatible with that of the child needing the transplant. Or the parent may be too ill to become a donor. Livers, unlike kidneys, aren't tissue-matched, so more distant relatives, if any, might be approached. But they might not qualify or might refuse. The child's sacrifice might be all that stands between her sibling and death.

Living Donors

In a Monty Python skit, two guys in white coats knock on the door of a house. When a man answers, they grab him and begin hustling him away. "Hey! What's going on?" he objects.

"You signed an organ-donor card," says one guy. "Well, we've come for them."

Part of the dark humor here comes from recognizing that people who sign donor cards can't be forced to give up their organs. Pretending they can is so absurd as to be funny.

But the laughing stops when we realize children can be compelled to give up an organ. Perhaps this is the most disturbing aspect of using children as donors. Lacking the capacity to consent, their fate depends on the decision of others. Even if they are willing to be donors when asked, their dependent status makes their situation inherently coercive.

Thomas Starzl, who pioneered both kidney and liver transplants, has made the strongest case against living donors of any age. Starzl claims that, in his experience, the weakest or least valued member of a family typically becomes targeted as the donor. Others in the family then manipulate the person into volunteering.

Surveys of living donors show they are most often pleased with their decision and would decide the same way again. This doesn't count much against Starzl's position, though. The surveys reflect only how donors feel after the fact. They don't prove consent wasn't coerced. Even people shoved out of an airplane with a parachute may turn out to enjoy the drop.

Renee Fox and Judith Swazey point out in their classic sociological study of transplantation that, where living donors are concerned, the potential always exists for "moral blackmail." This is the basis of Starzl's argument, and the potential is particularly strong where children are concerned.

Children not only lack the ability to understand what's involved in becoming a donor, they are under the total control of their parents. They are thus powerless to resist the pressure inherent in situations in which they are asked to donate an organ to help a dying family member. They can be hustled into the hospital without even having signed a organ-donor card.

Tasks

Shielding children completely requires excluding them as donors. Yet the cost of this can be too high, even judged by the interest of the child. A better solution is to permit children to be donors, but devise requirements and procedures to protect them from exploitation.

The tasks of broadening the concept of benefit and devising protective requirement can both be approached by asking what factors ought to be considered in deliberating about whether it's in the best interest of a child to donate an organ. The factors can serve as the basis for rules or guidelines. Some of the early court decisions involving kidney transplants are helpful in identifying what determines a child's best interest and who should decide when it justifies making the child into a donor.

Medical Benefit

Leon Marsden was dying of glomerulonephritis, the kidney disease that had affected Richard Herrick. But the year was 1957, and by then the Brigham group had performed a number of successful twin transplants. Leon was unlucky to have a fatal disease, but lucky to have an identical twin.

Leonard Marsden, Leon's brother, was in good health and willing to donate a kidney. Yet because he was 19 and the age of legal majority was then 21, he was unable to consent. Eager to have Leon's life spared, his parents readily gave their consent for the Brigham group to remove a kidney from Leonard and transplant it into Leon.

The surgeons weren't willing to accept the consent of the parents as sufficient. They pointed out to the Marsdens, as they had done to other parents, that in subjecting Leonard to surgery they wouldn't be providing him with any *medical* benefit.

The group was also concerned about themselves. Because Leonard would be receiving no medical benefit, they thought it possible that, under

Massachusetts law, they might be open to a charge of battery for "deliberately inflicting bodily harm" on Leonard. The hospital administrators thus
asked the Marsdens to go to court and seek a declaratory judgment. The
parents would petition the court (in effect) to order the surgeons to operate
on Leonard for the sake of Leon.

The Marsdens did as they were asked, and on June 12, 1957, Justice
Edward A. Counihan, sitting in the high-ceilinged chambers of the Supreme
Judicial Court of Massachusetts, delivered his ruling on their petition. The
two brothers and their anxious parents sat quietly as Justice Counihan
rendered his decision.

"I am satisfied from the testimony of the psychiatrist that grave emotional impact may be visited upon Leonard if the defendants [i.e. the Brigham
group] refuse to perform this operation and Leon should die, as apparently
he will . . . ," the judge read. "Such emotional disturbance could well
affect the health and well being of Leonard for the rest of his life. I therefore find that the operation is necessary for the continued good health and
continued well-being of Leonard and that in performing the operation the
defendants are conferring a benefit upon Leonard as well as upon Leon."

Justice Counihan's reference to Leonard's "continued good health and
continued well-being" suggests he's concerned to show that, appearances
to the contrary, the surgery on the healthy Leonard satisfies the traditional
legal notion that when a child is subjected to a medical treatment, the
treatment must be for the sake of the child. If Leon gets Leonard's kidney,
Leon can be expected to benefit, yet Leonard benefits as well.

The judge agrees, in effect, that what's at issue is a *medical* question
about Leonard's health. Because Leonard might be able to keep Leon from
dying by contributing a kidney, if the surgery to remove the kidney isn't performed and Leon dies, Leonard's health will suffer serious and lasting consequences. Hence, the surgery can justifiably be performed, not for Leon's
sake, but for Leonard's. The Brigham group thus originally construed
"medical benefit" too narrowly.

Something Important at Stake

I suggest, following Counihan, that the first and most basic requirement to
be met in justifying a child's becoming an organ donor is that the child must
have something important at stake in the use made of the organ. Becoming a donor must be in the child's best interest.

This can be understood as the child's having a stake in the welfare of the
organ's intended recipient. Leonard Marsden, with respect to his brother's

welfare, had at stake something that might affect his own "health and physical well-being" for the remainder of his life.

A child, following this line of reasoning, cannot be required to donate an organ to help a stranger, even if the organ would save the stranger's life. The child has no direct stake in the stranger's welfare, and so the donation wouldn't serve the best interest of the child.

Interest in Doubt

The Marsden brothers, like the Herricks, had a warm personal relationship. But what if such ties don't exist? What if the potential donor is a family member, but isn't capable of having a personal relationship? Can the family member still be thought of as having an interest in the welfare of the recipient and ordered to donate an organ?

These are issues raised by the Pescinski case.

In 1958 Richard Pescinski was diagnosed as a catatonic schizophrenic and admitted to the Winnebago (Wisconsin) State Hospital. He was withdrawn, unresponsive, and distant. Although apparently aware of his surroundings and of other people, he was indifferent to them. His mental age was estimated as comparable to a 12-year-old's, and he needed constant supervision and care. Effective antipsychotic drugs had not yet been introduced.

Pescinski was eventually transferred to the Good Samaritan Home, a long-term care facility. Dr. William Hoffman, the medical director, described him as having no lucid intervals and being completely impaired in decision making. In Hoffman's words, Pescinski was "insane seven days a week."

In 1974 Richard's 38-year-old sister, Elaine Jeske, was facing a crisis. A long-term glomerulonephritis sufferer, her damaged kidneys had been removed in 1970, and since then she'd been kept alive by twice-weekly dialysis. But after four years, she'd become so weak and debilitated she was confined to a wheelchair. Her physician, Dr. H.M. Kauffman, had outlined her alternatives starkly—get a kidney transplant or die.

Elaine's chance of surviving in 1974 was much better with a kidney from a living donor than from a cadaver. Her six children were all rejected as potential donors by Dr. Kauffman on the basis of his own "moral conviction" that they were too young. Elaine's parents both volunteered to contribute a kidney, but both were over 60, and Dr. Kauffman rejected them as too old.

Her sister, Janice Lausier, was a diabetic and so not a suitable donor. Her

43-year-old brother Ralph, a dairy farmer with ten children, was in uncertain health and had so many family obligations he was unwilling to risk giving up a kidney.

Tests showed, as fate would have it, that Richard, the only adult in the family incapable of giving consent, was a good match for Elaine. Janice, acting on Elaine's behalf, petitioned the county court to issue an order allowing Richard's kidney to be removed and donated to Elaine. The court refused on the grounds that Richard hadn't consented and, besides, the court had no power to approve such an operation.

Janice appealed to the Wisconsin Supreme Court.

Chief Justice Wilkie, author of the majority opinion, held that "absolutely no evidence" had been presented during the hearing to demonstrate Richard's interest would be served by donating a kidney. Richard showed no concern about Elaine (or anyone else), and whether she lived or died was a matter of indifference to him.

An incompetent "should have his own interests protected," Wilkie concluded. In the absence of Richard's consent and in a situation in which "no benefit to him has been established," the Court failed "to find any authority" to order the transplant.

Elaine Pescinski Jeske was out of luck.

Dissent: Moral Benefit

Wilkie's ruling was in keeping with the principle that to become a donor someone not capable of consent must gain something important to justify the risk. Richard wasn't capable of enjoying the "continued well-being" Counihan thought warranted Leonard Marsden's donating a kidney to his brother. Leonard could gain a personal "medical benefit" by becoming a donor, but Richard couldn't.

But was there some other benefit Richard, despite his mental impairment, might be capable of enjoying? Justice Day, in his dissenting opinion, claimed one had been neglected.

Given "the normal ties of family," Day wrote, Richard "would most probably consent," if he were competent. But in construing benefit as "only those things which financially or physically benefit the incompetent," Richard is "forever excluded from doing the decent thing." He must "be always a taker, never a giver."

Day, unlike Wilkie, held that courts have the power to substitute their judgment for that of legal incompetents. Thus, in making a decision for an individual, a court ought to "give the incompetent the benefit of the doubt, endow him with the finest qualities of his humanity, [and] assume the goodness of his nature, instead of assuming the opposite."

The benefit Richard stands to gain from the transplant, Day suggests, is a *moral* one. Someone who can "express humanity" gains a benefit. Donating a kidney is thus a way for an incompetent person to manifest human dignity. The court, in refusing to order Richard to help his sister, denied him an opportunity to express his dignity. Thus, the court denied him the chance to do something to benefit himself.

Personal Importance

Day's opinion calls attention to the importance of considering human dignity in making decisions affecting those incapable of consent. "Incompetents" have dignity by virtue of being human and are thus entitled to treatment that recognizes this. That's why we consider it wrong to shut up in back wards those who, like Richard Pescinski, are isolated from the world because of their illness. Such segregation denies people meaningful human contact and so involves treating them as hardly more than defective machines.

Day goes too far, however, in assuming "the normal ties of family" make it likely incompetent family members would, if competent, agree to donate an organ. If in making decisions for people incapable of consent, we do as Day recommends and assume "the goodness of [their] nature" and "give [them] the benefit of the doubt," we expose them to exploitation.

It would be too easy to claim when a child or cognitively impaired person could serve as an organ donor that the person *ought* to, because his dignity demands it. This would give grounds to the old fear that orphanages and psychiatric hospitals might become de facto organ warehouses.

Not everyone with the opportunity to help a family member by giving up a kidney leaps at the chance. (Elaine's brother Ralph refused her request.) Recognizing the dignity of those incompetent to consent doesn't require we assume that, if competent, they would be moral heroes and ready to surrender an organ to any family member (or maybe anybody at all) needing it.

We can respect the dignity of those who are incompetent by requiring of them what we reasonably expect of others. Under what conditions, then, do we expect those able to consent to decide to become organ donors? That the risk to the donor's health and safety be small is an obvious requirement.

Scarcely less obvious is that the recipient be someone important to the donor. Being a first-degree relative like a sister or mother may be a prima facie indicator of importance, but it's by no means determining. Everyone knows of cases of closeness and devotion in which the people are neither biologically related nor spouses. We know also of contrary cases, where brothers or sisters, children and parents, are virtual strangers or even bitter enemies.

What sort of sister was Elaine? Did she visit Richard at Good Samaritan Home? Did she talk to her children about him? Had they been close as kids, before Richard's illness manifested itself? Or did Elaine ignore him until she needed a kidney?

We don't expect people to donate a kidney to strangers. When it happens, we consider it an example of extraordinary altruism.

Even accepting Day's notion that Richard would gain in moral dignity by becoming a kidney donor, this would be a weak basis for ordering him to donate a kidney to a stranger. It would be ridiculous to claim the donation would be right for Richard, while remaining an extraordinary act for the rest of us. Expressing dignity, to repeat, doesn't require moral heroism.

We don't know much about the relationship between Elaine and Richard. But Justice Wilkie pointedly commented that Elaine's attorney had presented no evidence to show it was in Richard's interest to donate a kidney. Presumably, then, Richard couldn't plausibly be said to have a stake in his sister's welfare.

If Elaine failed to make herself an important person in her brother's life, she paid dearly for it. With no kidney available for transplant, she died of her disease within a year of the Court's ruling.

Forced Risks

If becoming an organ donor involved zero risk, whether children (or other incompetents) should be donors wouldn't be a question with much moral bite. But donating an organ involves (at least) the risks of infection and death from surgery. It's this that forced the Brigham group to think hard about the issue from the beginning.

Children may promote their interest by becoming donors, but only when this doesn't subject them to considerable risks. Because of the low-to-moderate risks involved in blood, skin, and bone-marrow donation, requiring children to become donors in these cases is relatively unproblematic. But what about kidney donations?

Here the risks are more serious. Three in every 10,000 kidney donors die (about one every four years) from the surgery. The mortality rate may be dropping with improved care, but it will always be higher than the rate for, say, skin grafts. Is the rate low enough for us to decide to put a child at risk?

Perhaps. It's appropriate to subject a child to some risk to protect her best interest. Thus, in cases where the life or well-being of an important person in the child's life is at stake, it's reasonable to put the child at risk for the benefit she may gain. We do this in other medical contexts, even when the child's life isn't endangered—surgery to correct clubfoot, cleft palate, or amblyopia, for example.

Where the chances of a child's dying or suffering harm are considerable or unknown, we don't have adequate justification to put a child at risk, even to save the life of a person important to the child. We're free to decide to risk our own lives for another, because we're capable of understanding our alternatives and the consequences of our actions. Children aren't. Hence, when we decide for them, we must take the most conservative stance compatible with their interests.

Day's notion of "substituted judgment" would have us make every child a hero. We know, however, it's not always in the best interest of someone to be a hero. It can be dangerous or downright deadly.

What we know of risks at present indicates it's sometimes justifiable to make children kidney donors, but not liver-segment or lung donors. We don't yet know enough about the operative and long-term effects and risks of such donations to subject children to them, even when a child has an important stake in the life and well-being of a recipient.

The AMA's Council on Ethical and Judicial Affairs puts the point with characteristic terseness: "Children should not be used for transplants that are considered experimental or non-standard."

Donors of Last Resort

When identical twins alone could be transplanted successfully, only a sibling could be a donor. But tissue crossmatching and more effective immuno-suppressive drugs allowed the donor net to be cast wider to snare family members, friends, and even complete strangers.

Into the 1980s, however, most transplant centers allowed only family members to be donors. This helps explain why, during the earlier decades of transplant surgery, children and incompetent adults were so often seen as the only hope for desperate family members. Elaine Pescinski was forced to turn to her brother, because everyone else in her family was either medically unacceptable or refused her request.

The rule underlying donor selection from the beginning has been that children and others incapable of consenting ought to be donors of last resort. Those able to consent are (by definition) capable of looking out for their welfare, but those incapable are open to exploitation. Hence, we have a duty to protect them.

This means, in practice, that children should become donors only in cases in which their risks and sacrifices may preserve the life of someone important to them and no other medically appropriate donor is available.

Exactly this sort of situation led a Kentucky court in 1969 to rule that surgeons could transplant a kidney from an institutionalized mentally retarded man into his older brother.

Strunk

Although Jerry Strunk was 27, he had the mental age of a child of 6. He was in excellent health, but his brother Tommy was dying of a kidney disease. Jerry was the only family member who was a good tissue match for Tommy.

Unlike Elaine Pescinski and her brother, Tommy Strunk was Jerry's best friend. A psychiatrist testified that Tommy's death would have "an extremely traumatic effect on Jerry," and a social worker observed that Tommy was Jerry's "role model." She also pointed out that when the brothers' aging parents died, Tommy would be Jerry's only close family member.

The court decided, after hearing arguments, that it was in Jerry's interest to donate a kidney to Tommy. Jerry, the court said, "was greatly dependent upon Tommy, emotionally and psychologically," and "his well-being would be jeopardized more severely by the loss of his brother than by the loss of a kidney."

But when is a child or incompetent adult the "donor of last resort?" Jerry was Tommy's, but was Richard Pescinski really Elaine's? Her uncle was a good match, but he refused, for his own reasons, to give her a kidney.

With cases like this we're back to the Monty Python asymmetry between those competent to consent and those who aren't. Children aren't competent to decide to become donors, but they're also not competent to decide *not* to become donors. A decision belonging to competent people belongs to someone else in the case of incompetent people.

This asymmetry has a built-in potential for exploitation. Suppose Mary Logan needs a kidney transplant. High blood pressure eliminates Harold, her husband, as a donor, but their healthy 22-year-old son Carl, now in his first year of law school, has the same blood type and is a good tissue match. The Logan's mentally retarded 16-year-old son, Donald, is also a good match, however. So who should be the donor?

Carl is willing, but he's the pride and joy of the Logan family, and his parents don't want to interrupt his education and subject him to the pains and risks of surgery. Carl is their investment in the future. Donald, however, is a constant source of worry and difficulty. "Now he has a chance to do something to help the family," Harold (sounding a bit like Justice Day) says to his wife.

Harold and Mary instruct Carl to refuse to donate a kidney to his mother when he is interviewed by the social worker at the transplant center. Harold is medically unacceptable, Carl refuses, and no one else steps forward. Thus, Donald becomes the donor of last resort.

Who is looking out for Donald? The duty to protect incompetent people from exploitation rests with whoever has the responsibility to decide what is in their best interest.

Who should that be?

Who's to Say?

Parents are the obvious candidates, but I think two considerations rule them out. First, parents like the Logans can conspire to sacrifice the weakest member of the family to promote the welfare of a more valued one. In either an unconscious or deliberate process of gaming, they can transform a child into the donor of last resort. The person who needs the most protection thus becomes, ironically, the one who is the most vulnerable.

The situation isn't improved if, as Lanie Ross recommends, the family as a whole is given the power to decide. While this could (as she says) promote intimate relations in the family and allow the family to draw upon its own values, religious beliefs, and sense of itself in deciding whether a child should become a donor, it leaves children with no protection from family pressures. Indeed, Ross's process of family decision-making describes exactly the situation Starzl considered so inherently coercive as to lead him to recommend against the use of even adults as living donors.

A second difficulty is that parents can be forced into Sophie's-choice situations requiring them to help one child (or family member) only at the expense of another. This faces them with a conflict of interest, so that whatever decision they make will be suspect (even to themselves) and open to charges of unfairness and favoritism.

Committees

Decisions about accepting patients as candidates for transplants are now made by hospital committees. The same approach might be taken to decide when children ought to become organ donors.

Rodney Williams, for one, advocates the use of ad hoc groups to make decisions about children as potential bone-marrow donors. He describes the way these groups operate at a Honolulu hospital.

A committee composed of a child psychiatrist, a pediatrician, and a third staff member with no direct interest in the case interviews children in an informal way and determines if they understand "their role in the transplant procedure" and if their willingness to be a donor is "free from duress and based on adequate information."

Depending on the judgment of the committee, a child is either accepted or rejected as a donor. The committee process, as Williams observes, is inexpensive, efficient, and offers a way to consider the best interest of a child.

But a committee approach to deciding whether a child should be an organ donor is beset by difficulties. First, committees work effectively only when children are old enough to grasp what's being asked of them and agree to it. They must be able, that is, to give informed assent. But how should we deal with younger children or incompetent adults incapable of assent?

Committees are also limited in their powers to obtain data relevant to the decision they must make. If a family member refuses to provide information or lies to the committee (claiming he has a close relationship with a child, for example), the committee can impose no sanctions and must make its decision on the basis of whatever data it can gather or surmise.

More is at stake, furthermore, for an organ donor than for a bone-marrow donor. Harvesting bone marrow requires the discomfort of having a large needle jabbed into the hipbone, but no significant danger is associated with it. For a kidney donor, surgery is more extensive and more painful; it involves greater risk of infection and a chance of dying. The long-term effects are also permanent; bone marrow is replenished within a few weeks, while kidneys and lung segments are gone forever. Because more is at stake for organ donors, more protection for vulnerable potential donors is required.

Courts

Williams observes that, unlike committee deliberations, court proceedings are "time consuming and costly." This can be true, but the issue of protecting people from exploitation is important enough to warrant spending additional time and money. More than any other institution, the courts are in the best position to guarantee that stringent criteria for a child's becoming a donor are satisfied and that the best interest of the child is served.

Courts of law, unlike committees, however constituted, operate within a tradition of protecting the rights of individuals by invoking a variety of procedural and substantive safeguards. Should a 5-year-old boy contribute a kidney to his adult sister? A court, to put itself in a position to answer this question, can conduct discovery proceedings and gather relevant medical and personal information.

Experts can be called on to offer opinions, and family members required to testify under oath. Rules of evidence, relevance, and proof can be brought to bear on the basic question. Most important, a court can appoint an attorney (a guardian *ad litem*) to represent the 5-year-old to make sure everything recognized as relevant to the child's interest is brought forward for the court to consider.

Because courts have powers that committees lack, committees are never able to delve so thoroughly into issues affecting the welfare of potential donors. At the end of hearings, when the evidence and arguments for and against a child's becoming a donor have been presented, a court's deliberations offer the best chance of getting an independent and objective decision. A committee might have arrived at the same decision, but where protecting the vulnerable is concerned, process and safeguards matter.

The point of view I'm supporting mirrors that expressed in the 1977 decision of a Massachusetts court asked to decide who should make serious medical decisions affecting mentally incompetent patients. As the presiding justice wrote, handing down the decision in the Saikewicz case:

> We take a dim view of any attempt to shift the ultimate decision-making responsibility away from the duly establish court . . . to any committee, panel, or group, ad hoc or permanent . . . . [Q]uestions of life and death seem to us to require the process of detached but passionate investigation and decisions that would form the ideals under which the judicial branch of government was created. Achieving this ideal is our responsibility . . . and is not to be entrusted to any other group proposing to represent the "morality and conscience of our society," no matter how highly motivated and impressively constituted.

Courts have the power to protect vulnerable individuals and are suited to dealing with the subtleties and variations of every case. No one can say exactly how old and cognitively able a child must be to grasp what's involved in becoming an organ donor. A court, however, can determine whether a particular child understands it. Thus, a court can give appropriate weight to a child's assent to becoming a donor.

Giving appropriate weight, doesn't mean treating assent as equivalent to consent. In the case of a well-educated 16-year-old, the difference may be insignificant. But in other instances, assent may be meaningless, because it results from ignorance, confusion, or family pressure.

Courts may also decide that a child's unwillingness to assent isn't reason enough to rule out the child as a donor. Donating an organ to someone of crucial importance in the child's life may be in the child's best interest, even if the child fails to realize it. Hospital committees, no matter what their composition, lack the legal power to order that a child become a donor. Court's don't.

Decisions about potential donors are ultimately decisions about people—what they're capable of understanding, how good their health is, what harm they might suffer, and how significant the intended recipient is to the donor. The texture of life is too rich to permit us to answer such questions by following an automatic procedure.

The answers must be based on evidence and analysis, but ultimately somebody must decide whether it's legitimate to subject a vulnerable person to risks producing no direct benefit to him. Since the beginnings of transplantation, the justice system has performed well in making these decisions. We'd be wise to continue to count on the courts.

Still Necessary

I've argued that a child (or other incompetent person) may become an organ donor when: (a) it's in the child's best interest to help extend the life of the recipient; (b) risk to the child is reasonable; (c) the child is the donor of last resort. I've also supported the idea that a court of law is best suited for making the decision.

No one is pleased that children must be organ donors. Because of advances in transplant medicine, they donate kidneys less often than before. But it's difficult to say whether they'll ever be called on to become liver- or lung-segment donors. If the surgery turns out to involve no more risk than donating a kidney, given the shortage of organs, chances are they will.

If the time comes when we can grow organs from stem cells, construct them by tissue engineering, or use ones from genetically altered pigs, we'll no longer need to recruit defenseless people to save the lives of hopeless ones.

But until then, the issues we've discussed won't go away.

7

Kurosawa in California

The Baby Fae Case and Unproven Treatments

The child known as Baby Fae was born on October 14, 1984, in Barstow, California, a remote town in the Mojave Desert. Weighing five pounds, blue-eyed and well-proportioned, with dark brown curly hair, Baby Fae, although three weeks premature, appeared completely normal.

Yet it soon became obvious to the delivery team at Barstow Memorial Hospital that something was seriously wrong. Her breathing was rapid and her body limp and unresponsive. Most telling, she gasped for air, and her skin, instead of being pink and rosy, had a dusky bluish tinge.

The obstetrician suspected Baby Fae suffered from a congenital heart defect and advised the mother to take her daughter to nearby Loma Linda University Medical Center for a more thorough evaluation.

Baby Fae's parents, known only as Teresa and Howard, were young, poor, and uneducated. Each had a police record for minor infractions—Teresa for passing bad checks, Howard for disorderly conduct. To start a new life with their 2-year-old son Beau, they had moved to California from a small Kansas town.

They were not married, and by the time Baby Fae was born, they were no longer living together. Teresa was then 23, Howard 35. Besides Beau, Howard had two children from an earlier marriage. He had met Teresa while she was flagging for a road crew and he was driving an asphalt truck. They were together for four years, but their fights eventually became so frequent they decided to separate.

When Howard moved out, Teresa signed up for welfare, and Henry, a friend who worked as a car mechanic, moved in to help her through the last weeks of her pregnancy. Teresa denied she and Henry were romantically involved, but his living with her made Howard stay away.

Teresa unhesitatingly accepted primary responsibility for her baby's care. Although Howard would later take part in the critical decision about her treatment, Teresa was the one who decided to act on the recommendation of the Barstow doctors and take Baby Fae to Loma Linda to be assessed.

Loma Linda

The town of Loma Linda ("beautiful hill" in Spanish) was little more than a sprawl of one-story tract houses, fast-food restaurants, gas stations, and parking lots. Sixty miles east of Los Angeles, on the far side of San Bernadino, Loma Linda stretched out along the edge of the Mojave Desert. While sharing the desert's heat, it didn't share its clean air, and on most days, a pall of acrid, yellowish smog hung over the town.

Loma Linda was settled by members of the Seventh Day Adventist Church. Adventism is an evangelical religion that grew out of a nineteenth-century American millenialist movement. It is committed to the personal, visible, and imminent return of Christ and considers the Bible the basis of faith and conduct. Church members dominated Loma Linda the way the Mormons dominated Salt Lake City. Adventists don't approve of using alcohol, for example, so Loma Linda had no bars.

Because Adventists view caring for the sick as part of the Church's mission, they founded the Loma Linda University Medical Center. The center's motto, "To make man whole," was taken very seriously. The medical school was the largest private medical college in California, and its pediatric intensive-care unit's reputation made it the major referral hospital in the region. The medical center, with its 500-bed hospital, was supported almost exclusively by Church contributions and medical fees.

The majority of physicians (85 percent) at the medical center were Church members, although the great majority of patients were not. Many of the doctors had received all their training, from undergraduate education through medical school and residency, at Loma Linda. The medical center also funded most of its own research. Thus, researchers had more freedom to do things their own way at Loma Linda.

Diagnosis

Teresa drove her daughter to Loma Linda on October 15 and rented a room in a cheap motel nearby. She had already had the baby baptized by a Roman Catholic priest. That same day, Baby Fae was examined and tested at the medical center by a cadre of neonatologists, pediatricians, and pediatric cardiologists.

The diagnosis wasn't complicated.

An echocardiogram revealed Baby Fae had a developmental anomaly called hypoplastic left-heart syndrome. The defect, which has an unknown cause, is a cardiovascular malformation in which the lower left chamber of the heart—the left ventricle—is almost completely missing. Also, the aorta, the main artery carrying blood from the left ventricle to the rest of the body, may be only one-tenth of its normal size, with a diameter more like a strand of spaghetti than a crayon. Because blood can't be pumped out of the heart effectively, the infant's skin turns blue and body tissues, including the brain, begin to die from oxygen starvation.

Two- to three-hundred babies a year are born in the United States with hypoplastic left-heart syndrome. The defect is responsible for about a quarter of the deaths occurring in the first week of life. Newborns with the anomaly who aren't treated with surgery die within the first month. Only one child is known to have lived beyond a month, and he died in the middle of his third year.

Staff physicians at Loma Linda explained Baby Fae's dire condition to Teresa and outlined some options. While they didn't mention the possibility of a heart transplant, they told her about an operation known as the Norwood procedure available in Philadelphia or Boston. The surgery, developed by William Norwood at Philadelphia's Children's Hospital, was performed in two stages: the first to repair the aorta, the second to improve the pumping action of the left ventricle. The doctors told her the procedure was only palliative, meaning that at best it would only buy the baby a little time.

The usual option, the physicians explained, was to keep the child as comfortable as possible until she died. She would sleep for longer and longer periods, then eventually not wake. Teresa could take her baby home to die, leave her at Loma Linda where the nurses would care for her until the end, or take her back to Barstow Memorial Hospital.

Baby Fae spent the night of October 15 at the Loma Linda medical center, but the next day Teresa took her to the motel. She had decided it was better for Fae to die there, rather than at home. She wanted to avoid upsetting Beau, who was hardly more than a baby himself. Also, she couldn't bear the idea of continuing to live in a house where her baby had died.

Leonard Bailey

While Teresa was watching over her doomed child in a motel room, Leonard Bailey and his two sons were vacationing in San Francisco. Bailey was a pediatric cardiac surgeon at Loma Linda Medical Center with a long-standing interest in hypoplastic left-heart syndrome. At 41, he was a fit man with deeply hooded eyes, thinning hair, and a bushy moustache that gave him a vague resemblance to Peter Seller's Inspector Clouseau.

Bailey, a Seventh Day Adventist, had received most of his medical training at Loma Linda, but he had spent a year as a resident in cardiovascular surgery at Toronto's Hospital for Sick Children. While in the residency program, he had cared for many seriously ill infants, but he had been particularly moved by the hopeless plight of those who were wholly normal except for having a defective heart.

"Again and again," Bailey recalled, "we would be presented with newborns with hypoplastic left-heart syndrome. The presiding doctor would say, 'Well, it's too bad, but we haven't had much success treating these babies. I suppose we can try this or that, but. . . .'" On one such occasion, Bailey had a sudden insight. "That baby needs a cardiac replacement," he blurted out, "and we should be looking to solve that problem."

Bailey was then only 31, and he was expressing what he later called "the kind of naive dream you would expect from a young surgeon piping up to his mentors." Yet Bailey didn't forget his dream. "I know that my thought that day has helped keep me alive over the years," he recalled.

Research

Within two years of returning to Loma Linda, Bailey initiated a research program in heart transplants. His project was markedly different from Norman Shumway's at Stanford, as well from studies taking place at hospitals in Denver, Boston, and elsewhere.

Bailey's research was the only project at the time to involve cross-species heart transplants—xenografts. Why Bailey chose to work on heart xenografts, rather than human-to-human transplants, he never directly explained.

The primary reason may be that his awareness of the severe shortage of donor human hearts prompted him to look for an alternative. While hundreds of adult heart transplants had been performed by the mid-70s, an effective system of organ procurement and distribution had yet to be developed. Hearts, in particular, couldn't be transported for long distances, and their local availability was a matter of chance.

Donor infant hearts were (and are) particularly rare. A donor heart, as well as having the right blood type, has to be an appropriate size for an infant. Relatively few infants suffer brain death, and those that do seldom die in ways that leave their hearts undamaged and suitable for transplant.

The shortage of organs for infants was underscored by the fact that the first infant heart transplant didn't take place until August 1983. Hollie Ruffey, 9-days-old and born with hypoplastic left-heart syndrome, was given a new heart in London, although she died three weeks later from kidney failure.

A baby hadn't been transplanted earlier because surgeons hadn't been able to match up a newborn needing a transplant with a donor heart of the right blood type and size. Bailey, like other cardiac surgeons, was aware of the scarcity of hearts.

Bailey was also influenced by the much publicized xenografts carried out by other researchers. In 1964 James D. Hardy of the University of Mississippi transplanted a chimpanzee heart into Boyd Rush, a 68-year-old deaf mute. Rush's stepsister had signed a consent form permitting "the insertion of a suitable heart transplant," but the form didn't mention that the heart might come from an animal. Rush lived only two hours after the transplant.

Hardy justified his use of the chimp heart on the grounds that it was impossible to obtain a human heart, but he was criticized so severely for experimenting on an incompetent patient and not securing proper consent that he never performed another xenograft. Years later, speaking of Hardy, Bailey told an interviewer, "He's an idol of mine, because he followed through and did what he should have done [and] took a gamble to save a human life."

The South African surgeon Christian Barnard, who had performed the first human-to-human heart transplant in 1967, experimented with animal hearts in a piggy-back procedure. In 1977 he hooked up a baboon heart to the failing heart of a 26-year-old Italian woman to boost its power, but the woman died within four hours. That same year Barnard piggy-backed a chimp heart onto the heart of Benjamin Forbes, a 59-year-old accountant, who lived for only three and a half days.

Barnard gave up his approach after these failures, "not because I'm convinced I'm on the wrong track," he said, but because he found it emotionally disturbing to sacrifice a chimp for its heart. Also, Barnard admitted, better antirejection drugs were needed before xenografts could be successful.

Bailey's Research

At about the same time Barnard gave up his research efforts, Leonard Bailey was starting his. During the first seven years of his project, Bailey, by his own account, performed more than 150 heart transplants between infant animals. His most successful case was the transplantation of a lamb's heart into a goat. The goat lived five and a half months, but its body eventually rejected the foreign organ.

Yet that was long enough to encourage Bailey to think a primate-to-human transplant might last much longer. Perhaps it might even last indefinitely, he thought, because human and primate tissues were more likely to be compatible.

Bailey established a breeding colony of baboons at Loma Linda and directed efforts to prepare them to become heart donors for human babies. His collaborators tested the baboons to make sure they were free of viruses, parasites, and the agents causing toxoplasmosis and tuberculosis. They gave the animals EKGs and lung scans to establish that they were healthy.

The researchers also tissue-typed the baboons as a means of predicting how compatible their organs might be with human tissues. Bailey believed that, for human newborns, a baboon heart might "prove to be the organ of choice, even if certain human hearts are available." Baboon tissue could be typed in advance of the need and so, with respect to tissue compatibility, might be a better bet than a human heart available only by chance.

"By late 1983, I was getting such good data on the compatibility of cross-species transplants between goats and sheep that I knew it was too good not to be partially true," Bailey told an interviewer.

Tissue-typing baboons to identify ones whose organs would provoke the least immunological response from a human was, Bailey thought, one of his lab's major research contributions. Another was determining how much of the antirejection drug cyclosporine could be given newborns without damaging their kidneys or harming other organs. His studies suggested newborns could tolerate cyclosporine better than adults and could be given larger doses. So far as he knew, Bailey told a reporter, his was the only group in the world studying the use of cyclosporine in heart transplants in infant animals.

Bailey's experiments also persuaded him that newborns would be good recipients of animal organs. Both his data and that of others, he thought, showed that the immune system of newborns was "underdeveloped." If so, then a transplanted heart had a good chance of being tolerated for a significant period of time. Also, Bailey had transplanted a goat's heart into an infant goat that had matured normally and even gave birth to her own offspring. Perhaps a heart transplanted into a human infant might increase in size as the infant grew.

Self-Funded

Loma Linda was not known as a leader in medical research, and most of the work carried out there was supported by internal funds raised from physician's fees and Church contributions. His research, Bailey said at a news conference, was paid for by more than a million dollars "out of our back pocket."

Outside funding agencies had rejected his grant proposals. "One was actually denied on the basis of my age," Bailey claimed. "I was apparently too old for a grant from that organization." (Journalists pressed him to name the organizations that had turned him down, but Bailey refused. When queried, a representative of the National Heart, Lung, and Blood Institute, the major funding agency in heart research, said he could find no record of any application from Bailey.)

Bailey also told reporters that the medical journals had rejected the papers he'd submitted reporting the results of his research. The grant and journal reviewers who turned him down, he said, "weren't watching babies die as I was." Bailey's work was thus virtually unknown to members of the medical and scientific community outside of Loma Linda.

IRB Approval

Bailey was so encouraged by his results that in the spring of 1983 he approached Loma Linda's Institutional Review Board (IRB) for approval to perform a series of five baboon-to-human heart transplants. Even though Bailey had no external grants, the medical center itself received federal support, and the law requires that institutions accepting National Institutes of Health financing establish a committee to review all research protocols involving human subjects. An IRB cannot direct an investigator's research, but it can play a powerful advisory role. It must approve the informed consent document that patients (or their surrogates) must sign advising them of the expected risks and benefits of participating in a research project.

The Loma Linda IRB, headed by Jack Provonsha of the medical faculty, reviewed Bailey's proposal and data, then recommended that outside reviewers be asked to evaluate the project. The sense of the group, Provonsha said, was that Bailey had not done enough work to determine how long a cross-species heart transplant recipient might survive.

Stuart W. Jamieson, a member of Norman Shumway's heart-transplant research group at Stanford, was brought in as a consultant. Jamieson paid a visit to Loma Linda in March and later admitted that when he first heard about Bailey's research, "it seemed somewhat ambitious and vaguely bizarre."

But after talking to Bailey and members of his group, Jamieson was impressed by the amount of "systematic and conscientious" research they had done. He became convinced Bailey was doing important work and that his proposed transplants should proceed. "We talked for a day," Jamieson later said, "and I suggested some other studies he might do."

In one of those studies, which Bailey carried out over the next few months, a baboon heart was connected to a heart-lung machine and human blood was circulated through the machine and the heart. The aim was to determine whether human blood was likely to have preformed antibodies that would attack the heart and lead to prompt rejection.

A second outside review was carried out in June of 1984 by Sandra Nehlsen-Cannarella, an immunologist from New York's Montefiore Hospital and Albert Einstein Medical School. She and Bailey soon began to collaborate. "I came to California believing such a transplant was possible," she later said, "and after a week of viewing the clinical literature and reviewing Dr. Bailey's experiments with animals, I was *convinced* it was more than feasible. It could be done."

Making the Decision

Because it was raining in San Francisco, Bailey and his two sons cut their vacation short and returned home. Later that day, a pediatric cardiologist at Loma Linda, knowing of Bailey's plans to perform a xenograft, mentioned Baby Fae to him as a possible candidate for the transplant.

The IRB, after what Bailey described as "fourteen months of agonizing," had finally approved his proposal only the week before. Bailey was authorized to carry out a series of five baboon-to-human heart transplants in newborns meeting the criteria of needing new hearts and having nothing else wrong with them. "We were prepared to move when a desperate situation presented itself," Bailey recalled.

On October 19, when Baby Fae was six days old, a neonatologist from Loma Linda called Teresa at the motel. He told her, for the first time, that there was one kind of surgery that might help her child. A heart transplant from an animal donor might be possible, and if Teresa were interested, she should return to the hospital with her baby and talk with Dr. Bailey about it.

Teresa, her friend Henry, and her mother spent several hours considering the almost incredible possibility presented to them. Then, at 11:30 that evening, Teresa readmitted Baby Fae to the hospital. She was put into a bed, but given no treatment, because a decision about the transplant hadn't been made.

She was still only waiting to die.

For almost seven hours, from midnight until well into the next morning, Bailey talked with Teresa, Henry, and Teresa's mother. He showed them slides and a film of his research and explained why he believed a baboon heart transplant might be successful. He told them about the Norwood procedure and said that its results had been disappointing. Besides, it was only a palliative procedure, not a curative one.

He also told them he could give no guarantee that a xenograft would be successful, because the type of transplant he would be performing had never been attempted in a newborn. He explained it was unlikely a human heart would be available for Baby Fae, because tissue- and size-matched donor hearts for newborns were quite rare.

If the xenograft took place, he said, they could expect Baby Fae to experience three rejection episodes. He believed these could be controlled by drugs, and none of the drugs would cause the baby to suffer brain damage.

Around 5:00 the next morning, Teresa agreed to allow an immunological workup of Baby Fae to determine whether one of the baboons at the research facility was compatible with her immune system.

Baby Fae's condition had deteriorated during the night, and as soon as Teresa permitted the compatibility testing, Baby Fae was put on life support and given drugs to boost her blood pressure and clear her lungs. Teresa left the hospital to talk to her estranged husband and explain the situation to him.

Teresa and Howard returned to the medical center the next day, and Bailey once again went through a detailed account of his research results and why he believed a baboon heart transplant offered their daughter the best chance for survival. Over the next few days, the couple had several other meetings with him.

Wheels in Motion

Once Teresa agreed to an immunological workup of her child, Bailey called Nehlsen-Cannarella with the news. She said she would catch the next plane to California.

The two researchers shared the view that, as she put it, "a newborn can, with its combination of an undeveloped immune system and the aid of the [immunosuppressive] drug cyclosporine, accept the heart of a baboon—if we can find one with tissue of high-enough compatibility." Thus, the key to a successful xenograft would lie in selecting a baboon with highly compatible tissue.

During the next six days, the researchers tested Baby Fae's lymphocytes against others from a variety of sources: parents, relatives, strangers, and six baboons from the breeding colony. Nehlsen-Cannarella reported that

Baby Fae's lymphocytes reacted weakly against her parents and strongly against strangers and a few baboons. Yet "amazingly, she had weak reactions against three of the baboons, and her reaction against one baboon was very, very weak."

Consent

By October 23, although the immunological testing was not yet completed, Bailey was ready to prepare Baby Fae for surgery by giving her injections of cyclosporine. Before taking this step, however, he needed the approval of her parents. On that date, Teresa and Howard signed a consent document giving their permission for Baby Fae to be transplanted with a baboon heart. For the consent to be valid, however, the parents would have to sign a second time, after a cooling-off period.

Eighteen hours after Teresa and Howard signed the first time, they were again asked to grant permission to allow their daughter to be transplanted with a baboon heart. They signed the consent document a second time.

Consent was then complete, but Bailey and others at the medical center explained to them that even the second signing didn't mean they had taken an irrevocable step. They could withdraw consent at any time before the surgery. Teresa and Howard later told reporters that at no time did they feel pressured into agreeing to the operation.

Surgery

On Friday, October 26, at 7:30 in the morning, Baby Fae was wheeled from the intensive care unit of the Loma Linda hospital to a surgical suite in the medical center. She was 15 days old and on "maximum support." Her life expectancy was being reckoned by her physicians in hours, not even days.

Earlier that morning, around 4:00, Bailey and Nehlsen-Cannarella had finally received the laboratory results they needed to select a baboon donor. Because of Baby Fae's worsening condition, pressure had been building for Bailey to operate as soon as possible. "The baby was dying, and we were running against time," Nehlsen-Cannarella recalled.

The feeling in the operating room was one of tense excitement. The surgical team was aware that a historic operation was about to be performed, and everyone behaved in an organized, highly professional manner.

Baby Fae was given anesthesia. Her body temperature was then lowered by an ice-water blanket to sixty-eight degrees Fahrenheit to slow her physiological processes and thus make the surgery less traumatic.

Bailey left the operating suite around 9:15 to remove the heart from the 5-month-old female baboon he and Nehlsen-Cannarella had selected. The baboon was already prepared in an operating room, and the surgery took hardly fifteen minutes.

Baby Fae's chest was then opened and her sternum spread apart. She was attached to a heart-lung machine to support her circulation, then her heart stopped with an injection of potassium. Her heart was removed. Bailey, in a procedure lasting about an hour, sewed the baboon heart into place. He had to transplant the aorta from the donor heart as well, because Baby Fae's defect was so severe her own aorta was unusable.

Bailey's performance as a surgeon, experts later agreed, demonstrated his technical brilliance. Operations on newborns are among the most difficult procedures. Organs are small, the veins and arteries minute, and the drugs employed can have unpredictable and potentially lethal effects. The baboon heart was about the size of an egg, and the aorta Bailey attached was no larger in diameter than a pencil. The operation, everyone agreed, was a superb surgical accomplishment.

Tension in the operating room ratcheted to a higher level when the time came to try to restart the baboon heart. Would it beat? Bailey applied the paddles, sending a small jolt of electricity through the motionless heart.

It started beating.

The monitor beeped. The EKG line began to rise on the screen. No one applauded, but team members clenched their fists and kept their eyes focused on the monitor. They punched each other on the arm like the winners of a soccer game and said, "It's going! It's going!"

Baby Fae was slowly weaned off the heart-lung machine, and soon the transplanted heart was carrying the full load of blood circulation. Her skin gradually lost its dusky blue-white pallor and turned a healthy pink.

The entire operation lasted five hours.

Baby Fae was moved to Loma Linda's surgical intensive care unit. In addition to standard support measures, such as being given higher concentrations of oxygen, she received regular injections of steroids and cyclosporin to suppress her immune response and prevent her new heart from being rejected. Her heart was monitored by repeated ultrasound tests intended to detect the delayed function associated with tissue rejection.

Word Spreads

Except to Seventh Day Adventists, Loma Linda University Medical Center was scarcely known beyond the patch of southern California from which it drew its patients. But the announcement on the afternoon of October 26 that a surgeon had transplanted a baboon heart into a human baby put the medical center at the focus of worldwide attention. Journalists and TV crews swarmed over the campus to gather details.

The previous year, in March 1983, the first recipient of an artificial heart, Barney Clark, had died, and the media were primed for the next breakthrough in the treatment of failing hearts. The Loma Linda staff were thrilled by what their medical center had accomplished, and the atmosphere was charged with excitement and exhilaration.

Leonard Bailey came directly from surgery to appear at a press conference. He answered reporters' questions about his animal research, his failure to get grants, his belief a xenograft had been the best treatment option available for Baby Fae, and his confidence in its chances of success. He spoke with straightforward candor, making no effort to dodge awkward or embarrassing issues.

It was, however, the only time Bailey appeared in an open forum. Later, he issued printed statements in response to criticisms, and the only interview he gave was to the generally uncritical trade publication *Medical World News*. Hospital representatives took over the job of briefing the press. They announced Bailey had no interest in publicity and was too busy caring for Baby Fae and conducting his research to make himself available for another press conference.

Reactions

Reporters soon began interviewing heart transplant surgeons and researchers and discovered that opinions about Bailey's decision to transplant a baboon heart into Baby Fae were sharply divided.

Both Michael DeBakey, an innovator in heart-repair surgery, and William DeVries, who implanted the first artificial heart, said they believed the surgery had the potential to buy patients time so that a donor human heart could be located. Thomas Starzl, the surgeon who pioneered liver transplants and had once transplanted primate kidneys into humans, endorsed Bailey and his group as "competent professionals carrying out an acceptable medical experiment upon an otherwise hopeless patient."

But many transplant researchers were critical of the xenograft, suggesting that little of either therapeutic or scientific value was likely to come from it. John Najarian, head of the Transplant Service at the University of Minnesota and a major figure in the transplant community, was blunter than most in his assessment. "The operation is doomed to failure," he said. "I am not aware of any finding in the clinical literature that suggests anything but this prevailing rule—that the human body will reject a transplanted animal organ."

Najarian suggested, by implication, that Bailey was an outsider doing little more than dabbling in an area in which he had little expertise. "If we thought xenografts would be successful, we would use them," he said. His estimate of the worth of Baby Fae's surgery as an experiment was similarly caustic. "This is not good clinical experimentation, because we are not yet at the point where we can cross the xenograft barrier."

A storm of criticism erupted when Bailey admitted he hadn't tried to locate a human heart for Baby Fae. He had assumed a donor heart wouldn't be available, but didn't ask the regional organ-procurement agency for specific data. Further, even though six days elapsed between the signing of the consent document and the surgery, Bailey made no effort to obtain a donor heart during this period.

Paul Terasaki, Director of the Regional Organ Procurement Agency, told reporters that if Loma Linda had notified him of the need for a heart, the agency could have provided one from a 2-month-old infant from Salt Lake City. The heart became available on October 26, the day of Baby Fae's surgery.

A hospital spokesman said Bailey's team had been unaware of the availability of a human heart at the time. But even if they had known about it, chances are they wouldn't have used it, because it would be too large for a tiny infant.

Bailey, responding in a printed statement to the criticism that he hadn't sought a donor human heart, emphasized his seven years of experimentation, the scarcity of appropriately sized infant hearts, and the IRB's approval of his proposal to perform a series of five baboon-human transplants. He said a prior decision had been made to perform a xenograft and that Baby Fae was the strongest of several candidates considered.

This response was in keeping with his view that a "compatible" baboon heart would be more likely to succeed in an infant than a poorly matched human one. It seemed to many to imply, though, that Bailey was more interested in conducting his experiment than in doing what was best for Baby Fae.

Bailey appeared to make this point explicit in his later interview with *Medical World News*. "We were not searching for a human heart," he told reporter Dennis Breo. "We were out to enter the whole new area of transplanting tissue-matched baboon hearts into newborns, who are supported with anti-suppressive drugs." Using an outsized, non-tissue-matched human heart might have "pacified some people," Bailey said, "but it would have been very poor science."

Bailey himself had provoked a third criticism when he told the news conference that no one had been able to duplicate William Norwood's results and that only 2 percent of infants treated with the Norwood procedure were surviving. Others quickly corrected Bailey, pointing out that the procedure was used by several surgeons and had been shown to benefit 40 to 60 percent of babies with hypoplastic left-heart syndrome.

Bailey later said what he had meant was that the procedure hadn't been successful in *his* hands. This led critics to speculate that the mistaken figures Bailey mentioned to the press were the same as those he gave to Baby Fae's parents.

Questions

These criticisms raised concern about the consent document Teresa and Howard had signed. Had Bailey informed them he wouldn't be seeking a human heart? Did they know about the chances of success with a human heart? Did he tell them the Norwood procedure would give their baby a 40-percent or better chance of staying alive for a longer time—perhaps long enough for a donor heart to be located?

And what about money? Loma Linda had agreed to pay all the costs of Baby Fae's xenograft, but what did the center tell the parents about paying for medical care, if they chose a human heart transplant or the Norwood procedure? Critics considered it possible that a lack of money might have pressured Teresa and Howard to agree to the xenograft.

Two years earlier, William DeVries had circulated copies of the consent document signed by Barney Clark and thus forestalled speculation about whether Clark realized what he was agreeing to. Also, because the clinical trial of the artificial heart was supported by federal money, the research protocol was a public document. Loma Linda, by contrast, refused to release either the consent document signed by Teresa and Howard or Bailey's xenograft protocol approved by its IRB. Thus, crucial questions about Bailey's clinical trial and the legitimacy of the parents' consent couldn't be answered.

First Days

Baby Fae was returned to the intensive care unit immediately after surgery. Her new heart beat well, and she was put on a mechanical ventilator to breathe for her. Steroids were administered to control inflammation, but additional cyclosporine was withheld for a while, because of its potential toxic effects.

Thirty or so members of People for the Ethical Treatment of Animals, condemning Baby Fae's xenograft as "ghoulish tinkering," picketed in front of the hospital. "It boils down to having killed a perfectly healthy baboon in order to prolong a child's suffering," a protester said.

Worried by the demonstration, Loma Linda posted security officers with dogs around the medical center and put Baby Fae's room under guard. "If you had the opportunity to see this baby and her mother, it would help convince you of the propriety of what we're trying to do here," Bailey said, explaining what he would say to the protesters.

Baby Fae's name was taken off the critical list three days after the surgery. She was breathing on her own and sucking water from a bottle. She appeared to be making rapid progress toward recovery, and in a few more days, although she was kept isolated, she was off all respiratory support.

She was also beginning to respond to her mother. Teresa rocked her in a chair, talked to her, and soothed her when she was upset or fussy. She graduated from IV feedings to baby formula taken from a bottle and began yawning, kicking, and stretching like any other infant. Loma Linda photographers videotaped her antics and made stills available to the press.

Teresa and Howard were delighted with her progress. They let it be known they were accepting bids from publications interested in the story of their daughter. Loma Linda said it had no intention of acting as a go-between to broker a deal.

Six days after the surgery, Loma Linda, apparently stung by persistent criticism, instructed a representative to tell reporters, "We are actively seeking a human heart" for Baby Fae. Using a baboon replacement "would be considered second."

Last Days

Eighteen days after the transplant, on November 13, Baby Fae took a turn for the worse. Her heart and kidneys began to fail, apparently as a result of immunological rejection. The team of twenty of so physicians concerned with her care discussed the best course of treatment.

They put her back on a respirator and administered drugs to strengthen her heartbeat. To control the rejection, they increased the amount of cyclosporin she was getting. Bailey and others in the team telephoned immunologists and transplant experts around the country to solicit their advice.

The medical team's regular 4:00 meeting ended on a hopeful note. The antirejection drugs seemed to be working. The antibodies circulating in Baby Fae's blood had declined, and her heart rate, rhythm, and blood pressure were normal. She was rosy-cheeked and active. Her urine output was down, but the team wasn't worried about that. By cutting out some antibiotics and adding more digitalis, they could strengthen her heartbeat, and the better blood flow should increase her urine production.

Then Baby Fae crashed.

By 6:00 she was approaching complete kidney failure. The medical team filled her abdominal cavity with dialyzing fluid and used peritoneal dialysis to try to clear the waste products, particularly potassium, from her blood. Despite their efforts, they couldn't eliminate the chemical imbalance caused by the kidney failure. Her heart, as a result, began to beat irregularly. The team administered drugs to try to reestablish a normal heartbeat.

Their attempt failed. Her heartbeat continued to slow, dropping from 160 beats per minute to 100, then to 75. She was exhibiting bradycardia, a slowed heartbeat.

She then developed a critical cardiac rhythm disorder called complete (or atrioventricular) heart block. In this condition, electrical pacemaking signals from the sinus node at the top of the heart travel to the upper chambers but are then disrupted ("blocked"). The heart muscle in the lower chambers, lacking prompting, begins to contract on its own. The upper and lower chambers are soon beating out of sync, and the heart loses its capacity to circulate blood. Bailey decided against implanting a pacemaker for "a variety of reasons," which he didn't spell out.

Baby Fae's heart stopped beating around 9:00 Thursday evening. The team attempted to restart it by closed cardiac massage, but they were unsuccessful. No further efforts were made, and she was declared dead.

She was 35 days old.

Bailey had remained with Baby Fae virtually around the clock since the start of her crisis. Friday morning, ashen-faced and shaken, he appeared at a news conference to announce her death and to pay tribute to her and her parents.

He thanked them for offering "a new ray of hope to babies to come" and said that despite the sad outcome, the parents still felt "the surgery was worth it." The last thing Baby Fae's mother said to him, Bailey reported, was, "Carry on."

Autopsy and Criticisms

Almost a year later, in October 1985, Bailey told interviewers that Baby Fae's death was the result of a failure to match her blood type with the baboon's. She was O, the baboon AB. He had believed cyclosporine and an incompletely developed immune system would allow an infant to tolerate unmatched blood. Deciding against matching was "a tactical error that came back to haunt us," Bailey said.

The recipient of incompatible blood produces antibodies that make red blood cells clump together. These clumps block blood vessels and eventually cause death by stroke, heart attack, or multiple organ failure. The autopsy showed Baby Fae's kidneys were filled with clots that destroyed their function.

"If Baby Fae had the type AB blood group, she would still be alive today," Bailey said.

But immunologists Olga Jonasson and Mark A. Hardy, in a review accompanying Bailey's account of the Baby Fae case published in *JAMA*, an *American Medical Association* journal, disagreed with Bailey's analysis of why the xenograft failed. They characterized as "wishful thinking" and incompatible with scientific evidence his assumption that the immune system in a newborn is immature and thus more likely to tolerate foreign tissue.

They also observed that Bailey's supposition that baboon cells can be typed to establish their relative compatibility with human tissue had no support from published studies. Hence, "the overall implication that this particular baboon was 'compatible' with the patient must be rejected."

Jonasson and Hardy's interpretation of the autopsy findings was that while cyclosporine had controlled cell-mediated rejection (attack by white blood cells), it didn't control humoral (antibody) rejection. It was this that produced the hemorrhaging and inflammation that led to Baby Fae's death. Bailey's view that these were due only to the incompatibility of blood types, they dismissed as patently "incorrect."

NIH Site Visit

Even though Bailey's research was funded privately, it involved human subjects and so had to be carried out in compliance with the regulations of the National Institutes of Health's Office of Protection from Research Risks (OPRR).

Shortly after Baby Fae's death, the OPRR director had several discussions with Loma Linda administrators and the head of the IRB that had approved Bailey's protocol. Loma Linda afterward invited the OPRR to conduct a site visit and review Bailey's research program and the consent procedures the IRB had followed.

The visitors found, as recounted in a March 5, 1985, report, that the IRB had behaved "appropriately" in reviewing Bailey's research protocol. However, they complained, records of board meetings were so sketchy it wasn't possible to reconstruct discussions of the central issues.

Also, while the IRB had spent much time on the informed-consent document, they had spent comparatively little on the consent *process*. They had focused on the form—the words on paper—and slighted the interaction between Bailey and the parents and the circumstances in which Bailey and other staff members provided information to Teresa and Howard.

Even so, the visitors said they believed the parents had been given "appropriate and thorough explanations of the alternatives available, the risks and benefits of the procedure, and the experimental nature of the transplant."

The visitors weren't so charitable in assessing the consent document. They called attention to three serious flaws, two of them directly relevant to Baby Fae. One was that the benefit that might reasonably be anticipated from a xenograft was exaggerated. The document explicitly mentioned "long-term survival" as an expected possibility, but the visitors considered this an overstatement.

A second shortcoming was that Bailey's protocol didn't include the possibility of seeking a human donor heart and, if one became available, transplanting it. The consent document, in the visitors' view, should be written to state whether a human-heart would be sought and, if so, the arrangements that would be made for a human heart transplant and an estimation of its chances of success. If a search is not planned, the reasons for this should be clearly stated.

Even given such shortcomings in the consent document, the visitors concluded, "the parents of Baby Fae fully understood the alternatives available, as well as the risks and reasonably expected benefits of the transplant."

(The report has its own difficulties. How was it possible for Baby Fae's parents to have understood "fully" the alternatives available, when Bailey underestimated the value of the Norwood procedure and made no effort to find a donor heart? How was it possible for the parents to have understood fully the "reasonably expected benefits," when the site visitors themselves viewed "long-term survival" as an overstatement?)

While Bailey's xenograft research and Loma Linda's oversight were not exactly endorsed by the OPRR report, neither were they condemned. The way was left open for Bailey to proceed with the four additional xenografts called for in his research protocol. Four other babies like Baby Fae were to get baboon hearts.

More than a year after Baby Fae's death, Bailey was still stating publicly that he planned to go forward with the additional xenografts.

IN *RASHOMON,* Akira Kurosawa's classic film, four people involved in a rape and murder give different and incompatible accounts of what happened. Each account is a perceived reality that, judged in its own terms, is wholly convincing. There is no way, however, to step outside these perceptions and say what *really* happened.

Baby Fae's case offers material for constructing two radically different versions of events. Leonard Bailey is the central figure in both versions, although Loma Linda University Medical Center, its IRB, and even the Seventh Day Adventist Church play supporting roles.

Medical Hero

In the first version, Leonard Bailey is a medical hero who deserves a place in the pantheon of pioneering physicians. His story is a compelling tale of concern, hard work, and dedication.

A young physician moved by the hopelessness of babies with an incurable heart defect resolves to find the means to save them. Unable to get his grant applications funded, he persuades his university to support his research. He works alone for seven years, performing experiment after experiment, but his papers are rejected for publication and he is virtually ignored by the scientific community.

He is eventually convinced his results demonstrate that a baboon-human heart transplant offers the best possibility for the long-term survival of babies with faulty hearts. He performs the surgery on an ideal candidate and makes the news public. He is met with carping criticisms that fail to recognize his dedication, his years of research, or the significance of his accomplishment.

This version of the facts was endorsed by Bailey and his colleagues at Loma Linda. They were sure they had made medical history and were pleased to see the university and its medical school recognized as a center of excellence. "I'm not reluctant to see Loma Linda thrust into the news," Bailey told a reporter.

While Bailey engaged in no self-promotion, the medical center and the Seventh Day Adventist Church were quick to laud his achievement. The pastor of the campus church, Louis Venden, expressed the pride felt by many. "I've been bemused by sports fans," he told his congregation, "who get all excited when their team captures a World Series, and they say, 'We're number one.' For the first time in my life, I know how they feel."

Bailey, for those who accept this first version, deserves to be mentioned along with Norman Shumway, Christian Barnard, William DeVries, and other heart-replacement pioneers.

Medical Adventurer

In the second version, Leonard Bailey is a medical adventurer, a daredevil researcher determined to conduct an experiment without regard for his patient's welfare. Most telling is that he never intended for Baby Fae to receive a human heart. He wasn't prepared to perform such a transplant, and at no time did he refer Baby Fae's parents to a medical center (like Stanford) that was. Further, he never considered using a baboon heart as a bridge to a human transplant. Bailey recruited Baby Fae, purely and simply, to be an experimental subject.

To get Teresa and Howard to consent, he downplayed the likelihood of finding an appropriate human heart, understated the value of the Norwood procedure, and overstated the potential value of a baboon transplant.

Bailey was a maverick researcher, isolated from mainstream science. Peer reviewers rejected his papers and grant proposals. This alone doesn't imply that his ideas were wrong, but it's a strong reason to suspect a research program is flawed, and Bailey's was.

Bailey was able to go forward with his work because of the funding he received from Loma Linda. But by operating without external overseeing, he was deprived of the on-going evaluations by outside reviewers that shape most research. Insulated from criticism, Bailey was inclined to accept as established, ideas others considered doubtful or wrong.

Bailey, to summarize this second version, was a medical buccaneer, concerned more with his research than with his patient. He was an isolated, obstinate experimenter who went to unacceptable lengths to try to prove to the scientific world that scorned him that his solution to the problem of hypoplastic left-heart syndrome was better than anyone else's.

Take Three

We live in a richer conceptual world than Kurosawa's characters. Hence, we aren't forced to endorse either version of the Baby Fae case. Combining both yields a picture of a physician-researcher who, although motivated by unimpeachable ideals, was too easily convinced by his experimental results and thus ended up ignoring the best interest of his patient.

Bailey undoubtedly wanted to find an effective way to save the lives of infants with lethal heart defects. His animal research persuaded him a baboon transplant would not only work, but be even better than a human transplant. It would also, he believed, offer the possibility of long-term success.

Bailey didn't see a need to seek a human heart for Baby Fae or think of a xenograft as a bridge. He believed he had more to offer Baby Fae than anyone else, including Norman Shumway and William Norwood.

If not sheer arrogance, this was (to borrow Jonasson and Hardy's phrase) wishful thinking. The scientific literature didn't support his belief that an infant's immune system would tolerate a foreign organ, nor that tissue-typing of baboons could establish "compatibility" with human tissue. Also, kidney transplanters a decade earlier had recognized the need to crossmatch the blood type of donors and recipients, because drugs couldn't overcome the body's response to incompatibility.

Best Interest

Giving Baby Fae a baboon heart was justified only if it was in her best interest in the circumstances. The crucial question then is: Was it the optimal medical treatment available?

Clearly not.

The facts suggest Bailey did what he *thought* was best for Baby Fae. But they also suggest he should have known better. Before Baby Fae, four primate hearts were transplanted into humans, and in each case the recipient died. The record for longevity was Christian Barnard's second patient, who lived for three and a half *days*. Even Bailey's best animal transplant lived only five and a half months.

A human heart transplant offered Baby Fae a better chance at life than a xenograft. Hollie Ruffie was the only infant prior to receive a human heart, and although she lived only three weeks, the cause of her death wasn't directly related to her heart. The evidence of hundreds of adult heart transplants, moreover, made the success of infant transplants likely.

Even the Norwood procedure offered Baby Fae more than a xenograft. The operation was risky and couldn't repair her heart defect permanently, but it might have extended her life long enough for a human donor heart to be found.

Under the Circumstances

The "circumstances" include the fact that Teresa and Howard were too poor to travel to a distant city for surgery or pay the hospital bills for a heart transplant. Consequently, although a human heart transplant or the Norwood procedure might have offered Baby Fae a better chance at life, if her parents couldn't pay for either, neither was a genuine option.

The only real option at the time was the one mentioned to Teresa by the physicians at Loma Linda—make her baby as comfortable as possible, then wait for her to die. It's no wonder Bailey's proposal was welcomed by Teresa, for in place of death, he offered the hope of "long-term survival."

But that hope wasn't based on a realistic foundation. Bailey believed he knew what was best for Baby Fae, and Teresa and Howard consented to the treatment he proposed. The result was that instead of Baby Fae's dying peacefully, her periods of sleep growing longer and longer until she finally failed to wake, she endured twenty-one days of aggressive, invasive treatment.

She was injected with powerful medications to keep her heart beating, subjected to heart surgery, given toxic antirejection drugs, and placed on a mechanical respirator. She was cut with knives, stuck with needles, and had tubes inserted in her nose and throat.

Surgery is harsh, and postoperative care is invasive and intense. What justifies such treatment is that the patient is likely to benefit from it. But there was never a genuine possibility Baby Fae would benefit from a baboon transplant. Rather than having her life extended, she had her dying prolonged.

Nothing of Value

Did Baby Fae's surgery at least contribute to the development of xenografts more likely to be effective? Teresa hoped it would when she told Bailey to "Carry on." But nothing of scientific or medical importance came out of the transplant. Although Bailey published his case report, it contained no useful new information and various dubious assumptions. Baby Fae's transplant was just another case of a treatment shown time and again to be doomed to failure. "We don't do xenografts," John Najarian said, speaking for the community of transplant researchers, "because they are not successful."

Source of the Problem

The Baby Fae case calls attention to a gap in the array of regulations designed to protect research subjects, particularly children. An IRB is supposed to shield children from the optimistic zeal of researchers, but in the Baby Fae case, the system didn't work. It failed to protect Baby Fae's best interest, because, in the final analysis, the Loma Linda IRB was dependent on Bailey's judgment about the value of the treatment based on his research.

A major task of an IRB is to review consent documents and make sure the risks and benefits of a treatment are spelled out so that patients (or parents) can make an informed decision. But such a spelling out cannot be divorced from estimating the scientific and medical value of the treatment.

And here's the source of the problem: it's not the primary job of an IRB to evaluate the scientific or medical worth of a project's research findings. Indeed, an IRB may not have among its members the expertise needed to make such an evaluation.

This is where expert reviewers for external granting agencies play a crucial role. They act as a brake on the enthusiasm (and hopes) of researchers and prevent them from overstating the expected value of a treatment. Without the counterweight of on-going external reviews, an IRB may be prone to endorse the researcher's estimate of a treatment's value.

This is what happened in the Baby Fae case. Because Bailey's research was internally funded, it was not subject to the continuous monitoring of a granting agency like the National Heart, Lung, and Blood Institute or the FDA. Thus, the informed-consent document the Loma Linda IRB approved reflected Bailey's own belief that long-term survival was a reasonably expected outcome of a baboon heart transplant.

A view not shared by anyone in the transplant community.

(Nothing suggests that Stuart Jamieson, the Stanford reviewer, ever saw the consent document. He reported he was shocked when, after the xenograft, he learned Bailey didn't plan to search for a donor human heart.)

If the Loma Linda IRB, which included experienced physicians, didn't recognize that long-term survival was an overstatement of what was likely, how could medically naive parents like Teresa and Howard?

Because parents must rely on what they are told about an experimental procedure, an over-enthusiastic estimation of its expected benefit can skew their decision in its favor. Teresa and Howard worked hard to decide what was best for their daughter, but they decided on the basis of faulty information.

No Private Funding?

One way of preventing the repetition of cases like Baby Fae's is to revise federal regulations and forbid research supported by private funding to involve human subjects. This would effectively put government granting agencies in charge of making judgments about the potential benefits of all experimental treatments.

This restriction would have a serious and unacceptable consequence, however. It would eliminate a vast amount of important research funded by medical foundations, the pharmaceutical industry, medical-device manufacturers, and a variety of biotechnology companies. Federally funded research would become the only game in town.

A New Rule for Experimental Treatments

A more acceptable and direct solution is to add some version of the following rule to federal regulations governing human subjects:

> Children may not receive an experimental treatment having the
> potential to produce a serious adverse outcome until it has been
> tested with adults and established as reasonably safe and effective,
> except when the treatment can be tested only in children.

With such a rule in place, no future Leonard Baileys relying on private funding would be free of the constraints on experimental treatments imposed by reviewers from external agencies. No IRB would be able to rely primarily on the researcher's assessment of the risks and benefits of a treatment.

This rule can also protect children when an experimental treatment is supported by public funds. While external reviewers may prevent IRBs from endorsing over-enthusiastic assessments of the value of a treatment, such protection is subject to failure. Some external reviewers may be more easily satisfied than others. Thus, it is better to institutionalize the protection of children by means of a stringent rule like the one I'm proposing.

Possibility Alone Not Enough

The rule forbids (de facto) the use of xenografts in children until they are relatively successful in adults. (Bailey wouldn't be able to proceed in the same way today, because xenografts must now be approved by the FDA, no matter what the source of funding.) It similarly rules out implantable artificial hearts and forms of surgery in which a reasonable balance of benefits to risks haven't been established with adults.

A consequence of the rule is that even when a procedure might be viewed by a researcher as offering the possibility of saving a child's life, parents aren't permitted to consent to the use of the procedure. Because parents are often prepared to try anything that might extend the life of their child, it will be difficult for them to accept that physicians aren't free to try a procedure they've heard is potentially successful. If the child is going to die if nothing is done, why not take a chance on the procedure?

The simple answer is that it wouldn't be in the best interest of the child. If a procedure isn't likely to be successful (or buy time needed for another that is), increasing or prolonging a child's suffering is never in the best interest of the child.

Helping Others Is Not Enough

But isn't the opportunity to gain knowledge lost? Maybe so and maybe not. Mere repetition of a procedure doesn't necessarily lead to understanding. Experiments with blood transfusion began in the seventeenth century; Samuel Pepys's diary describes an early attempt. Hundreds of people over the years were given animal and human blood, and, while a few benefitted, a great many died. Not until Karl Landsteiner worked out blood groups in 1907 did transfusion became a reasonable treatment. Xenografts are still waiting for their Landsteiner.

Even if useful knowledge might result from an experimental treatment, that doesn't justify using the treatment on a child. The duty of parents is to make consent decisions by considering the best interest of their child. Period.

Parents violate this duty if they decide to sacrifice their child to further science or help other children in the future. If a child's treatment turns out to benefit others, this is all for the good. But the benefit must be a byproduct of what is done with the aim of doing what is best for the child.

Children-Only Therapies

The last clause of the rule I've proposed addresses experimental therapies that can be tested *only* in children. The Norwood procedure, for example, cannot be proven effective in adults before it is used on children, because the problem it's intended to solve doesn't occur in adults. Similarly, treatments of extremely premature infants for problems associated with undeveloped lungs cannot be tested first in adults.

Protecting children when adult patients cannot serve as a firewall seems best accomplished by amending NIH regulations to require IRBs to include outside members with expertise in the area of the proposed therapy. Their role would be to assist the IRB in making a realistic assessment of the benefits and risks of a treatment proposed in a research protocol.

The IRB could then determine whether the treatment is sufficiently promising to be permitted in principle. If so, the IRB would decide, with the help of the outside experts, whether the language of the consent document properly informed parents about the treatment and its reasonably expected risks and benefits.

The consent document (but not information about individuals) should also be made public. In refusing to release the document in the Baby Fae case, Loma Linda hid behind its private status. But when the lives and safety of research subjects are concerned, the public is entitled to know what parents were told about the expected risks and benefits of an experimental treatment. We shouldn't permit private money to buy protection from public scrutiny of human research.

Even when a therapy is part of a clinical trial supported by grants from an outside agency, the IRB should include experts who have no institutional ties to the hospital where the therapy is to be used. The outsiders, in this case, are to protect children from an *institution's* enthusiasm and wish to enhance its reputation.

Inherent Risks

New treatments are inherently risky. Children can be protected from a researcher's zeal or a medical school's desire to shine in the public's eye, but when children have a problem for which there is no established therapy, a novel treatment is likely to threaten them with dangers that cannot be foreseen.

But denying children such treatments, when they are reasonable, is withholding from them perhaps the only available means to extend their lives. The mistake in the case of Baby Fae was not that a xenograft was a novel treatment, but that xenografts were already known to fail. A human heart transplant for Baby Fae would have been novel but justifiable.

Success

Leonard Bailey never announced publicly that he'd given up the idea of doing four more baboon-to-human heart transplants. He never did them though.

Nor has anyone else performed a primate-to-human heart transplant. Even now, nearly two decades later, it's still not reasonable to believe such a xenograft would be successful. We are still unable to control adequately the basic mechanisms that cause the rejection of foreign tissues.

Bailey did not, however, surrender his dream of saving the lives of babies condemned to inevitable death by hypoplastic left-heart syndrome. The shortage of infant hearts was as severe as ever, but Bailey found a source more promising than baboons—anencephalic infants.

In October 1987 he performed the first successful neonatal heart transplant. The heart given to Paul Holc was donated by the parents of an infant known to the public only as Baby Gabrielle.

Bailey's surgical skills, his daring, and his commitment to finding a remedy for hypoplastic left-heart syndrome thus paid off by saving the life of a child who otherwise would have died.

That's enough to make him a medical hero.

8

But Are They Really Dead?

Is No Heartbeat Enough for Death?

An intruder shot Pamela James in the head.

The 33-year-old mother of two small children was attacked by a man who broke into her house in Defiance, Ohio, on a Spring night in 1987.

James was rushed to the emergency room of the local hospital and treated to stabilize her condition. Because of her brain injury, the emergency physicians regarded her as a potential organ donor and transferred her to St. Vincent's Hospital in nearby Toledo. She was pronounced dead at St. Vincent's, and various tissues and organs for transplant were removed by a team of surgeons—skin, bone, liver, kidneys, and heart.

James's assailant was captured and confessed to the shooting. He was charged with aggravated homicide. While preparing for the trial, his defense attorney, Dave Williams, was looking through the James medical records when he noticed something that pulled him up short.

"I was stunned when I saw the coroner's report," Williams told an interviewer. "The time of death listed by the coroner was virtually to the minute coincidental with the time [the transplant team] removed the heart."

Williams engaged a neuropathologist to examine Pamela James's brain. The neuropathologist came to the conclusion that her brain was "startlingly normal" and she had suffered only a "lower-grade injury" from which it would be reasonable to expect recovery.

Williams decided the evidence showed Pamela James had been killed by the removal of her organs, not by the shot fired by his client. "She was managed for the purpose of harvest, rather than managed as a neurological patient," Williams held. "She never got a chance to survive."

St. Vincent's Hospital insisted James was dead when her organs were removed, but the Lucas County prosecutor dropped the murder charge against Williams's client. He was allowed to plead guilty to a lesser charge in a plea-bargain agreement.

"It would never have occurred to me that a person could be not fatally injured and still end up on an operating table for the purpose of having their organs harvested," Williams recalled, reflecting on his defense of his client.

Sixty Minutes

The Pamela James case served as the dramatic hook for "Not Quite Dead," a CBS *Sixty Minutes* segment produced by Walter Bogdonich and broadcast on April 13, 1997. The on-camera reporter, Mike Wallace, segued into the main story by suggesting that a *Sixty Minutes'* investigation had discovered the Pamela James case was not unique and that transplant surgeons are beginning to employ doubtful practices in their rush to acquire transplant organs.

"With each passing year as more people die waiting for organs," Wallace said, "we have found that transplant doctors have begun aggressively to take organs in ways that some distinguished doctors and ethicists say are highly improper and possibly illegal."

At the focus of the story were the issues and circumstances leading the Cleveland Clinic, one of the nation's most respected medical facilities, to became the target of a criminal investigation. Carmen Marino, an assistant prosecutor from the Cuyahoga County District Attorney's office, was at the time of the broadcast seeking to determine whether the Cleveland Clinic planned to implement a draft protocol for acquiring transplant organs that might, according to Marino, leave the surgeons open to a charge of homicide.

The attention of the legal authorities had been drawn to the Cleveland Clinic protocol by Peggy Bargholt, a woman with a deep and long-standing commitment to organ transplantation. When Bargholt's 4-year-old son Jeffrey died of a brain hemorrhage in 1987, she donated his organs for transplant, thus benefitting several people. Soon after his death, she began working at LifeBanc, a Cleveland organ-procurement agency, and part of her community-relations job was to encourage others to donate the organs of their newly deceased family members.

Yet while working at LifeBanc, Bargholt discovered something that shocked her. She was familiar with the ordinary practice of removing transplant organs from people declared brain dead, but the Cleveland Clinic, according to its draft protocol, was planning to take organs from patients who, though seriously brain damaged, were not brain dead. The organs would be removed after such patients were declared dead by what Mike Wallace described as "an older, less-precise method . . . , the absence of a heartbeat."

Under the Cleveland Clinic's protocol, according to Wallace, "with the consent of the family, life support would be withdrawn [from a patient], and a doctor not affiliated with the transplant team would declare death after just two minutes without a heartbeat." The hospital also planned to give patients who were potential donors what Wallace characterized as "massive doses of potentially harmful drugs solely to make their organs available for transplant."

Peggy Bargholt took her concerns about the protocol to Mary Ellen Waithe, a bioethicist at Cleveland State University and Bargholt's academic supervisor. "We investigated for a month," Waithe told Wallace, "and the response of everyone I consulted with was, 'What are they trying to do, kill them?'" She decided, after having been told this by "three or four people," that "if they are, we need to get the authorities involved."

Before taking such a step, however, Bargholt and Waithe, according to a New York Times story, wrote an academic paper about the Cleveland Clinic's draft protocol and submitted it to JAMA. When the paper was rejected, they wrote to the Attorney General of Ohio and expressed their concerns. He referred them to the county District Attorney's office, where responsibility for investigating the case was assigned to Carmen Marino.

Marino reviewed the documents from the Cleveland Clinic provided by Bargholt and Waithe. He was particularly worried by the part of the draft calling for administering doses of heparin and Regitine to patients who are potential organ donors. Heparin keeps blood from clotting, and Regitine, a vasodilator, keeps blood vessels open. Thus the combination helps promote blood flow through organs and prevents clots from forming. Without the flow of blood, the organs will die, and if clots form inside them, they may become useless for transplantation.

"But aren't these patients going to die anyway?" Mike Wallace asked Waithe. "Aren't they as good as dead?"

"As good as dead is not dead," Waithe replied. "It's not up to physicians . . . to determine what our legal criteria are." Waithe also told New York Times reporter Gina Kolata before the Sixty Minutes broadcast that if physicians at the Cleveland Clinic followed the procedure outlined in the protocol, they would be "murdering patients to get their organs."

Waithe's view was shared by Carmen Marino. After reviewing the documents supplied to him by Bargholt and Waithe, he informed the Cleveland Clinic that "This sort of protocol results in a homicide." He said he would insist his office approve any protocol for removing organs from donors whose hearts have stopped beating but who are not brain dead.

The Cleveland Clinic assured him it wouldn't put the draft plan into practice. But it also released a statement denying that Regitine was harmful to patients and asserting that the protocol met "the highest legal and ethical standards."

The head of the hospital's ethics committee expressed outrage that Bargholt and Waithe hadn't come to the committee with their concerns but had, instead, involved the District Attorney's office and supplied Marino with unauthorized copies of internal documents.

Carmen Marino's investigation eventually came to an end when he found no evidence of legal wrongdoing on the part of the Cleveland Clinic or its physicians. Even so, by insisting that the District Attorney's office review any future protocol before the hospital implemented it, he put the physicians on notice that they were under continuing scrutiny.

"The chances of this happening to you or to a member of your family are already minuscule," Mike Wallace said in a closing statement. "And now that this controversy is finally out in the open, the chances are probably nil."

"NOT QUITE DEAD" infuriated the transplant community. It was denounced on web sites and in newsletters as unfair, biased, sensational, destructive, and wholly misleading.

The criticisms had merit. The Pamela James case wasn't a clear example of someone whose organs were illicitly removed. Had she been tested at St. Vincent's to determine whether she was brain dead? Had her family instructed the hospital to remove her from life support? Were her physicians following her advance directive? Did they wait a few minutes after her heart stopped before removing her organs?

By leaving such questions unanswered, *Sixty Minutes* invited viewers to endorse the defense attorney's claim that James wasn't killed by his client, James's assailant, but by the transplant surgeons.

Also, while the point of the story seemed to be that "aggressive" transplant surgeons were removing organs from patients who weren't really dead, Wallace's concluding remark undercut this claim. The chances were "minuscule" to begin with, he said, and "now that this controversy is finally out in the open, they are probably nil."

So should we accept Mike Wallace's invitation to treat the whole *Sixty Minutes* story as hardly more serious than a bad dream? Can we ignore it as merely another attempt by a television program to increase its audience share by sensationalizing an unfamiliar topic? First it was dental fillings causing neurological disorders, now it's illicit organ snatching.

We aren't free to shrug off "Not Quite Dead," however, because for all its flaws, it dramatically raised two crucial questions about the use of organs from donors who aren't brain dead: *When should we consider such a potential donor dead?* and *Is it morally acceptable to give drugs that help preserve a patient's organs but don't help the patient?* While the broadcast is now several years in the past, the questions remain as pertinent and in need of answers as before.

To approach them it's useful to begin with a case that proceeds according to a protocol probably similar to the draft the Cleveland Clinic was considering adopting. (We can't be sure how similar, because the hospital never made the draft public.) The case gives a better sense of the procedures actually followed at transplant centers than does the *Sixty Minutes* story. This makes it possible to ignore the razzle-dazzle and focus on the relevant issues.

The Dean Oliver Case

Dean Oliver (as I'll call him) was a fit 40-year-old tax accountant who had just completed his late afternoon run when he collapsed on the driveway of his house in suburban Baltimore.

Alice Rudman, his wife, was sitting on the patio and saw him fall. She rushed out and knelt beside him. She could feel Dean's heart beating, but he was unconscious. His face was pale, and his skin felt cold and clammy. He was also having trouble breathing, taking rapid, shallow gasps after long intervals.

Alice felt sure Dean would die if they had to wait for the ambulance. Because they lived only a couple of miles from Shoreside Medical Center, she wrestled his limp body into the front seat of her car and rushed him to the emergency room.

Dr. Clara Rosenberg and the ER team swarmed over Dean's inert body. They immediately inserted a breathing tube into his trachea and attached him to a mechanical ventilator, looked for bleeding, and checked his vital signs. Soon the oxygen level in Dean's blood was back to normal, his lungs were clear, and his arterial pressure steady.

The immediate crisis was over.

Dean still had not regained consciousness, however, and Dr. Rosenberg began to try to diagnose his problem. She ruled out the likelihood of a heart attack, then ordered a CT-scan of his head. He might have suffered head trauma, even though there was no outward sign of it. No blood, broken skin, or contusions.

What the scan showed was worse than Dr. Rosenberg had imagined. An exploded blood vessel in Dean's brain, a ruptured aneurysm, had caused massive damage, destroying large portions of the cerebrum. The hemorrhaging blood had formed an orange-sized spherical mass that had destroyed or compressed the surrounding tissues.

The bleeding seemed to have stopped, but because of the location of the mass, surgery would be of no use. Trying to remove the clot would destroy too much brain tissue. Dean wasn't able to breathe because of pressure on his brain stem exerted by the clot. A neurosurgeon screwed a device into Dean's skull to monitor his intracranial pressure. Although Dr. Rosenberg put Dean on drugs to help reduce brain swelling, no effective treatment was possible for his injury.

Dr. Rosenberg explained to Alice that the damage to Dean's brain was so severe he would never regain consciousness. Dean could be maintained on life support for an indefinite time, but he had no prospect of recovery.

"You mean he's brain dead?" Alice asked.

"Not in the technical sense," Dr. Rosenberg said. "He still has measurable brain stem activity, but if we take him off the ventilator, we expect him to die rather quickly."

"Dean's living will says not to keep him on life support the way he is now," Alice said. "He also wanted to donate his organs to help other people."

Dr. Rosenberg introduced Alice to Dr. Jarrel Hay. At Alice's request, Dr. Hay went over Dean's advance directive and explained Shoreside's protocol for removing Dean's organs when his death was declared. Alice then met with the hospital's attorney and signed a document stating she understood the procedure and agreed to its being followed in Dean's case.

Dean was moved to an intensive care unit and monitored overnight. Despite the drugs, his brain continued to swell, increasing the pressure on his brain stem. Yet he still didn't meet the criteria for brain death.

The following morning Dean was wheeled into a small recovery room adjacent to an operating room. Dr. Sara Stein, a surgeon Alice hadn't met before, in a minor procedure using a local anesthetic, inserted a small tube, a cannula, into an artery in Dean's groin and sewed it into place. Dean was given doses of heparin and Regitine through his IV line.

Alice arrived around 7:00. She sat in a chair beside Dean's bed for about an hour, talking to him and squeezing his hand. She then kissed him, smoothed the hair back from his forehead, and left the room.

She found Dr. Carl Greeley at the nurse's station. Dr. Greeley, who had no connection with the transplant unit, had assumed responsibility for taking care of Dean as soon as he was moved out of the ER. He was Dean's attending physician.

"He's ready to go now," Alice told Dr. Greeley.

"You're doing something courageous," Dr. Greeley told her.

"Dean did it." Alice walked toward the elevator.

Dr. Greeley, Dr. Hay, and a group including physicians, nurses, and technicians wheeled Dean from the recovery area to the operating room. He was prepped for surgery. A technician painted the upper part of his body with a brown antibacterial solution (to protect his organs from bacterial contamination) and covered him with strategically placed green surgical drapes.

Dr. Greeley weaned Dean off the ventilator by steadily reducing the volume of the oxygen mixture forced into his lungs. Dean's heart rate increased, a sign of respiratory distress, and Dr. Greeley injected him with morphine to ease any discomfort he might be feeling. When the weaning was completed, Dr. Greeley pulled out Dean's breathing tube.

Dean's heart began to beat irregularly, then fluttered out of control, going into fibrillation. Then his heart stopped completely, reaching the state known as asystole. His blood pressure continued to fall, and his blood stopped circulating.

Dr. Greeley made no attempt to control Dean's flailing heart or to restart it. Instead, he glanced repeatedly at the machines monitoring Dean's heart and arterial blood pressure, then at the clock on the wall.

Two minutes elapsed. Three, four. Then five.

"This patient is dead," Dr. Greeley said, making a formal pro-nouncement.

Dr. Greeley moved away from the operating table. Dr. Vinge and his organ recovery team came forward. Dr. Zho attached a line to the cannula in the groin and started a chilled fluid flowing through Dean's body. It would help preserve the organs and slow the process of deterioration.

Dr. Zho took out the kidneys, liver, and pancreas. Other members of the team would later recover the corneas, blood vessels, bone segments, and patches of skin.

More than a dozen people would ultimately benefit from Dean's organs and tissues.

Recognizing Death

Dean Oliver became what the transplant community calls a *non-heartbeating donor*. These are patients with disorders (usually brain injuries) so severe recovery is impossible, but who don't satisfy the criteria for brain death and are declared dead according to cardiopulmonary criteria. That is, they cease breathing and their hearts stop.

If Dean Oliver was dead, removing his organs was quite all right. But was Dean, to borrow the *Sixty Minutes* segment title, "not quite dead" when his organs were removed? Or, as Mary Ellen Waithe's view implies, was Dean *murdered* by Dr. Vinge to take his organs? Dean was pronounced dead by Dr. Greeley, but was he *really* dead?

Background

Human beings, unlike some of their machines, aren't equipped with a light that blinks off when they cease functioning. Thus no society has ever been quite sure when to declare someone dead. Some cultures in the Middle East, even now, don't consider people dead until three days after their hearts have stopped beating.

Science has done about as much to confuse the situation as to solve the problem. The rise of physiology in the seventeenth century, with its studies of suspended animation and organs functioning outside the body, blurred even further the line between the living and the dead.

William Harvey in 1627 kept a headless rooster's heart functioning by blowing air into its lungs with a bellows, and generations of physiologists demonstrated that the hearts of frogs and chickens could be kept beating outside the body for extended periods. The development of techniques for artificial respiration showed that people pronounced dead could sometimes be resuscitated, and Dr. Frankenstein's pathetic creature suggested how science might be powerful enough even to reanimate an assemblage of organic parts.

Doubts about whether death could be correctly determined became widespread during the nineteenth century. "The difference between the end of a weak life, and the commencement of death, is so small," London surgeon G. A. Walker wrote in 1839, "that we can scarcely suppose under-takers capable of distinguishing an apparent from a real death."

At a time when victims of cholera or typhoid were rushed to their graves to avoid spreading disease, it's likely a number of comatose people were buried alive. Franz Hartmann, a physician practicing in the last decade of the century, estimated that in Germany a thousand premature burials occurred each year.

Fear of premature burial became so common that various devices were invented to prevent it. In 1874 Vienna built a morgue with electrical sensors in the slabs. If a body moved, the sensors would send a signal to ring a bell in a central office. Patents were issued in the United States for gadgets permitting an awakened "corpse" to signal for help from the grave, and Mary Baker Eddy, the founder of Christian Science, supposedly ordered that a telephone be installed in her tomb.

Concern about premature burial found its way into literature. Edgar Allen Poe's "The Fall of the House of Usher" and "The Premature Burial" expressed Poe's own worries. They were shared by other writers. Hans Christian Anderson, who died in 1875, habitually left a note on his bedside table saying "Am merely in suspended animation." A few days before Anderson died, he instructed a friend to open his veins before he was buried.

Terms of the Contemporary Debate

"When is someone dead?" is clearly an old question, but the advent of artificial ventilation and the success of organ transplantation starting in the 1950s gave it a uniquely modern urgency and sharpness. If machines and medicines can keep a patient's body functioning indefinitely, is the person still alive? If a surgeon removes a beating heart, has the surgeon killed the patient?

Our cultural intuitions are that it can be morally legitimate for physicians to discontinue life support and surgeons to remove vital organs. Either is acceptable undeniably when the patient is dead. So we are faced with two basic questions: *What counts as death?* and *How do we recognize when it has occurred?*

The terms of the contemporary debate were set during the 1970s when most states, under the influence of the federal Uniform Determination of Death Act, passed laws introducing the concept of brain death. The Act's definition followed the formulation of a Presidential Commission appointed to study the issue, and its definition was modeled on the one in the 1968 report of the Harvard Medical School's Ad Hoc Committee to Examine the Definition of Brain Death.

The Harvard Committee was explicit about why a definition was needed. "Our primary purpose," the report stated, "is to define irreversible coma as a new criterion for death," because "obsolete criteria . . . can lead to controversy in obtaining organs for transplantation." Also, the Committee, under the influence of its chair, Henry K. Beecher, wanted to avoid wasting resources on patients no longer able to benefit from life-support measures and to save families from the financial and emotional costs of supporting such patients.

The Committee's concern about the controversy in obtaining transplant organs wasn't unrealistic. The only source for cadaver organs from the 1950s into the early 1970s were donors determined to be dead according to traditional cardiopulmonary (heart-lung) criteria, and surgeons during this pioneering phase of transplantation sometimes waited several hours before removing organs. Results were usually unsatisfactory, because the deteriorated organs were not likely to function effectively, if at all.

Surgeons who tried to reduce the time between death and transplantation sometimes found themselves in legal difficulties. David Hume in Virginia, Denton Cooley in Texas, and Norman Schumway in California were among the surgeons accused during the 1960s of causing the deaths of donors by removing their organs too quickly. Schumway was even charged with homicide.

The Pamela James case, used as a story hook by *Sixty Minutes*, is a sharp echo of this past controversy, and while Dave Williams wasn't the first defense attorney to argue that it was really the surgeons, not his client, who killed a homicide victim, he may be the only one to have succeeded.

Brain Death

The legal criteria for brain death adopted by all fifty states are for *whole-brain death*. Death is defined in the model act as "the irreversible cessation of all functions of the entire brain," which is supposed to mean activity in the brain is completely absent—no neurons firing, no integrated processes occurring. Neurological tests and EEG data don't define death, but they provide evidence that brain functions are permanently absent and therefore that the definition of death is satisfied. The data answer the question, "How do we know that death has occurred?"

Defining death as the loss of *all* brain activity helped the whole-brain notion gain rapid public acceptance. Considering the old problem of distinguishing life from death, the speed with which the concept was endorsed and became part of the law suggests most people welcomed it with relief as a scientific way of resolving doubts.

Yet those dealing with the concept professionally recognized from the start that it was fraught with problems. That its criteria don't apply to children under 2 or to anencephalic infants are limitations that have made it difficult to secure transplant organs. Some legislators have gone so far as to propose that anencephalic infants, because they have little or no brain, simply be *declared* dead (see Chapter 4).

Further, some critics consider the whole-brain concept unreasonably stringent and favor the loss of *higher* brain functions as sufficient. Thus, those like Karen Quinlan or Nancy Cruzan, existing in a persistent vegetative state with permanent loss of consciousness, might be considered dead.

Other critics view the whole-brain definition as missing the point and propose defining death as the loss of status as a *person*. A knowledge of brain functioning is thus relevant to determining death, but it's not essential. Hence someone might be declared dead in terms of the criteria we accept as determining who should be considered a person. The criteria might include an inability to interact in any way with others, a permanent loss of consciousness, and an inability to plan for a future life.

A variety of definitions of death have been proposed and all are offered as superior in various ways to the whole-brain concept. But the notion of death as brain death—as whole-brain death—appears to most people so simple, so intuitively *right*, as to need no argument. (No brain function, no life. Period.) Surveys show the public considers the question "When does death occur?" answered correctly and isn't concerned in the least with the issues raised by critics.

Cardiopulmonary Death

Mike Wallace claimed the Cleveland Clinic proposed to declare severely brain-injured people dead according to "an older, less-precise method . . . , the absence of a heartbeat."

The method for determining the absence of a heartbeat is no less "precise" than that for determining the absence of brain activity. But what Wallace seems to have had in mind is that the lack of a heartbeat isn't a precise indicator for the lack of brain activity. This is true. What isn't true, however, is the implication that death is equivalent to brain death.

The brain-death concept has been so strongly embraced and become so deeply ingrained that people are often surprised to learn it didn't *replace* the old cardiopulmonary concept. Rather, the brain-death definition supplemented the traditional one, so that we now operate with two distinct but equally legitimate sets of criteria.

Someone is dead, according to the model statue, either when all brain functions come to an end *or* when the "irreversible cessation of circulatory and respiratory functions" occurs.

The use of brain criteria for determining death is actually quite uncommon. About 98 percent of deaths are determined by cardiopulmonary criteria. This is because most people don't die from brain injuries but from various sorts of organ failure due to diseases like cancer, diabetes, or pneumonia. These failures trigger a series of biochemical and physiological events causing breathing to cease and the heart to stop functioning.

Someone whose heart is no longer circulating blood may be declared dead. But because brain-death criteria require that no electrical activity be taking place in the brain, those meeting the cardiopulmonary criteria don't simultaneously meet the brain-death criteria. Some form of brain activity may continue for minutes or even hours. It won't consist in anything so basic as responding to a needle jab or noxious odor, but will involve only disorganized neuronal firings—electrical noise.

Dead is Dead

The two sets of criteria make it easy to fall into the pattern of speaking as if there are two *kinds* of death—brain death and heart death. This invites people to consider only individuals meeting the brain-death criteria as *really* dead. Prosecutor Carmen Marino made this error in insisting it would be wrong for the Cleveland Clinic to remove organs from patients who were not yet brain dead. (Had he gone to court on an actual case, he probably would have lost.) Mary Ellen Waithe believed physicians were redefining death, whereas they were really using the cardiopulmonary criteria for determining death.

Holding that only those who are brain dead are *really* dead is like saying that although you can either drive or fly to Chicago, the *real* Chicago is the one you reach by plane. Dead is dead, no matter which set of criteria is employed. Or to put the point formally, satisfying either set of criteria is sufficient for determining death.

Controlled and Uncontrolled Donors

The transplant community divides non-heartbeating donors into *uncontrolled* and *controlled*. Consider someone who suffers a devastating brain injury in a car crash and is rushed to a trauma center. She dies before she reaches the emergency room, and her husband immediately consents to donate her organs. She is an *uncontrolled* donor, because she died without prearrangement.

Dean Oliver was a *controlled* donor. He was on life-support and was expected to die when he was taken off. The conditions under which he died were arranged in a way that would provide the best protection for his organs.

While the Cleveland Clinic, faced with a criminal investigation, backed away from its plans to remove organs from controlled non-heartbeating donors, medical centers like the University of Wisconsin and the University of Pittsburgh have followed similar protocols for several years. Indeed, more than half the nation's sixty-three organ procurement organizations have procedures and rules for recovering transplant organs from non-heartbeating donors, and it's likely that all such organizations will soon adopt a uniform policy.

Nearly 99 percent of transplanted organs from dead donors come from people declared brain dead. But about 98 percent of people declared dead are ones satisfying the cardiopulmonary criteria. Thus, if even a small percentage of those pronounced dead by these criteria became donors (disease and debilitation would rule out many), a substantial number of transplant organs would become available. Currently, only about sixty donors a year are non-heartbeating ones, so the potential for adding additional ones is considerable.

Organ transplants save thousands of lives every year, and many more could be saved if organs weren't in such short supply. New names are added to the waiting list at the rate of one every fourteen minutes, and at any moment, about 70,000 people are on the list. Sadly, about 5,000 people a year die before the organ they require becomes available.

The demand for kidneys is particularly pressing, and researchers doubt that even if all suitable ones were acquired from those declared brain dead, the need could be met. But kidneys are the organs most likely to be recovered in usable condition from non-heartbeating donors.

The need for more organs is thus the driving force behind the decision to employ controlled non-heartbeating donors. But every transplant center knows that in formulating its protocol it's walking on moral eggshells. Not only must it do what is right, but it must avoid creating the impression of greedily snatching organs from people who aren't really dead.

When some people believe they hear the eggshells crunch, even slightly, they bail out of the donor system. This is what happened because of the Cleveland Clinic inquiry. Even before the *Sixty Minutes* story, the *Cleveland Plain-Dealer* published a news story about the District Attorney's plans to investigate the Cleveland Clinic's draft protocol. Over the next ten days, organ donation in the area dropped from an expected thirty donors to just one. Figures aren't available to show the impact of the broadcast of "Not Quite Dead," but it's likely to have lowered organ donations nationwide.

Such episodes alarm some in the transplant community. Many people are already reluctant to donate the organs of a family member, and some don't trust physicians to give them a fair shake at recovery if they're viewed as potential donors. Thus critics worry that although implementing controlled non-heartbeating donor protocols will recover more organs, a backlash might damage the entire procurement system. Trying to acquire extra organs might result in a massive net loss.

The risk can't be eliminated, but it can be minimized by making sure such protocols meet explicit moral principles. This is basic to satisfying the public that Mike Wallace's "aggressive" surgeons are not, in Mary Ellen Waithe's words, "murdering people to get their organs."

The Determination of Death

The Dead-Donor Rule requires that a donor be dead before the vital organs are removed. Organs necessary for life can't be taken before death, even if a patient consents.

Someone conscious and competent may decide to terminate life-support and become a non-heartbeating donor. But if she asks a physician to end her life by removing her organs, her request can't be granted. The surgery would constitute physician-assisted suicide or active euthanasia, and while the surgery might be morally acceptable, it is definitely illegal.

It was the Dead-Donor Rule that defense attorney Dave Williams claimed surgeons at St. Vincent's Hospital had violated, killing Pamela James. An acceptable non-heartbeating donor protocol must not violate the Dead-Donor Rule. The protocol must thus provide criteria for determining when death occurs.

Death is a diagnostic category, similar to measles or diabetes. A physician makes a diagnosis on the basis of data relevant to determining whether a condition (red itchy rash, fever) fits into a disease category (measles). A diagnosis is, ultimately, a clinical judgment.

While data may sometimes virtually dictate a diagnosis (rash, fever, presence of the measles virus), most often they provide only evidence supporting a conclusion. A clinician must thus decide when the evidence is strong enough to establish a particular diagnosis. This is a reason doctors can disagree.

Additional information may make a diagnosis less or more likely. Ideally, physicians would like to gather enough information to establish a diagnosis beyond a reasonable doubt. But the realities of medicine often don't allow this, because sick people need to be treated. Hence, diagnostic decisions may have to be made on the basis of inadequate information.

In non-heartbeating donor protocols, the pertinent diagnostic criteria are for cardiopulmonary death, rather than brain death. The legal definition from the model act is straightforward enough: the "irreversible cessation of circulatory and respiratory functions."

But definitions have to be applied to cases, and it's here that matters get sticky. Determining that breathing has ceased and the heart has arrested isn't problematic. Clinical observations alone have been used for centuries to establish death—no detectable heartbeat, no misting of a mirror by the patient's breath. While such clinical observations remain the primary data in low-tech settings, in high-tech hospitals devices like oximeters, EKGs, and cardiac and arterial pressure monitors supply supplementary information.

The problematic aspect of applying the cardiopulmonary criteria for death lies in determining when the cessation of circulatory and respiratory functions are *irreversible*.

Irreversible

This is not ordinarily an issue, because establishing the precise moment of death isn't necessary. Most people expire, even in hospitals, under conditions in which the status of their organs after death is irrelevant. Thus, if a physician isn't sure whether someone is dead, waiting half an hour after the heart has stopped makes the diagnosis clear.

But when someone's organs are going to be removed for transplantation, establishing the moment of death becomes crucial. The organs can't be removed too soon without violating the Dead-Donor Rule. Yet they must be removed while they are still in good condition.

Organs begin to deteriorate the moment the blood stops flowing and delivering oxygen to them. Clots form in tiny blood vessels and tissues begin to break down. The longer the delay in removing or preserving the organs, the more damage they will suffer. Damaged organs when transplanted are less likely to function and more likely to be rejected. Considering the risks of anesthesia, infection, and major surgery, getting a bad organ may leave a recipient worse off. Hence, removing organs as near after the death of the donor as possible is critical.

So how is an attending physician to decide that when a patient's heart has stopped, it's stopped *irreversibly*? One way of answering the question is to attempt resuscitation (using drugs and electric shock) and fail.

But this isn't a morally defensible method in the case of non-heartbeating donors. They (or their families) have already decided against resuscitation, and to attempt it would violate their moral and legal right to reject medical treatment.

To make the decision about irreversibility, the patient's physician ordinarily must do nothing but wait. The reason to wait is that, even without intervention, spontaneous revival sometimes occurs. The heart starts pumping blood again, so the patient isn't dead according to the criteria.

But wait for how long? Long enough to rule out the possibility of spontaneous revival, but unfortunately, studies haven't been done relating time elapsed to the frequency of this happening. Anecdotal evidence suggests that after the heart stops, spontaneous revival, if it occurs at all, will occur within the first *ten to fifteen seconds* and almost certainly within the first *minute*.

Some non-heartbeating donor protocols are silent about the amount of time that must elapse after cardiac arrest before death can be diagnosed. The most widely debated protocol, the one at the University of Pittsburgh Medical Center (which has encouraged public discussion), requires two minutes, but others specify one, three, or five minutes.

The recommendations from expert committees don't provide a definitive answer either. The authors of the "Guidelines for the Determination of Death" in the 1981 *Report of the Medical Consultants on the Diagnosis of Death* recognized a need to wait "a few minutes." The Institute of Medicine in a 1997 report recommended that "at least five minutes" should pass but acknowledged this was on the conservative end of the range.

Data about spontaneous revival would help in deciding how much time should elapse after the heart arrests before death can be diagnosed with reasonable certainty. Without such data, selecting a particular time interval and making it part of a protocol borders on the arbitrary. As strong a case can be made for one minute as for five.

Clinical Judgment

A tempting and reasonable resolution is to require no set amount of time and leave it to the patient's physician (who can't be a member of the transplant team) to decide when the patient is dead. Death, in this respect, is simply another diagnostic category, and its determination is ultimately a clinical judgment.

Patients who have arranged to become non-heartbeating donors after their death expect a physician to make this judgment. By the time they are moved to an operating room to prepare them for surgery, they must have made three explicit and informed decisions: (1) they don't want their lives sustained by medical intervention, once recovery is recognized as impossible; (2) they don't want to be resuscitated when their hearts and lungs fail; (3) they want to donate their organs.

The patient's physician, with respect to treatment, has the duty of acting in accordance with the patient's decisions. Thus, these three decisions serve as guidelines for physicians, as reference standards for how they should treat their patients.

Consider the Dean Oliver case. Dr. Greeley (in keeping with decision 1) weaned Dean off the ventilator, even though the machine was keeping him alive. He gave Dean morphine when he was showing signs of distress, because treating him for the possibility of pain was compatible with the three decisions Dean and his wife had made. But when Dean began to go into respiratory failure, Dr. Greeley was constrained (by decision 2) from putting him back on the ventilator.

Dr. Greeley continued to monitor Dean's vital signs. Thus, he was aware of when Dean's heart arrested and his blood pressure fell so low his circulation collapsed. Dean was at that instant in a vague state of existence. He could not be known, even in principle, to be either alive or dead, because it was impossible to know whether his condition was reversible.

Dr. Greeley, under other circumstances or with some other patient, could wait an indefinite time before pronouncing death. But in Dean's case, he was constrained by Dean's third decision, to donate his organs. Waiting too long would frustrate Dean's intention and instructions.

Dr. Greeley waited five minutes, then declared Dean dead. But he could have legitimately resolved the vagueness of Dean's state by waiting however long it took for him to be satisfied Dean was dead according to the cardiopulmonary criteria. In making that determination, though, he would have to consider as a factor Dean's decision to donate his organs.

Dr. Greeley, under this scenario, wouldn't have to tick off the minutes. Rather, he would examine Dean and read the numbers from the relevant monitors. Believing, reasonably but not beyond the possibility of doubt, that Dean's heart wasn't going to start again, Dr. Greeley could declare him dead.

The elapsed time might be forty-five seconds, one minute, two, six, or whatever. Dr. Greeley would be acting in keeping with the way a physician often must act in diagnosing a disorder so that treatment can be initiated. Time and incomplete information are factors in both kinds of cases.

A Decisive Practical Consideration

Relying on a physician's clinical judgment to resolve the question of when a potential donor should be declared dead can be defended on both medical and moral grounds. No physician who exercised such a judgment would be doing anything wrong, and a surgeon who removed a patient's vital organs after death was declared would not be (contrary to Waithe) "murdering" the donor.

Even so, making unfettered clinical judgment the accepted way of determining death in the case of non-heartbeating donors would not be good public policy.

Episodes like the legal and media flap over the Cleveland Clinic's draft protocol reveal in the starkest way the tenuous nature of the public's commitment to organ donation. Because many people already fear that doctors are inclined to be premature in declaring patients dead to acquire their organs, it's especially crucial to counter the perception that someone declared dead by cardiopulmonary criteria is still alive when organs are removed.

The Dead-Donor Rule must not only be satisfied technically, it must be accepted by the public as satisfied. To make this happen, all organ retrieval protocols need to adopt a national standard. In lieu of data about spontaneous revival, almost any given elapse of time after the heart stops might be a reasonable candidate. But the Institute of Medicine recommendation of a five-minute wait has the most going for it.

The recommendation is based on the judgment and experience of experts and thus isn't completely arbitrary. If it errs, it errs (as the authors of the recommendation admit) on the side of conservatism. Most people are likely to believe someone whose heart hasn't beat and who hasn't breathed for five minutes is genuinely dead.

Data currently available show that after three to five minutes without oxygen, the brain becomes irreversibly damaged. Such damage isn't likely to meet the criteria for brain death at that instant, but revival isn't likely to occur either. (Most people, Waithe aside, probably do consider those who have suffered severe brain damage "as good as dead," not because they believe it's okay to treat them any way we want, but because they think it's wrong to try to resuscitate them. W.W. Jacobs's "The Monkey's Paw" and Stephen King's *Pet Sematary* reflect this popular attitude toward trying to bring people back after a certain point.)

Finally, while organs begin to deteriorate when the blood supply to them is interrupted, five minutes is not so long that the organs will become unusable. It's a good compromise between haste and waste.

The five-minute standard should be regarded as only a provisional rule. Once research has answered the question about the correlation between elapsed time and self-revival, the public may come to accept a shorter waiting time, depending on the data.

Also, once people become familiar with the idea of recovering organs from non-heartbeating donors, the public's uneasiness about the protocols is likely to weaken. Brain death has become so tightly linked with organ donation it will take time and education for people to realize that the Dead-Donor Rule can also be satisfied when brain death isn't the diagnosis.

Treating the Organs

Organs need to be in good condition to justify transplanting them. The Cleveland Clinic's protocol aimed to protect the organs of donors by giving the patients injections of heparin and Regitine.

It was this provision of the protocol that spurred Mary Ellen Waithe and Peggy Bargholt to take their documents to the prosecutor's office ("'What are they trying to do, kill them?'"). The hospital's intention to use, as Mike Wallace put it, "massive doses of potentially harmful drugs solely to make [a patient's] organs available for transplant" was also the aspect of most concern to prosecutor Carmen Marino.

These worries prompted our second question: *Is it morally acceptable to give a patient drugs not to benefit the patient, but to protect the organs?* The answer depends on how a second question is answered: *Could the drugs harm the patient?*

Medicine is committed to the principle that harming a patient deliberately is always wrong, no matter what benefits may result. Thus, it would be wrong to use drugs that would hasten a patient's death but protect the organs, even if the organs could be used to save the lives of half a dozen people.

Also, it would be wrong to harm a patient, even at the patient's request. Hence, a woman can't engage a surgeon to remove her heart and give it to her husband. (It's not just the Dead-Donor Rule or laws against homicide that stand in the way of taking people's organs before they're dead.) Thus, if injecting patients with heparin and Regitine would harm then, giving them the drugs would be wrong.

The drugs are definitely of no advantage to patients, but whether they can cause harm is another vexed issue. Some experts, but by no means all, believe they can hasten the deaths of some who receive them. People with severe head injuries may experience more bleeding into the brain if given heparin. Regitine may reduce the likelihood of a body's restoring its own heartbeat, because the drug may block the synthesis of adrenaline, which can cause a stopped heart to kick back into action.

No actual case of either drug accelerating the death of a donor has been reported. Even so, the possibility they might shorten some donors' lives suggests their use shouldn't be an automatic provision of any protocol. But this doesn't mean it would be wrong to use them in all cases.

The patient (or the family) intends for the donor's organs to be used to benefit others, and while this intention doesn't warrant active euthanasia, it permits the patient's physician to do what is necessary to realize that intention, so long as it doesn't hasten the patient's death. Hence, when the physician judges that a drug won't shorten the patient's life, administering it would be morally acceptable.

Dr. Greeley injected Dean with heparin and Regitine, because the bleeding in his brain appeared to have stopped. If it hadn't, the drugs might have increased the bleeding and so shortened Dean's life. Under those circumstances, Dr. Greeley shouldn't have used them.

But if it's true, as critics charge, that Regitine also reduces the likelihood of spontaneous revival, wouldn't it *always* be wrong to use it? No, because the patient has already rejected resuscitation, and giving a drug that suppresses the synthesis of a chemical that might produce revival isn't morally different from refraining from using a defibrillator. The patient has chosen not to be resuscitated—by any means.

End Notes

Dean Oliver, five minutes after his heart stopped, met the cardiopulmonary criteria in the judgment of Dr. Greeley. He thus was dead when his organs were removed and certainly wasn't "murdered" by Dr. Vinge, the transplant surgeon. His organs were protected by drugs that, while they didn't benefit him medically, either caused him no harm or, at worst, allowed him to realize his intentions of not being resuscitated and becoming an organ donor.

If the procedures outlined in the Cleveland Clinic's draft protocol paralleled those followed in the Dean Oliver case, the protocol was morally unobjectionable.

Carmen Marino, the prosecutor, Mary Ellen Waithe, the bioethicist, and the producer of the *Sixty Minutes* segment "Not Quite Dead" were thus all barking up the wrong moral tree. The root of their confusion was their tacit assumption that death can occur only when the criteria for *brain* death are satisfied.

Perhaps it's now time for a *Sixty Minutes* segment called "Quite Dead," showing how the recognition of the cardiopulmonary criteria for death and the adoption of morally acceptable non-heartbeating donor protocols could increase the supply of transplant organs.

The thousands of people waiting for organs to save their lives would find the story particularly compelling.

9

Xenotransplantation, Part 1

Chasing the Dream

January 15: Republic of Costa Linda, Esperanza City, Cookstone XenoCenter

"Our facilities exceed those of the Mayo Clinic, Stanford, Pittsburgh or any place in the States you care to name," Dr. Thomas Cookstone said. "My investors have great confidence in what we're doing here, and they support us well. That's why we've been able to build a world-class institution on this island."

"They told us in Seattle you don't have XRA oversight," Susan Lawton said. She glanced at her husband in the wheelchair beside her. His face was grey and his breathing labored, even though he was receiving pure oxygen from the clear plastic tube clipped to his nostrils.

"The Xenotransplant Research Agency doesn't have jurisdiction over us," Dr. Cookstone said. "Costa Linda's an independent republic. Quite frankly I'm glad we don't have to contend with the bureaucrats and their endless paperwork and petty rules. I'm sure they also told you in Seattle that Mr. Lawton couldn't get a new heart unless he was one of the lucky few chosen under some center's experimental protocol."

"He wasn't chosen." Susan nodded. "That's why we came down here. We heard your center took people needing transplants, if they can pay cash in advance."

"Our business office requires that now," Dr. Cookstone said. "Insurance companies are slow to change, but we think when they study our track record, they'll realize it's cheaper for them to send patients like Mr. Lawton to us than to keep them hospitalized while waiting for a human donor heart."

"Quality." Tom Lawton gasped the word. "What about quality." He took several quick breaths, almost panting.

He'd been coping with heart failure for the last thirteen months, waiting for a donor heart that never arrived. He refused to go on a heart pump, because he couldn't stand being tethered to a machine. A xenograft would give him the freedom he needed, and he could stop thinking of himself as a cardiac cripple.

Being turned down by the Seattle program was a bitter disappointment. Worse, it was the only one in the country that had been recruiting volunteers. He'd be dead before any of the other research centers accepted new patients.

"Not having the XRA looking over our shoulders actually helps us improve quality," Dr. Cookstone said. "Most important, we can use primate organs. The XRA has banned them, but they're more likely to be tolerated than pig organs."

"But you do follow the basic XRA guidelines for safety?" Susan asked. "You're not going to give Tom a transplant that will make him sicker?"

"Oh, not at all." Dr. Cookstone frowned. "We use only organs from healthy chimps or baboons. We breed our own baboons, and the chimps are carefully screened before and after we buy them from dealers. Our animals are then kept in special housing to protect them from exposure to harmful bacteria and viruses." He nodded. "We've already done more than two hundred xenos. Livers, kidneys, and lungs, as well as hearts. And no unanticipated problems with our patients, either. We've got a better than seventy percent success rate."

"How much does it cost?" Tom asked. He inhaled the oxygen deeply. "And when?"

"Four-hundred-thousand for a chimp heart," Dr. Cookstone said. "It would be more, but you're lucky, because we've got patients lined up for the kidneys and liver." He paused. "We can arrange a wire transfer for you. As soon as the money is in our account, we can go forward with the surgery."

"The doctors in Seattle said Tom's heart might fail at any moment," Susan said. "You've got all their records and test results. So if we pay today, when can you do the transplant?"

"Day after tomorrow." Cookstone smiled.

"Thank God," Tom said.

Monday, May 1: Two Years Later, St. Louis, MO

Clara Henderson entered the kitchen through the carport door and sat down at the table. She hadn't been sure she could complete the five-mile drive home from work.

She lowered her head, resting it on her folded arms, then closed her eyes. She didn't move except to breathe. Better. But her face felt like it was on fire. And the wide, blood-red ribbon of rash running across her stomach prickled. It felt like a band of biting ants. She rubbed at it through her clothes.

The movement made her head swim. She seemed to be rocking in a rowboat on the water. A wave of nausea washed through her. Sour saliva flooded her mouth, and she swallowed hard.

She was sick. She couldn't deny it any longer. She'd felt it coming since last night. She'd noticed the rash when changing into her nightgown, and she'd already felt tired. Like she was getting the flu. The fever hadn't started until around three, an hour before she got off work.

She'd been checking out books for Mrs. Lawton.

She asked her how Mr. Lawton was doing, as always. Everybody working in the library knew Tom Lawton had gotten a chimp-heart transplant in Costa Linda. He was the first in St. Louis, so he'd been interviewed locally a dozen times. But that was a couple of years ago, and people didn't pay much attention to him anymore. He was old news.

But she talked to him and his wife often, because they were in the library four or five times a week. He seemed fine, like a completely normal person. He was only forty or so, and it was sad somebody so young had needed a transplant. He was the same age as her husband Bill.

"He's been under the weather the last day or two," Mrs. Lawton told her. "Probably getting a spring cold."

"I might be getting one myself," Clara said.

Shortly after Mrs. Lawton left, Clara had suddenly felt hot all over. As if she'd been dropped into an oven. Even her feet were hot.

"You'd better go on home, Clara," Jeanette, the head librarian, told her. "You don't look well."

She'd planned to stick out the half hour until her shift ended, but she'd taken Jeanette's suggestion with relief. By the time she'd walked to her car, she was burning up and too weak to concentrate on driving. The road, the traffic lights, and the cars whizzing around her had a vague, dreamlike quality.

But she'd made it. Bill would be home at four-thirty. He'd take care of her.

Another wave of nausea swelled up from her stomach. She swallowed hard, but this time she knew she was going to vomit. She struggled out of her chair. The bathroom was too far to go, but maybe she could make the few steps to the sink.

She staggered. Her stomach heaved.

A mass of blood and undigested food forced itself into her throat, then exploded from her mouth. Red matter stained and streaked the white porcelain.

Clara Henderson slumped to the floor unconscious.

June 10: Atlanta, Centers For Disease Control

Jane Chen clicked on the first slide.

A man's torso with a heavy, red rash filled the screen.

David Simcoff, the agency's congressional liaison officer, shifted in his chair to get a better view. He exchanged a nervous glance with Margaret Paterson, the head of the agency. Both were edgy and tense, as if waiting to witness an execution.

While they had a sense of what was coming, only Jane Chen and Brady Williams grasped the full picture. They'd been developing it for four feverish months, directing their teams to ferret out data from Africa, Japan, Europe, and virtually every country in North and South America. Now they were briefing the two people most responsible for recommending to the government the course of action the nation ought to follow.

"Esperanza fever begins with a raised, red, papular rash across the torso," Chen said. "The rash is accompanied by lassitude and a mild temperature elevation. People report feeling like they're getting the flu."

Next slide. A graph of temperature plotted against time. The line was steep and almost straight.

"Within twelve hours, their core temperature rises, becoming a raging fever spiking at highs of 106 or 107 Fahrenheit." Chen used a laser pointer to trace the line. "Then comes swollen lymph nodes, vomiting of blood, and bloody diarrhea. The lining of the GI tract sloughs off, making swallowing painful. With the high fever, the patient experiences apathy, delirium, and often loss of consciousness."

Click. A chart of symptoms and therapies.

"Antibiotics and antivirals have no discernible effect. The patient is treated empirically to get the symptoms under control." She flashed the pointer at the chart. "Bringing down the fever with cooling blankets and acetaminophen, pain control with morphine, keeping the patient hydrated with IV fluids, and providing respiratory support." She shook his head. "We don't have much else to offer."

Click. Another chart. Numbers scattered along a line.

"We've identified a core group of a thousand patients," Chen said. "More than seven hundred have already died from Esperanza fever, and we're expecting maybe seventy-five or a hundred more deaths. Death occurs within fifteen days after the onset of the first signs. The throat swells, the lungs fill with blood and collapse. Ventilator support becomes impossible, and respiratory failure causes death."

"Only twenty percent survive?" Simcoff asked. He shook his head and frowned. "Isn't that about as bad as an infectious disease gets? What's the best guess about the origin?"

"I'll let Brady tell you about that."

Chen handed the remote to Williams and sat down at the conference table beside Margaret Paterson.

Williams called up a world map marked with scores of tiny white dots. Many dots formed sizeable clusters. Most of the clusters were in large U.S. and European cities. Smaller ones were in major cities in India, China, Russia, Argentina, and Japan. A number of dots were scattered across the Middle East and Africa. Rio de Janeiro, Sao Paulo, and Mexico City were heavily dotted. A thick cluster surrounded the small Caribbean island of Costa Linda.

"Each dot represents a confirmed or probable case," Williams said. "But we don't consider the count reliable. Not only did we have trouble getting information from many countries, the clinical criteria are too imprecise for us to be sure physicians are always seeing the same thing."

"If they're not, we've got more than one raging pandemic," Paterson said.

"We considered that possibility, but it didn't seem probable," William said. "It also seemed unlikely after we did contact traces and began to discover that at one, two, or three nodes back up the tree, patients had a connection with someone who had undergone a primate xenograft."

"A transplant using a primate organ?" Simcoff stood up. "You're kidding!" He sat back down heavily. "But you can't do them in this country. Or in Britain or Europe, for that matter. And the World Health Organization bans them everywhere."

"Look at this." Williams tapped the cluster of white dots around Costa Linda. "The population of the entire island is no more than five million, but they've got more than a hundred cases. The great majority of them in or around Esperanza."

"You think that's point zero?" Paterson asked. "That EF originated there, then spread?"

"We're sure of it," Chen said. She turned toward Williams. "Tell them why, Brady."

Williams clicked the remote and a low, white, concrete-block building with a red tile roof appeared on the screen. Behind it was another structure connected by a covered breezeway. Both buildings were surrounded by a clipped green lawn. Lush tropical plants, many with large bright flowers, grew in beds along the foundations.

"Cookstone XenoCenter," Williams said. "A private, for-profit xeno-transplantation center headed by Thomas Cookstone. Cookstone is an American M.D. trained in transplant surgery who decided to make some money. He pulled together a group of investors and set up this off-shore facility to provide xenografts to anybody who could meet his price."

"Nothing illegal about it." Simcoff sighed. "So long as they conform to the laws of their own country, they can ignore every other country's regulations. Ours, the Brits', German, French, Italian . . . whoever. And the World Health Organization has no enforcement powers, so its rules are only recommendations."

"I'm sure Dr. Cookstone explained to officials of the Costa Linda government that it was good for them and their country's economy to have a xenotransplant industry," Paterson said.

"Exactly," Williams said. "The Cookstone XenoCenter has been in business three years, and it's Costa Linda's major source of foreign revenue. They've done over four hundred solid organ transplants, taking people who can pay from all over the world."

"We think there are one or more founders of infection in most of the countries represented," Chen said. "And we've got evidence to show the index cases are xenograft recipients operated on at Cookstone XenoCenter."

"Where do they get their animals?" Paterson asked.

"Cookstone maintains a colony of baboons, and they buy chimps and orangutans from animal dealers in Africa," Williams said. "Jane and I made a site visit, and their vet showed us the precautions they take to prevent infections from parasites, bacteria, and viruses."

"They do a good job without any oversight," Chen said.

"Apparently not good enough," Paterson said. "Has the agent responsible for Esperanza fever been identified?"

Williams clicked the remote. A fuzzy white image of what could have been several starfish appeared.

"This is an electron micrograph of the viral particle we think is the causative agent," Williams said. "We're calling it EFV—Esperanza fever virus. Nobody has ever seen anything that looks like it before."

"We've had the viral screens done too," Chen said.

"We've recovered EFV from the blood of twenty people with florid symptoms," Williams said.

"We would expect to find it in every case," Chen said. "We've sent a dozen bloods to Yale and the NIH Infectious Disease labs. They've screened the samples against three hundred known viral antibody types and gotten no hits."

"Unknown virus," Paterson said.

"Looks like it," Chen said. "Our virologists think it's probably an endogenous retrovirus. One that's incorporated into the DNA and passed on from generation to generation."

"So even raising primates under rigorously controlled conditions couldn't eliminate it?" Simcoff asked. "It's part of the animal's genetic material."

"Exactly." Williams clicked the remote. "Here are the possibilities." He directed the pointer at the screen. "First, the virus is endogenous and has been read directly out of the primate's DNA. While it's harmless to the animals, it's deadly to humans. Second, the primate's original virus was dormant, but now has mutated into a lethal agent. Or last, the virus's genetic material has combined with fragments of human DNA and a new infectious virus has emerged."

"But what about the spread?" Simcoff asked. "Even if this center transplanted five hundred primate organs, that's not enough to account for the number diagnosed with EF. The disease has got to spread some way."

"It does," Williams said. "We think the organ recipients transmitted it to people in close or frequent contact with them. Then those contacts transmitted it to others."

"Maybe like the flu virus," Chen said. "Maybe a cough or a sneeze and the viral particles are inhaled. Or maybe they're deposited on the surface of a table or a book, then somebody touching the surfaces picks them up on a finger. All it would take then would be for the contact to do something like rub his eye to get the particles into the body."

"Then this could be worse than AIDS," David Simcoff said. "You could get the disease just by being in the same room with somebody who's infected."

"A worldwide pandemic is possible," Margaret Paterson said. "It could be like the Spanish Influenza or the Black Death. Tens or even hundreds of millions of people could die."

All four fell silent at once.

GIVEN THE horrifying specter of risk raised by this scenario, how could anyone dare to consider carrying out clinical trials of xenotransplantation?

The answer is simple—the potential benefits of xenotransplantation are so enormous it can't be ignored.

Forget for a moment the gloomy doomsday scenario sketched above and imagine a Brave New World of the immediate future. It's a world in which xenotransplantation is an established and effective therapy for a variety of potentially fatal diseases resulting from sick organs—emphysema, poly-cystic kidney disease, congestive heart failure, and cirrhosis to name only a few. Specially bred pigs are a ready source for new organs.

Organs Off the Shelf

The old dream of spare-parts surgery would be realized.

Xenotransplantation, in our imagined world, is elegantly simple. When a vital organ begins to show signs of failure, surgeons replace it with a suitable pig organ. We thus don't need to wait until people are knocking at death's door before intervening. We're able to take action early and minimize a patient's suffering and prevent her physical deterioration.

Instead of waiting until a patient in heart failure risks pneumonia from the fluid accumulating in her lungs, sleeps propped up in bed to avoid drowning in her own secretions, and gasps for breath when she walks up the stairs, the transplant surgeon can give her a new heart and restore her to health.

A miracle cure not requiring a miracle.

Acting early by giving such people a xenograft—an organ from an animal—is much like replacing the fuel injector in a car that has an engine that splutters, runs rough, and doesn't accelerate. The new injector solves those problems, and the early action prevents others from developing.

Having suitable spare parts available off the shelf marks the difference between old and new transplantation. Consider how frustrating it would be if whenever you needed a fuel injector, you had to wait until a car like yours was totalled in an accident. The injector would also have to be undamaged and the model fit your car's engine. You'd also have to be able to pay for it, and even then you could only become a *candidate* for the injec-tor, because other people also need one.

Because (in our imagined world) transplantable pig organs are as readily available as engine parts, patients can rely on getting the treatment they need when they need it. Centers support their own breeding facilities, thus giving surgeons access to off-the-shelf organs. Their patients need not suffer the debilitating and depressing experience of waiting for a donor organ, wondering if they will be dead before one becomes available. Organs from the same donor can be transplanted into half-a-dozen people during a brief period of time.

The quality of the organs is also higher. They don't have to be severed from the blood supply keeping them healthy and functioning until just before transplantation. They can then be taken from one operating suite to another without spending several hours in transit. This reduces the tissue damage human organs sustain while being transported from one city to another.

Also, the pig organs are healthier. The pigs are bred, fed, exercised, and protected from disease with an eye on producing organs that are as perfect as possible. Human donor organs may come from people who haven't taken good care of themselves. A liver may be fatty, the arteries of a heart clogged, or a lung damaged by smoking or pollution.

Using pig organs drains the urgency from transplantation. It becomes elective surgery. Like hip or heart-valve replacements, heart, liver, kidney, and lung transplants remain serious surgery, but the procedures are carried out routinely and the outcomes can be counted on to be good.

No Organ Shortage

Human donor organs are hard to come by. At any given time in the United States, about sixty-five thousand people are on the waiting list for an organ. The list is also growing at a rapid rate. In 1998 a new name was added every eighteen minutes, but by 2000 one was added every sixteen. With an aging population, the list is likely to grow longer even faster.

Organs available from people declared dead by brain-death criteria aren't adequate to meet the present need. Nor can it be met when kidneys and liver segments from living donors are added. The total number of organs available, even with these additions, comes to around twenty thousand.

This leaves forty-five thousand people in need of an organ. Depending on their disease and medical condition, some are able to wait for a year or two for a donor organ. Dialysis helps those in kidney failure, and a mechanical pump assists some with heart disease. But those needing a liver or a lung have no medicines or machines to turn to for anything more than immediate support.

Being on the waiting list for an organ doesn't guarantee getting one. Five thousand people a year die while waiting—more than a dozen a day. Children, teenagers, wives, husbands, brothers, and sisters. Friends and relations.

The majority who die while waiting are people whose lives could be extended not merely for a few weeks, but for *years*, sometimes decades. Their deaths could be prevented—if enough donor organs were available. Xeno-transplantation eliminates the shortage by making human donor organs unnecessary.

And even more people than those on waiting lists could be saved if more organs were available. A significant number of people who might benefit from a transplant, never make it to a waiting list. Although it's astonishing, estimates suggest there may be as many people who could benefit from a transplant who aren't on a waiting list as there are who are. This means another sixty-five thousand who might have their lives extended by transplants don't get one.

Some may be people who aren't referred to a center for evaluation by their physicians. Their physicians may consider them too old, too poor, or too sick to qualify. Or perhaps their physician doesn't know how successful transplants can be.

If organs were in abundance, getting a transplant would be cheaper, and maybe people with inadequate insurance or even none could qualify. Maybe our society would consider life-saving transplants part of basic health care and offer them to all. Xenotransplants could make that possible.

Ethical Problems Evaporate

With transplantable hearts, livers, kidneys, and lungs as readily available as pork chops, most of the gnarled ethical problems associated with acquiring and allocating human donor organs fade away. Debates over issues determining who lives and who dies become hypothetical discussions.

- Organs from anencephalic infants are no longer needed. Thus, we don't have to wrestle with the problem of when to declare such infants dead.
- We no longer need to consider when it's morally legitimate to remove organs from people declared dead by cardiopulmonary criteria who don't yet meet brain-death criteria. Because we don't need the organs to save lives, we can abandon the hairsplitting physiological and philosophical debates about non-heartbeating donors.
- Living donors are no longer necessary. Thus, we don't have to face some vexing questions about informed consent. We don't have to determine, in particular, whether it's ever acceptable to make organ donors out of people incapable of consenting. Problems raised by children and the mentally impaired can thus be neatly sidestepped. We also don't have to worry about whether adults who decide to donate a kidney, liver- or lung-segment have been pressured into it by their families.
- We can, if we like, give livers to alcoholics, hearts to the overweight and underexercised, lungs to cigarette smokers, and kidneys to anybody needing a new one.

We don't have to wrestle with such questions as whether those needing a transplant as a result of a lifestyle disease (alcoholism, obesity, emphysema, drug use) should be kicked off the waiting list or, at best, assigned a lower ranking than others. Whether people need a transplant because of their careless lives or as a result of factors outside their control (such as a viral infection or a genetic disease) becomes a matter of moral indifference.

We don't have to ask whether such "social worth" factors as being the mother of small children or an accomplished pianist should play a role in organ allocation. If we commit ourselves to providing a basic standard of medical care to convicted murderers, even they can have the organs they need without competing with soccer moms, Nobel Prize winners, or secular saints. We also don't need to decide whether organs should go to the sickest person or to the person who might medically benefit most. An organ can go to each.

We don't have to ask, when a transplanted organ is rejected, whether the recipient is entitled to a second, a third, or even a fourth. We can re-transplant somebody as many times as is medically useful. By giving someone a third heart, we won't be depriving someone who's been waiting a year for the first.

- We don't need schemes to increase the supply of donor organs. Hence, we don't have to debate policies of presumed consent that allow the state to take organs without permission or proposals to reward potential donors by promising to put them, in case of need, at the top of the transplant list.

  We can, likewise, ignore plans to buy insurance for potential donors or defray their funeral expenses. With human organs no longer needed, plans to secure more are pointless. Who needs more buggy whips when everybody's driving a car?
- We don't, finally, have to wrestle with the thorny issue of whether it's morally okay for a healthy person to sell a kidney. We thus needn't consider whether organ selling cheapens human life and society by transforming body parts into marketable commodities.

THE MORAL and social problems that disappear (as practical ones) are all generated by a need for donor organs. Because they can be used to save lives, pressure to increase their supply is intense, and competition to acquire them is fierce. But when organs are available in abundance, when the supply equals or outstrips the demand, the pressure and competition disappear.

This doesn't mean Utopia has arrived.

Breeding and raising special animals to supply organs, performing transplant surgery, and providing drugs and medical care costs a lot of money. Whether xenotransplants could become cheap enough to be available to everyone able to benefit remains an open question. Even non-exotic medical care can be too expensive for everyone to afford.

Xenotransplantation offers an elegant solution to the supply and allocation problems that have made debates about them the intellectual equivalent of blood sports. The problems simply evaporate. At least that's what happens in our imagined world.

In the real world problems abound. Not the least of them is whether xenotransplantation can ever be made to work.

Is It Possible?

As a crude estimate, about three hundred animal-to-human xenografts have been performed. What may have been the first attempt to use an animal organ to save a human life occurred as early as 1902. Emerich Ullmann, a Viennese physician who had been experimenting with animal-to-animal transplants, attached the kidney of a pig to blood vessels in the arm of a young woman dying of kidney failure.

Like so many early attempts at transplantation, this was a desperate effort to prolong the life of someone who was healthy, except for the disastrous fact that her kidneys weren't working. Kidney failure, in the absence of dialysis, condemned her to a prolonged and agonizing death.

If desperate diseases require desperate cures, it's no wonder physicians were prompted on numerous occasions to attempt kidney transplants. The spread of anesthesia and improvements in surgery during the nineteenth century made replacement-parts surgery an obvious avenue to explore at the beginning of the twentieth.

Ullmann had earlier reported to a meeting of his local surgical society the results of an experiment in which he transplanted a dog's kidney into the neck of a goat. He brought the goat with him for a demonstration, and his discussion was published in the *Vienna Clinical Weekly*. "You can see that the kidney is functioning completely normally," he told the surgeons, "and that urine is flowing in drops from the end of the protruding ureter."

Ullmann's pig-to-human transplant failed utterly. The woman died soon after the surgery. While we have no first-hand account of what happened when Ullmann hooked up the pig kidney to her blood vessels, the details are easy to reconstruct. We can also understand why Ullmann had at least temporary success with his dog-to-goat transplant.

What happened to the pig kidney has to do with the human immune response. An understanding of this response helps explain some of the steps recently taken to realize the dream of using animal organs to perfect spare-parts surgery.

A Pig Kidney

When Ullmann transplanted the pig kidney into his patient, he must have been stunned by the result. He never tried the experiment again and abandoned his research. Ullmann left no account of what he saw, but the consequences of such a xenograft are sudden and dramatic.

Once the human blood vessels are hooked up, the pig kidney turns pink and begins to function. Urine may drip from the ureter. But even as the human blood flows through the kidney, specific molecules or antigens on the surface of the endothelial cells lining the kidney's blood vessels activate the body's immune system. The kidney is recognized by the recipient's body as alien, and the immune system targets it for destruction.

Tens of millions of antibodies circulating in the blood latch onto the antigens, destroying the cells' ability to prevent clotting. Within *minutes*, as a rule, every vein and artery in the pig kidney, including those too tiny to see without magnification, choke up with coagulated lumps of blood. With the flow of oxygen-carrying blood shut off to the kidney's tissues, its cells begin to die and rupture.

The locking of the antibodies onto the pig antigens also signals the body's complement system to release defensive waves of more than thirty sorts of protein molecules. The release occurs in sequence—the complement cascade—like a line of tumbling dominos, and the last protein in the series leads an attack on the pig kidney, gnawing holes in the membranes of its cells and breaking down its tissues into a sort of organic slop.

The recipient's own cells are protected from this kamikaze strike by an array of complement-regulating proteins exposed on their surface. Molecules like DAF (decay accelerating factor), CD59 (one of a group of surface molecules), and MCP (membrane cofactor protein) act as recognition flags to avert attacks by the body's antibody and complement proteins.

Under the onslaught of the humoral immune response (antibodies and complement proteins), the pig kidney swells in size and is quickly, if not immediately, reduced to a black pulpy mass of dying tissue.

Surgeons have witnessed such destruction taking place before their very eyes, before their patients could even be sewn up and wheeled out of the operating room. The devastation can occur in minutes and never takes longer than a few hours.

Hyperacute Rejection

This violent and definitive process of annihilation is called *hyperacute rejection*. Emrich Ullmann was among the first to witness it, and his unfortunate patient would have died only a short time afterward.

If other alternatives weren't available, she would be as certain to die today as she was in 1902. Immunosuppressive drugs, even in high doses and ordinarily effective combinations, are as useless in preventing the process as an upraised hand is in stopping a tidal surge. Hyperacute rejection is a force of nature currently beyond our power to control.

It occurs when the immune system has encountered the alien antigens before and is already primed to assail them with pre-formed antibodies. If the recipient of a human kidney rejects it, then receives a second kidney from the same donor, the rejection will be hyperacute. Her body has become *sensitized* to the antigens, and the antibodies against those specific antigens continue to patrol her blood.

But why do humans have antibodies against pig antigens? We don't encounter pig organs in the course of ordinary life, except maybe as ham, spare ribs, and bacon, but what goes through our digestive system doesn't come into contact with our immune system.

The question of why we have preformed antibodies against pig antigens was first raised in the 1960s. It's only recently been answered, however. While the answer shows the subtlety of nature's workings, it also points to a problem no one has yet succeeded in solving.

Pig Antigens

Antibodies are formed when the immune system encounters alien molecules. (These are, by definition, antigens.) The molecules on the surfaces of invading viruses and bacteria thus provoke the immune system to churn out antibodies against them. Once formed, these antibodies continue to circulate in the blood, patrolling and prepared for another alien invasion.

If an invasion comes, the circulating antibodies can attack at once. The immune system doesn't have to take the time needed to fabricate a new kind of antibody. The body, in its version of off-the-shelf engineering, needs only step up the production of an existing model. That's why once we've been infected with the measles virus, if it comes around again, we don't get sick. Our immune system targets and attacks it immediately. We're immune to it.

Pig organs produce hyperacute rejection, but most cells from pig tissue and bone marrow don't. Organs have blood vessels running through them, and it's the clogging of these vessels that lead to the tissue damage characteristic of hyperacute rejection. Pig bone marrow and tissue cells don't sneak past the immune system unnoticed, however. They provoke an immune response and are attacked by antibodies, but usually immunosuppressive drugs can prevent their being rejected.

Pig heart valves are yet another story. They've been used for years to replace defective human ones, and they evoke almost no immune response. This is because they are made of cartilage and so are mostly nothing but assemblages of dead cells possessing none of the molecules that attract antibodies.

What happens with pig endothelial cells is quite different.

GAL

A strange fact of nature is that the endothelial cells lining the inside of a pig's blood vessels have on their surfaces complex molecules of a sugar called galactose-alpha,1,3-galactose (GAL, for short). Molecules containing this GAL component are also found on the surfaces of many common bacteria and viruses. Thus, the antibodies we develop against these organisms also turn out to be ones programmed to attack pig endothelial cells.

Pigs aren't the only animals to have GAL as a component of the molecules on their cells' surfaces. Cows, sheep, goats, deer, dogs, and other mammals have it, and humans, chimps, baboons, and other primates are the exception.

A kidney from a sheep thus also triggers a hyperacute rejection in humans, but one from a chimpanzee doesn't. Humans share a relatively recent evolutionary history with chimps. Hence, we resemble them more biologically, right down to the cellular and molecular level, than we do sheep. Humans and primates carry the gene for the GAL molecule, but it's not expressed. Rather, it's one of those segments of genetic material that don't get translated.

Primates, in the jargon of xenotransplantation, are *concordant* species, whereas the farm animals are *discordant* ones. A pig kidney transplanted into a baboon will also provoke hyperacute rejection, but a baboon kidney transplanted into a human won't. The immune reaction it triggers resembles the one caused by a badly tissue-matched human kidney—powerful and ultimately destructive but not violent.

The same sort of reaction would have resulted from Ullmann's transplantation of a dog kidney into a goat. Dogs and goats are concordant species, and neither has antibodies against GAL. We can be sure, though, that Ullmann's success was only temporary.

Continuing the tradition initiated by Ullmann, during the 1960s researchers used chimp and baboon kidneys and hearts several times to support desperately ill patients while human donor organs were sought. Most patients died after several days or even hours, but a few lived for weeks or months. One of surgeon Keith Reemtsma's patients survived for nine months with a baboon kidney, and that was in 1964 when drugs controlling the immune response were less effective than now. Twenty years later, Baby Fae lived for only twenty days with a baboon heart.

By using powerful immunosuppressive drugs, physicians can delay the rejection of a primate organ, but eventually the immune system wins the contest. No xenotransplant has ever been successful in the way a human-to-human transplant has. The baboon kidney that for weeks was pink and functioning eventually fills with clotted blood, blackens, and dies.

Acute Rejection

The process that destroys the baboon kidney is *acute rejection*. It's the process we can be sure eventually led Ullmann's goat to reject the dog kidney.

Because acute rejection is orchestrated by the T-cells of the immune system (T-cells come from the thymus gland in the torso, B-cells from the bone marrow), it's also called *cell-mediated* or *cellular rejection*. The T-cells recruit and activate other immune cells that assault the alien antigens marking a transplanted organ. Cells called natural killer cells, macrophages, and neutrophils ravage its tissues, rupturing its constituent cells and causing them to fall apart. This results in clots forming in the organ's veins and arteries, blocking blood flow and leading to its rapid death.

The effectiveness of cellular rejection in getting rid of a transplanted organ shows why making xenotransplantation work requires more than sneaking an organ past the barrier of hyperacute rejection. Elaborate experiments show that even when the processes of hyperacute rejection are kept in check, when a pig kidney is transplanted into a baboon, acute rejection will destroy it.

The experiment involves filtering from the baboon's blood the antibodies that attack GAL, then depleting the baboon's store of complement proteins. This renders impossible the usual immediate rain of destruction on alien antigens by the processes of hyperacute rejection. Even so, the pig kidney will function for no more than a few days before choking up with blood clots and showing signs of tissue deterioration. Presumably, this would also happen to a pig kidney transplanted into a person.

Acute rejection also occurs in human-to-human transplants. It appears typically during the first three months after surgery, but increased doses of immunosuppressive drugs can usually bring it under control. But these same drugs, so effective in preventing the rejection of human organs, are unsuccessful in preventing the rejection of primate organs. Within seven to ten days, a primate kidney or heart follows the usual path of rejection—it swells, blackens, and dies.

Why don't the drugs do the job? One factor may be that the incompatibility of human and animal tissues is simply too great to be overcome. Or perhaps mechanisms of the immune system we don't yet understand are at work. Whatever the cause, some researchers believe new drugs capable of overcoming the human body's acute rejection of primate organs might be possible.

None is currently available.

Chronic Rejection

Organ transplant recipients may do well for several months or even years, showing no signs of rejection. Then bodily peace is suddenly shattered and their immune system begins to attack the organ, assaulting it as if it had just been transplanted.

This is the phenomenon known as *chronic rejection*, and it remains a constant threat to transplant recipients. Usually when an episode of chronic rejection occurs, it can be brought under control by increasing the recipient's dose of immunosuppressive drugs or by adding another drug to the regimen. But if the drugs don't work, life-sustaining steps (such as another transplant) have to be taken immediately. Otherwise, patients who had been doing well for so long quickly develop organ failure and die.

Why this unexpected rejection occurs is another transplant mystery. Some researchers suspect that, as with the acute rejection of primate organs, more immune processes may be involved than the ones we now know about.

The pig kidney experiments show that even when baboons are deprived of the means to mount a hyperacute-rejection attack, *acute* rejection soon takes over and destroys the alien kidney. Acute rejection does what hyperacute rejection was kept from doing. So if acute rejection could be defeated, does this mean *chronic* rejection would emerge and destroy the kidney?

No one knows for sure, because no pig organ has survived long enough in any human or primate to determine whether chronic rejection would occur. Even so, researchers experienced in the power of the immune system don't doubt it would. But they won't be able to investigate the question until someone succeeds in holding acute rejection at bay for at least a few months.

Why Not Primates?

Hyperacute rejection destroys pig organs so rapidly it would seem to make sense for researchers to focus on primates as donors. They could avoid the problem of GAL's triggering the most destructive of the immune responses and concentrate on discovering why primate organs are tolerated at first, then rejected.

The strategy is appealing, and in earlier years it might have been pursued. The chimpanzee is the primate most appropriate to serve as a donor. Genetically chimps are the closest to humans, the species sharing more than ninety-eight percent of their genes, and in size, chimps are the best match.

But chimps are an endangered species and don't breed well in captivity. Most important for many people, chimps display the intelligence, personality, and social behavior that make them a sibling species. Killing chimps for their organs thus seems a serious wrong. While only some philosophers are willing to attribute rights to chimps or other animals, nearly all believe the intelligence of chimps requires us to recognize they have interests and an inherent worth we ought to respect.

Hence, we aren't free to kill chimps or cause them suffering for any purpose that suits us, but must have compelling reasons for setting aside their interests. This holds for animals in general, some thinkers claim, but it is particularly true for primates that have a high level of intelligence and an apparent sense of self.

Baboons have been the favored primate donor in a number of experimental transplants. (Baby Fae received a baboon heart.) Baboons don't have the almost-human quality of chimps, and they breed well in captivity. Most ethicists (but not all) would consider it acceptable to rely on baboons as a source of transplant organs. They would consider sacrificing a baboon to save the lives of several humans justifiable. The seriousness of the purpose would warrant overriding the interest of the baboon, if there were no reasonable alternative.

Baboons aren't large enough to be ideal donors, however. Even adult males rarely weigh as much as eighty or ninety pounds, and their hearts and lungs aren't large enough to function effectively in an adult human. Baboon kidneys would work well enough, though, and the liver would grow in size to serve the needs of a human.

On the minus side, huge colonies of baboons would have to be established to provide the fifty or sixty thousand transplant organs a year currently needed. Baboons don't reach sexual maturity until around the age of five, and pregnancy lasts six months. Multiple births are rare. The costs of raising the necessary number of animals would probably be prohibitive.

Perhaps the most decisive reason for not using baboons (or any sort of primate) as a source of organs is the threat of disease they pose. Because of their genetic similarity to humans, viruses hidden in primate organs might mutate and cause a disease like AIDS. Thus, as the opening scenario suggests, by trying to help relatively few people, we would be risking the safety of the whole population. This risk is discussed in detail in Part II.

Why Pigs?

Pigs, though intelligent and social, don't display these traits at the same level as primates. Pigs produce litters of as many as ten, gestation takes less than four months, and the offspring grow rapidly. Within six months, a pig reaches the size of a human adult. Varieties of pigs can also be bred, permitting transplant organs to be matched in size.

Most important, pigs are already bred and raised for food throughout the world. The United States alone produces a hundred million a year. Pigs are cheap to maintain, and their biology resembles human biology. Because of their economic importance, we know a lot about their genetics and physiology.

That pigs are raised to be eaten isn't likely to convince those opposed to killing animals to benefit humans that it's acceptable to raise pigs as a source of transplant organs. But most people are more comfortable with taking organs from pigs than from primates. Also, it seems more justifiable to exploit pigs to save lives than to raise them for food when other sources of food are readily available.

Researchers, faced with such considerations, have generally decided to focus on the pig as a potential source of organs. They have then taken it as their job to find ways to make pig organs acceptable to human bodies.

Knockout Pigs

The major challenge to using pig organs is to do something about GAL in the lining of pig blood vessels. It's the trigger for hyperacute rejection that destroys the transplanted organ.

If the GAL molecule could be eliminated or replaced by another, antibodies would no longer have a target to home in on. Thus, the GAL antibodies would circulate harmlessly, and the death squad of complement proteins wouldn't be called out. The donor organ would be secure from attack.

The *knockout* mouse is an example of what could be possible with pigs.

Scientists for more than a decade have used the techniques of molecular biology to alter the DNA of mice by *knocking out* particular genes. Mice can be bred, for example, lacking a particular enzyme, and the consequences of this can be studied as the mice develop. Because a human disease may involve the lack of just that enzyme, the knockout mouse serves as an animal model of the disease.

Knocking out the gene encoding GAL in pigs would make xenografts feasible by eliminating the antigen triggering hyperacute rejection. So if knockout mice can be bred, why not knockout pigs?

The problem with this strategy is that it requires modifying pig embryonic stem cells. Stem cells are the undifferentiated cells produced after a fertilized egg has divided several times and become a hollow ball of cells called a blastocyst. As development proceeds, the stem cells differentiate into 120 or so cell types that make up such tissues and organs as blood, bone, brain, and liver.

Embryonic stem cells, before differentiation, have the potential to become any of these cell types. Afterward, their fate is sealed, and they can't go back to their previous state. When they divide, they produce only cells of the same kind—bone cells make bone cells, brain cells make brain cells. Stem cells are thus like clay before it's fired. (Cloning shows, however, that the DNA in a body cell can be manipulated into returning to the default position. It's as if fired clay could be made malleable again.)

If the techniques of molecular genetics are used to knock out a gene in the DNA of a stem cell and the altered cell is inserted into a developing embryo, the offspring will lack the trait encoded by the knocked-out gene. Thus, just as we knock out an enzyme in the mouse, we can knock out the troublesome GAL sugar in the pig.

Except we can't do it.

And for the most basic reason—no one has been able to identify the stem cells in pig embryos. Only mouse and human stem cells have so far been recovered from embryos. Perhaps before long, pig stem cells will be discovered and someone will then produce knockout pigs. But until that happens, research must proceed along other lines.

Mouse Models

One of those lines involves developing knockout-mouse models. Researchers realized the whole GAL-sugar molecule wouldn't have to be eliminated to make pig organs acceptable to the human immune system. Only the GAL component of the molecule would have to go, and it wouldn't have to be knocked out itself. It would be enough to knock out the enzyme that *attaches* the GAL to the sugar base. A light bulb that doesn't get screwed into the socket can't serve as a beacon.

The enzyme GT (short for alpha-1, 3-galactosyltransferese) is the relevant one, but researchers couldn't eliminate it in pigs, because that too requires tinkering with pig stem cells. But they could attempt it in mice and see what happens to them. If the mice developed cancers or leaky or clotting blood vessels, there would be little incentive to develop pigs with the gene encoding GT knocked out.

Knockout mice lacking GT have been bred. Sure enough, their cells aren't marked with GAL. What's more, they show no sign of developing diseases more often than ordinary mice.

This suggests organs from pigs genetically modified to lack GT will also have cells unmarked by GAL and so won't be the target for hyperacute rejection. Such good news suggests we should search for pig stem cells and knock out the gene for GT.

But like everything else about xenotransplantation, the result isn't exactly what anybody had in mind. When the mice with GT (and no GAL sugar) are exposed to the antigens in human blood serum, they *still* sustain considerable damage.

Some investigators speculate this may be because when the GAL component is left off the end of the molecule, it exposes *another* molecule that was masked by it. The exposed molecule then serves as a target for antibodies in the way GAL did.

Studies of knockout mice thus suggest knockout pigs might not be the elegant solution to the GAL problem researchers imagined. The immune system is a weasel, capable of quick and unanticipated moves.

GAL Substitute

Getting rid of the trigger for hyperacute rejection means getting rid of GAL. If it can't be eliminated, some researchers reasoned, maybe it could be *replaced* by another sugar, one that doesn't attract antibodies. Park your new BMW on the street, and it's a target; substitute a rusty Volvo, and thieves ignore it.

Scientists have conducted some small-scale genetic-engineering experiments with pigs in which the GAL sugar has been replaced with the sugar found in people with type-O blood. About ninety percent of the GAL sugar, in some experiments, has been replaced by O-type sugar. But as successful as the replacement is, it's not successful enough.

Numbers make clear why.

In a single gram of the epithelial tissue lining a pig's blood vessels, there are about one *trillion* (1 followed by 12 zeros) molecules still containing GAL. (An ounce equals about twenty-eight grams.) This is such a large number of molecules that even ten percent of them are more than enough to trigger the hyperacute rejection response.

The experimental results have convinced many researchers this approach isn't one to invest much hope in. Substituting a new sugar for all (or even virtually all) the GAL molecules looks like a practical impossibility. Yet achieving anything less probably isn't going to eliminate hyperacute rejection.

Long Enough to Help?

If hyperacute and acute rejection can be overcome, can chronic rejection be fended off long enough to justify xenotransplantation? If the upper limit on the functioning of a pig organ turned out to be three or four months, nobody could say xenotransplantation had solved the problem of treating people with failing vital organs. Other modes of treatment, including transplants from human donors, would still be preferable.

Yet even less-than-perfect xenografts would be an important accomplishment. They could be used to bridge the gap between a failing organ and a human-donor transplant. Where livers and lungs are concerned, such a bridge might be the only hope available for a dying patient.

Transgenic Pigs

A more promising strategy than trying to eliminate GAL, some researchers believe, is to concentrate on preventing the damage to transplanted pig organs caused by the cascading complement proteins triggered by antibodies.

Transgenic pigs may offer a way of shielding organs.

Transgenic animals are produced by using genetic engineering to take genes from the DNA of one species and insert them into the DNA of another. The process is already used to make important biological products. Human genes have been incorporated into sheep, for example, causing them to produce in their blood a protein called AAT (alpha 1-antitrypsin). AAT is important in protecting the lungs and is useful in treating emphysema.

Substances like human insulin and growth hormone have been produced for more than a decade by genetically engineered bacteria. The next step in *pharming* (as the enterprise is waggishly called) is to breed large animals like sheep and cattle to become efficient and cheap pharmaceutical factories.

Thus the economic motive behind cloning Dolly was to eventually produce herds of transgenic sheep able to manufacture useful biological substances.

Given our ability to insert genes into other animals, the best way to prevent hyperacute rejection may be to produce transgenic pigs carrying the human genes that encode complement regulating proteins. If the proteins DAF, CD9, and MCP are expressed on the surfaces of the pig cells, they should put a brake on the activation of the cascade of destructive complement proteins. They would camouflage the pig cells as human ones, and this should let the pig escape the damage inflicted by hyperacute rejection.

Transgenic pigs with DAF displayed on their cells have been bred in Britain by the biotech company Imutran. Ten hearts from these pigs were transplanted into monkeys, and in two of the monkeys, the hearts were still beating after sixty days.

This was success, but only of a limited sort. The hearts were eventually rejected by all the monkeys, and in a second round of experiments, hearts from transgenic pigs transplanted into baboons met a similar fate. Also, the heavy doses of immunosuppressive drugs needed to delay rejection were highly toxic, causing such suffering and debilitation that some experiments were ended for humane reasons. Imutran, in more recent experiments, set a record when it succeeded in keeping pig hearts beating in baboons for as long as ninety-nine days.

The presence of more complement-inhibiting proteins on the surface of pig cells would probably help slow the rejection process. But no one believes it would stop it. Most researchers think that even if pig organs were wholly protected by their false colors from the destructive powers of complement proteins, this wouldn't be enough to prevent rejection.

The human body has evolved intricate mechanisms for protecting itself against invading microorganisms and multicellular parasites. Its defenses don't depend on a single, massive Maginot Line, and invaders breaking through one perimeter are faced with another, then another, then yet another. Defeating or tricking the immune system may be, at the moment, a practical impossibility. Some scientists believe, though, it may be possible to find a way to work with the immune system to achieve the same end.

Acquired immunological tolerance holds just that promise.

Owen's Calves

Raymond Owen, an agricultural researcher at the University of Wisconsin, published a paper in 1945 giving an account of a peculiar phenomenon he had observed in cattle.

Owen noticed that when cows have fraternal twins (a rare occurrence), the calves have *mixed* blood types. Instead of each calf having a single blood type, both have a blend of two different types. Owen suspected this was a result of the calves' placentas being connected via the mother's circulatory system. During the time of development, blood-forming stem cells from one calf would end up in the bone marrow of the other and vice versa. These cells would then produce different blood types, and each calf would end up with blends of both.

This phenomenon, Owen recognized, was contrary to the rules of blood mixing. When people are given transfusion of unmatched blood, the foreign blood is attacked by the immune system. It forms clots that block blood vessels, causing strokes, heart attacks, and kidney and liver damage. But the bodies of the twin calves functioned as well with blended blood types as other calves did with a single type. Most surprising, the calves also didn't make antibodies against either type.

The presence of two difference cell types in the same individual is called *chimerism*. The phenomenon is named after the Chimera of Greek mythology, a fire-breathing creature with the head of a lion, the body of a goat, and a tail that is a serpent.

Chicks That Don't Get Flu

McFarlane Burnet, an eminent Australian scientist, was engaged in war work when Owen's paper appeared. Burnet, as part of a government assignment during World War II, was trying to develop a flu vaccine. But he was also intrigued by Owen's observation and wondered how to make immunological sense of it.

Burnet injected viruses into fertilized chicken embryos to grow the quantities he needed to develop his vaccines. Acting on a hunch prompted by Owen's report, Burnet injected chicks hatched from the embryos with the virus that had been present during their embryonic development. He then examined their blood for antibodies to the virus.

He couldn't find any.

But the chicks should have produced antibodies to the virus. What was going on? Why should the chicks tolerate the virus?

Burnet decided the most likely explanation was that during the period when the chicks were developing and for a short time after hatching, they didn't produce antibodies to the flu virus, because their immune systems didn't distinguish between their own cells and the antigens to which they were constantly exposed during development.

The chicks had an immunological *tolerance* for the virus. This would also explain why Owen's chimerical calves didn't produce antibodies to the "foreign" blood in their veins. They too were immunologically tolerant of the antigens they were exposed to during development.

Patchwork Mice

Burnet's theory was of particular interest to the British immunologist P.D. Medawar. Medawar, at the beginning of the war, at the behest of the British War Wounds Committee had set up a research unit to study problems of skin grafting. Fighter and bomber pilots were suffering lethal and disfiguring burns from exploding fuel when their planes crashed, and often so much of their skin was destroyed, they needed skin from donors. Yet skin grafts worked only for a short time, if at all.

Medawar showed that a second skin graft from the same donor would be rejected faster than the first had been. He called this the "second-set response," and we now recognize it as hyperacute rejection due to pre-formed antibodies. Medawar was unable to solve the problem of graft rejection, but at the end of the war, he continued his research at University College in London.

Medawar set out to test Burnet's theory of immune tolerance as soon as he heard about it. Instead of viruses, though, he focused on cells injected into mice, the animal model for studying skin grafts.

Medawar focused on two strains of mice—one white, the other brown. He bred a brown mouse, and on the sixteenth day of her pregnancy, injected .01 milliliter of tissue (about five million cells) from an adult white mouse into the six fetuses. Only five of the six were born, but the mouse pups seemed healthy and normal. After they matured in eight weeks, a patch of skin from a white mouse was grafted onto each of them.

The grafts were inspected eleven days later.

Two showed classic signs of rejection. Yet three looked completely healthy, and as time passed, they became incorporated into the skin of the mice. The only thing peculiar about the brown mice was the white patch of fur marking their pelts.

Fifty days later, one of the mice was given another graft from a white donor. The second graft behaved just as the first had, showing no signs of inflammation or rejection. Medawar had created for the first time a healthy patchwork mouse, one that would accept a skin graft from another mouse.

Medawar had also demonstrated by the creation of the mouse the phenomenon he called *actively acquired tolerance*. Without drugs or radiation, the immune system of one animal could be conditioned to tolerate a graft from another.

Tolerance

The dream of some scientists is to find a way of treating humans that will make their immune systems tolerate pig organs. This goal shifts research away from modifying pigs to modifying humans. Human organ recipients, in fact, need to become chimeras, like Medawar's mice. Except, unlike the mice, recipients must become chimeric with another species.

A tolerance for pig organs must be *actively acquired*, and in practice this demands employing brutal methods. Some successful experiments with monkeys suggest a likely strategy.

A monkey is exposed to full-body radiation to destroy his bone marrow, which is the source of a variety of immune-system cells. He's next treated with chemotherapy drugs to knock out circulating antibodies, then high-dose radiation is used to shut down his thymus gland. The thymus (the source of T-cells) plays the major role in programming lymphocytes to distinguish between self and not-self, so its work has to be halted.

The monkey, its immune system wiped out, is injected with bone marrow from a donor monkey, and the marrow cells find their way to the inside of the monkey's bones. Once the donor marrow is established, it begins to make the usual variety of immune system cells. The host monkey's marrow recovers from the radiation and begins making stem cells that also turn into the usual immune system cells. The monkey now has a chimeric immune system—two systems in the same body.

When a kidney from the bone-marrow donor is transplanted into the monkey, his altered immune system shows no signs of rejecting it. Chimeric monkeys have lived for years with transplants and with their immune systems functioning. Thanks to bone-marrow chimerism, they have acquired immunological tolerance for the transplanted organs.

People and Tolerance

A few people have followed, by necessity, the path of the experimental monkeys. Some unlucky individuals have undergone a bone marrow transplant as a treatment for a disease like leukemia, then later needed a kidney transplant. The results can be gratifying. When a kidney comes from a donor who was also the bone-marrow donor, the recipients tolerate the transplant without needing immunosuppressive drugs. They seem to have actively acquired tolerance and show no signs of even chronic rejection.

But both the chimeric monkeys and the rare human cases involve donors who are members of the same species. Will cross-species chimerism also produce tolerance? More to the point, will chimerism allow humans to tolerate pig organs?

Humans haven't yet been tested, because the immune-system-destruction technique for producing chimerism hasn't worked even in baboons. The problem is the old enemy GAL. Researchers haven't been able to switch off the production of antibodies that attack this pig antigen. They've produced chimerism in mice by engineering GAL-knockout mice that don't produce GAL antibodies. Whether this approach can ever be made to work for baboons, not to mention humans, remains an open question.

Molecular Chimerism

Xenotransplantation researchers are nothing if not inventive, and the most recent effort to achieve immunological tolerance uses pig genes, rather than bone marrow, to produce chimerism. This is called *molecular chimerism*, because it's at the molecular level that alterations are made.

Baboons are again the experimental model.

Pig genes for some of the more important antigens primates react to are cloned into multiple copies. The copies are attached to (weakened) viruses, and the viruses are incubated with bone marrow cells taken from a baboon. The viruses enter the cells and insert the pig genes into the cell's DNA. The modified marrow cells are then injected into the baboon.

So the baboon's immune system won't destroy the altered cells, the animal must first have its immune system wiped out by radiation and chemotherapy, just as is done for an ordinary bone marrow transplant.

Once the baboon's immune system is up and running again and the pig genes are making the pig proteins, a kidney from a pig with the same blood and tissue type as the one from which the genes came is transplanted into the baboon.

Is the transplant successful?

Yes and no, as usual. The good news is that the cellular immune response isn't triggered by the organ. But the bad news is that the baboon's anti-GAL antibodies still rage uncontrolled and quickly destroy the organ.

Can anything be done about this? Maybe if the pig gene for the enzyme (GT) that's needed to make the GAL sugar were incorporated into the baboon's cells, the baboon's chimeric immune system would treat GAL as "self" and not attack it.

That's where matters are at the moment with molecular chimerism. The experimental results are too tentative for even its proponents to draw any solid conclusions. But we can be sure researchers will keep trying.

A Dream Unrealized

Since 1902, when Emrich Ullmann attached the pig kidney to the forearm of a dying patient in a desperate attempt to save her life, we've come a long way toward understanding in minute detail exactly why Ullmann's effort was doomed to failure.

That understanding has been the foundation for several immensely sophisticated and imaginative attempts to make xenotransplantation work. We've looked at strategies based on knockout pigs, a GAL substitute, transgenic pigs, chimeric pigs, and molecular-chimeric pigs.

While this isn't a full catalogue of even the more plausible attempts, it represents the major contemporary efforts to control or outwit the human immune system. None of them has succeeded, even judged by the limited standard of human-to-human transplantation.

The dream of replacement-parts surgery using off-the-shelf animal organs is no more at hand than is quantum computing or implantable memory chips. The dream is still intact and for some researchers it's almost an obsession, but its realization remains where it has always been—just over the horizon.

Practically speaking, despite our enhanced understanding of the immune system and impressive accomplishments in human transplantation, we're not much farther down the road toward successful xenotransplantation than was Emrich Ullmann.

But are we at least far enough along to start transplanting animal organs into people in an experimental way? Or, whatever the likelihood of success, are such clinical trials so risky, so threatening to the safety of us all, that we should forbid them?

The dream of xenotransplantation has a dark side we ignore only at our peril. Exactly what it is needs spelling out, and how we should deal with it requires making some hard decisions.

IO

Xenotransplantation, Part 2

Fearing the Worst, Hoping for the Best

In W.W. Jacob's classic horror story *The Monkey's Paw*, an elderly couple coming into possession of a mummified monkey hand with magical properties realize with a thrill of excitement that by using its power they can resurrect their recently dead son.

But when the mangled corpse of their boy lurches up the walk and starts pounding on the front door, the father sees they have made a terrible mistake.

Unintended Consequences

An obvious lesson of the story is that we should be cautious about translating our dreams into reality. The unintended consequences of getting what we wish for may face us with the prospect of desperately attempting to reverse a horrible result.

Many critics are opposed to seeing the dream of xenotransplantation realized. Some reject it for exploiting animals, while others spurn it for blurring the line between humans and beasts. Both criticisms express legitimate ethical concerns (although I find neither persuasive), but they and similar worries pale in significance when compared to the question of the public-health hazard posed by xenotransplantation.

An unusual aspect of xenotransplantation as a therapy is that the risk associated with it isn't limited to the patient. In the middle decades of the twentieth century, when surgeons were experimenting with transplanting human donor organs, only the recipients were taking a chance. If someone believed getting a donor liver might save her life, she could decide to take the gamble. When the liver failed, the outcome was sad, but only the recipient died.

Xenotransplantation can potentially affect an indefinite number of other people. If a recipient becomes infected with a lethal virus, the infection could spread, striking others not directly involved. Transplanting animal organs into people may thus put us all at risk. It would be irresponsible for us to follow the pattern of the past and leave decisions about xenografts to surgeons and their patients.

Everyone has a stake in the outcome.

The Basic Ethical Question

The fundamental ethical question about xenotransplantation, in my view, is whether we should proceed with it. Imagining the problem of hyperacute rejection brought under control, do we want to risk the public-health consequences of putting animal organs into people? Should we even go forward with clinical trials?

The scenario beginning Part I is pure fiction. But could something like the event it depicts happen? Could it happen not as a mere speculative possibility, the way Tom Cruise *might* be elected President, but as a realistic possibility?

To be blunt, could transplanting animal organs, tissues, or cells into humans trigger a worldwide epidemic of a deadly infectious disease? Could xenotransplants give rise to a disease capable of destroying as many people as have been wiped out by the bubonic plague, smallpox, cholera, or AIDS?

Because researchers regard pigs as the best source of animal organs, considering the potential dangers of transplanting pig materials into human recipients is a good place to start.

Viruses Unknown

The onset of the illness was always sudden.

It began with sharp pains in the head and an intolerable burning sensation, a feeling of being consumed by fire from the inside. Sweat poured from the victim's every pore, running down his face and drenching his clothes. Most people suffered only a short time, because within hours of becoming ill, they slipped into a coma and died.

The disease became known as the English Sweating Sickness. It first appeared in August 1485, the month Henry Tudor fought and killed King

Richard III on Bosworth field. It disappeared after five weeks, then returned briefly in 1517, 1528, and 1551. It broke out in Germany in 1529 and spread to the Netherlands, Lithuania, and Poland. Then it disappeared from history as completely and mysteriously as the Roanoke Colony.

The best guess of contemporary infectious-disease experts is that the English Sweating Sickness was a cholera-like illness caused by a mutated virus. The virus wreaked havoc episodically for four decades, then mutated again, turning benign. An influenza virus, experts say, is the most likely candidate for behaving this way. They have a high mutation rate, and a harmless strain could have changed into a deadly variant.

Now flash forward.

In August 1998 while the FDA was meeting in Washington to draft guidelines for xenotransplantation, in Hong Kong hundreds of thousands of chickens were being slaughtered to prevent the spread of a potentially fatal flu virus designated H5N1. The virus started out killing only chickens and ducks, but then began killing humans. Many fell ill, and at least four died. H5N1, fortunately, turned out to infect only people coming into direct contact with poultry and didn't spread from person to person.

But that was only luck.

If H5N1 had been spread by coughs and sneezes, it might have infected hundreds of millions of people and killed tens of millions. It could have resembled the Spanish Influenza pandemic of 1918–1919, which killed perhaps forty million people worldwide, twelve million in India alone. Twenty-eight percent of the civilian population in the United States fell sick with the flu, and half a million died from it. The disease, appearing in the midst of the First World War, killed 24,000 American soldiers, only ten thousand fewer than battlefield casualties.

A new and deadly strain of an influenza virus can appear at any time. No one knows where the ones causing the English Sweating Sickness or the Spanish flu originated, but the new flu viruses that spread across the world every winter are typically mutated forms originating in the Far East. There pigs and poultry are raised in close proximity on thousands of small farms, and pigs are often fed human waste, exposing them to human viruses.

When the genes of a virus infecting pigs recombine with those of a virus infecting chickens or ducks, the result is a new viral variant. Because many people live close to their animals, they're easily exposed to the virus. Once someone is infected, the virus then spreads from person to person, the speed of the outbreak amplified by modern transportation.

Soon a viral strain originating in Hunan Province is making people sick in London, New York, Dallas, and Los Angeles. Our immune systems have been primed to attack last year's viral variants, but they lack antibodies against a new one. If we're lucky, the variant produces nothing but a relatively mild, short illness.

The genetic recombination taking place between pig and poultry viruses could also occur in recipients of pig organs. A harmless virus present in a pig kidney has the potential to recombine with human viruses or, once inside a cell, with human DNA segments. The recombination might change the pig virus into a raging, virulent strain that kills its host and moves outward. The new virus might turn out to be more deadly than the English Sweating Sickness or the Spanish Influenza.

Pigs harbor a range of ordinary viruses. Those causing pig diseases most of us have never heard of—porcine influenza, parainfluenza, swine vesicular disease, encephalomyocarditis, parcovirus, and pseudorabies—can also infect humans. Some of the diseases can be fatal, and someone with a compromised immune system would be likely to die from them.

If transplanting organs from pigs presents so many risks, it's tempting to think we'd do better using primates as donors. But primate organs present even greater risks.

Primates?

The close genetic connection between primates and humans means organisms infecting primates are also likely to infect us. People coming into contact with monkeys, for example, risk infection from the monkeypox virus (similar to smallpox) and SIV (simian immunodeficiency virus). Baboons also carry several other viruses capable of infecting humans: SA8, simian cytomegalovirus, herpes papio, baboon endogenous retrovirus, STLV-1, and foamy viruses.

Those who work with primates sometimes fall ill with primate diseases. One study showed three out of 472 workers tested were positive for SIV antibodies, proving they were exposed. If more people don't become infected, it's only because most of us have little or no contact with primates.

Limits

The most obvious way to prevent the transmission of an infectious disease from an animal donor to a human recipient is to screen the animals and exclude those harboring microorganisms. This is an explicit precaution in guidelines framed by (among other groups) the National Institutes of Medicine and the British Nuffield Council.

The precaution is good in theory, but virologists argue that no matter how well primates are screened, they still pose too great a risk of causing infection to be used as donors. Even though screening may detect no active viruses, primates harbor at least thirty endogenous retroviruses in their DNA. It's possible, perhaps likely, one of these dormant viruses might be reactivated in the new environment of an organ recipient's body. Primates thus should be excluded as donor animals.

What about pigs, then?

The best way to produce disease-free pigs is to screen them to make sure they're not infected with bacteria and viruses, then breed them under sanitary conditions. Their offspring ought to be as disease-free as animals realistically can be. Recent studies, however, suggest that producing virus-free pigs is harder than previously believed. Indeed, it might be impossible.

British researchers Robin Weiss and David Onions discovered that pigs have multiple copies of three viruses of a type called *porcine endogenous retrovirus* (PERV) woven into their DNA. These viral genes are probably the result of an infection of the pig's ancestors, perhaps thousands of years ago. Copies of the virus are passed from one generation to the next through sperm and egg cells. PERV is dormant and doesn't seem to make pigs sick, but Weiss's experiments show PERV can infect colonies of human cells.

This suggests that if pig organs are transplanted, recipients could become infected with PERV. If this happens, no one knows how serious the result might be. Possibly the viral material might change into an active retrovirus, a sort of molecular Godzilla causing a disease. The disease might be a form of cancer and affect only the organ recipient. But it might be as deadly as smallpox or as terrible as HIV, the retrovirus that causes AIDS.

Whether PERV can be eliminated from pigs by breeding isn't certain. Biotran, a biotech company, reported that nine of its pigs didn't pass on PERV to the next generation, and both Nextran and Imuran, competing companies, claimed their herds showed no evidence of active infection from PERV. What's not clear, though, is whether current tests for PERV are sufficiently sensitive to detect it. (Because the light's too dim to see anything in the closet doesn't mean the monster's not there.)

As matters stand, so far as anyone knows, transplanting pig organs may expose recipients to undetectable and uneliminable retroviruses. This exposure carries with it a risk of infection and contagion no one can calculate. Thus, while pigs may be better candidates for donors than primates, they too pose unforeseeable hazards.

And hidden viruses are only part of the danger.

New Diseases

Most people have seen the situation dramatized on TV or read about it in thrillers—an unknown virus attacks its victims, striking them down in a rush of pain, fever, bloody hemorrhages, and physical debilitation, then killing them with kidney and heart failure.

The names of the diseases are familiar to us as words splashed across movie posters and book jackets—Ebola, Lassa Fever, Marburg. But despite their familiarity, the words make people shudder in the special way that words like *diphtheria, polio*, and *tuberculosis* did in earlier generations.

Shuddering is appropriate, because not only are the new diseases deadly, they appeared from nowhere, aren't well understood, and can't be treated effectively. Also, they all pose a similar difficulty when it comes to screening.

The initial outbreak of Marburg disease illustrates the problem. In August 1967 three workers involved in vaccine production at a facility operated by Hoeschst Pharmaceuticals in Marburg, Germany fell ill with muscle aches and low-grade fevers. Hospitalized, the patients soon suffered from nausea, their throats swelled, and their eyes turned bloodshot.

Three more workers from the facility fell ill, then so did a physician who had been caring for the first three. By September, twenty-three patients were hospitalized in Marburg, and fifty miles away in Frankfurt, six more people developed the same symptoms. Four were pharmaceutical workers, one the pathologist who had handled their biopsied tissues, and the last a physician who had cared for them. Then, far away in Belgrade, Yugoslavia, two more people fell ill, a veterinarian and his wife.

The initial flu-like symptoms were soon followed by swollen lymph nodes, a drop in white blood-cell count, and a depletion of blood platelets and factors controlling bleeding. By day six, the patients' bodies were covered by a painful red rash, and their throats were so swollen they couldn't swallow and had to be fed intravenously. Severe diarrhea appeared.

The rash was replaced on day eight by the death of the entire epidermis, an event caused by blockages in the network of capillaries supplying it with blood. The patients began vomiting blood on the tenth day, and around the three-week mark, the dead skin began to slough off. "Blood is pouring from all apertures," one patient's physician wrote in his notes.

By December 7, thirty-one patients had died. Most had succumbed during the first sixteen days, some after slipping into a coma produced by brain swelling. Two died of cardiac infarcts, their hearts unable to cope with the burden of pumping against blocked capillaries. Several suffered liver damage, and one became psychotic and never recovered.

The disease had a twenty-three percent mortality rate.

The Marburg medical team used molecular probes to search for known viruses, but none could be found. Convinced by the symptoms they were dealing with a viral disease, the team investigated the background of the patients and found all had been exposed to a group of Vervet monkeys imported from Uganda.

Investigators traced the monkeys to shipments sent to Belgrade, Marburg, and Frankfurt. Everyone who had fallen ill, including the veterinarian, had been exposed to the monkeys or monkey tissues, or had cared for someone with the illness. All three shipments had included sick or dead monkeys.

The Marburg team eventually discovered two strains of an unrecognized virus in the surviving monkeys. Comparing the recovered virus with recognized viruses, they found it was unknown before the 1967 outbreak.

The Marburg virus, to be transmitted, required direct contact with a sick animal or person. This lucky fact kept the number of fatalities low. If the virus had turned out to be like a flu virus, it might have spread like wildfire and killed thousands of people, if not tens or hundreds of thousands.

While Marburg claimed relatively few victims, its unexpected occurrence is a warning relevant to the decisions we must make about proceeding with clinical trials of xenotransplantation. We know now that a previously unrecognized animal disease may suddenly spread to humans with deadly results.

If the Marburg virus had remained dormant for months or years after infecting its victims, connecting it to the Vervet monkeys might have taken a long time. Thus, a much larger number of people might have died from the disease.

The Marburg outbreak illustrates why even the most advanced forms of screening aren't able to prevent an organ recipient from becoming infected with an unknown virus. Even though the Marburg team was sure they were dealing with a viral illness, their molecular probes failed to detect the virus. Viruses in humans are discovered only when they cause disease, and even then it may not be possible to locate them.

New diseases infecting humans don't emerge only from primate viruses either. In 1997 a pig farmer in a Malaysian village fell ill with what seemed to be the brain inflammation encephalitis. A year later, 258 pig farmers in Malysia fell ill with the same disease, and more than a hundred died. Not until 1999 did scientists at the Centers for Disease Control identify the cause of the illness. It was a new virus they called *Nipah*.

Virologists have catalogued about forty thousand species of viruses, and undoubtedly, thousands more are waiting to be discovered—or to discover us. Some thirty thousand viruses are known to cause diseases; probably more actually do, but we haven't discovered which ones. Given our relative ignorance, then, we can't be sure that even our most sophisticated screening processes will detect disease-causing viruses.

This means a virus we don't even suspect exists could be transmitted from an animal to a human in a xenograft and trigger a devastating plague. Consider HIV.

HIV

In 1999 Beatrice Hahn announced she and her research team had established a close connection between a primate virus and human immunodeficiency virus (HIV), the virus that causes AIDS. Simian immunodeficiency virus.chimpanzee (SIV.cpz) resembles HIV so closely that differences can easily be explained as mutations occurring *after* SIV.cpz crossed to the human species. SIV.cpz infects only a subspecies of chimpanzee known as *Pan troglodytes troglodytes* that inhabits areas of western Africa where AIDS made its first appearance. The oldest documented case of HIV infection is in a Bantu man from what is now Kinshasa in the Democratic Republic of Congo. Hahn speculates SIV was transmitted to humans when people slaughtering chimps for meat were exposed to their blood.

Molecular analysis of the HIV from a 1959 blood specimen and comparison of it with other HIV samples show AIDS probably first appeared in the late 1940s or early 1950s. The opening of roads into isolated areas of Africa eventually allowed the virus to spread from rural settlements to population centers.

With the advent of drugs known as protease inhibitors, for those in rich countries, HIV/AIDS became a chronic disease. Statistics show the story is otherwise for people in poor countries. North America has around a million cases and Latin America a million-and-a-half. Africa, with more than twenty million cases, has become the scene of a public health crisis.

THE AIDS STORY involves a harmless virus that becomes deadly when, as a result of unintentional human intervention, it crosses the species barrier. The Marburg outbreak involves a virus we aren't able to screen for, because it's unknown. Thus, the AIDS story is, in a sense, what could have happened had the Marburg virus taken several months or years to make people sick.

AIDS is more alarming as a warning about what could happen than the Marburg outbreak, because AIDS involves a new version of an animal gene, either a mutation or a recombination. Someone receiving an animal heart, liver, lung, or kidney will have the organ *inside her body*. The protective barrier of the skin will be breached, and the donor organ will be in direct contact with the recipient's organs. Perhaps for years, animal cells will nestle against human cells, and human blood will flow through the organ. The organ and any viruses harbored in it will thus be exposed constantly to the recipient's body and the viruses it harbors.

The exposure will also take place in the presence of a deliberately weakened immune response, because the recipient's immune system will be damped down by antirejection drugs. These factors create a laboratory for promoting genetic recombinations between animal and human viruses. The chances of a new and perhaps deadly virus emerging are increased.

A Big Unknown

It's *possible* an AIDS-like disease could emerge from transplanting animal tissues into humans. That AIDS itself emerged demonstrates that the possibility isn't merely speculative.

But even granting it is realistic, we still don't know how *likely* it is that xenotransplantation would produce a disease similar to AIDS. Perhaps it would never happen. What's the probability of an animal virus turning into a killer?

Past Xenografts

We can try looking to the past as a guide to determining future risks. We're not completely without experience. Perhaps three hundred or so transplants of animal organs have been performed since the start of the twentieth century, most using primate donors. So have these animal organs produced an infectious disease in any of the recipients?

Apparently not.

This seems reassuring, because transplants of human donor organs are known to produce infections. Hepatitis B, C, and G, herpes viruses, a single-stranded DNA virus called TTV, and HIV are among those that have slipped through the screening process and been transmitted to patients.

The most recent virus known to be passed on by infected organs is HHV-8, which causes Kaposi's sarcoma, a cancer of the skin and organ-linings. For those infected with HIV, because of weakened immune systems, Kaposi's sarcoma is often the first visible sign of AIDS.

Yet the lack of disease in xenograft recipients may be false reassurance. The recipients have usually died quickly, the animal organs remaining in their bodies only a few hours or days in most cases, a few weeks or months in a handful of others. Such times may be too short for mutations or recombinations to occur. Past cases thus can't tell us much about what might happen if an animal organ stays in contact with human cells for several years.

But another part of the past that might guide us is the human contact with pig viruses.

Pig to Patient

Humans have been exposed to pig viruses in numerous cell-to-cell contacts. Pig skin has been used for decades to cover serious burns, pig pancreatic islet cells are implanted to treat diabetes, and pig livers periodically serve as bridges for patients waiting for donor livers. Pig kidneys have been employed for external dialysis and spleens used in attempts at immunotherapy. Several hundred people have also been given implants of pig neural tissue to treat them for neurological damage or diseases, including Parkinson's.

Scientists are only now studying the consequences of such pig-to-human exposure. German researchers, in the most worrisome cases, discovered that PERV particles can be released from pig endothelial cells. What's more, when the pig cells are cultured with human embryonic kidney cells, the human cells become infected with PERV.

But other results tell a different story. In a study of ten patients given islet cells between 1990 and 1993, Swedish scientists found swine influenza virus in all ten. Although five tested positive for pig parvoviruses and five for other pig viruses, only one person had become ill and tests for PERV were negative.

In a study in St. Petersburg, Russia, 23 of 100 patients whose blood had been perfused through a pig spleen for one hour as long as eight years previously still had pig cells in their blood, although none tested positive for PERV. Researchers from Imutran, in another study, examined 160 patients treated with pig tissue implants at hospitals throughout the world and discovered no infections caused by pig viruses.

The studies so far are generally reassuring. But there's a limit to their usefulness. HIV may have crossed into humans only once, and no study of pig viruses in people can demonstrate that such an event will never happen again. It may even have happened already without our knowing about it yet.

Prions

Viruses aren't the only worry, and here too the past may serve as a guide. In 1956 injections of human growth hormone became a standard therapy for children failing to develop properly. The hormone was extracted from the pituitary glands of people recently dead.

Not until thirty years later, when a few patients developed the symptoms of the brain disorder Creutzfeldt-Jakob disease (CJD), did researchers realize that the extracts used to treat them must have been contaminated with an infectious agent with a long incubation period.

The agent causing CJD is a protein structure called a prion. It's the same sort of agent that causes mad-cow disease (bovine spongiform encephalopathy, or BSE), the brain disease which has particularly affected the cattle herds in European counties, Britain in particular, and been responsible for the death of more than a hundred people.

No one could have screened for prions in 1956, because their existence wasn't suspected. Also, the long lapse between infection and the occurrence of symptoms made it impossible to stop or modify a therapy that was infecting more and more people. We know now that Creutzfeldt-Jakob disease is also associated with the transplantation of corneas and dura mater (the tough tissue covering the brain) from infected donors. Only if the signs of CJD have appeared in a potential donor, however, is it possible to avoid transmitting the disease to a recipient.

Pressures

Pressures are building, even in the midst of debates about safety, to initiate clinical trials of xenotransplants. Why the hurry? One persuasive answer is that people are dying every day whose lives might be saved by xeno-transplants.

While this is true, critics see the rush toward clinical trials as driven by pressures exerted by multinational corporations. Imutran (a subsidiary of the Swiss company Novartis Pharm AG) and Nextran (owned by Baxter International, a medical-products manufacturer) are among those that have invested large sums in trying to develop xenotransplantation into a reliable therapy.

The shortage of human donors, an aging population, and the needs of cultures like Japan's that discourage organ donation add up to a huge potential market for transplantable pig organs. The market, by some estimates, is worth six billion dollars and can be expected to grow. With so much money in prospect, critics charge, corporations may be tempted to minimize public-health risks and push ahead with clinical trials.

Nor are the corporations alone in this. Patient advocacy groups and some transplant surgeons are also eager to initiate clinical trials. Pressure may be greatest from people pressing for cell transplants. Parkinson's, Huntington's, and Alzheimer's diseases, multiple sclerosis, diabetes, stroke, and brain injury are among the disorders that could benefit from implants of the right sort of animal cells.

Clinical trials of cell transplants have been underway in the United States (with FDA approval) since 1996, and some results have been encouraging. Parkinson's patients, in particular, have shown marked improvement when treated with injections of pig neural cells. Treatments for diabetes haven't been successful, though, and the results from the Huntington's trials are still being assessed. The other treatment possibilities remain at the stage of animal studies.

Transplanted cells lack the GAL-sugar found in the lining of blood vessels. Thus cells, unlike organs, don't have to cope with hyperacute rejection and are more likely to be tolerated. Yet, although cell implants may benefit patients, the public health risk from animal cells (whatever it is) seems the same as that posed by organs.

Monkey's-Paw Position

The basic ethical question about xenotransplantation, I said earlier, is whether to proceed with it. Are we, as a society, willing to take unknown risks to offer the potential benefits of xenografts and cell implants to those who have a serious, perhaps even life-threatening, need?

Some researchers and ethicists say no. Worried about unintended and unforseen consequences, they favor what I call the monkey's-paw position. That is, they consider going forward with xenografts as too dangerous and advocate a moratorium. Two strong arguments support their position.

THE TRIGGER ARGUMENT

Premise 1 The risk of triggering an epidemic of an AIDS-like disease is unknown but real.

Premise 2 Transplanting animal materials (organs or cells) into humans, even if successful, would help relatively few people.

Conclusion We are risking the lives of millions of people to help (at best) only a comparative few.

Given that the prime justification for using xenografts is to save lives, the trigger argument suggests that continuing to test xenografts would frustrate this end. It would be like trying to put out a fire with kerosene. While it might be possible, we risk losing a great many more lives than we save. The argument thus supports the further conclusion that we should declare a moratorium on xenografts until we can assess the risk we're taking to help the people who might benefit.

CONSENT ARGUMENT

The consent argument, like the trigger argument, invokes our ignorance of the risk xenografts pose.

> *Premise 1* The risk of triggering an epidemic of an AIDS-like disease is unknown but real.
>
> *Premise 2* Clinical trials of xenografts subject the entire population, not just the patients, to risk.
>
> *Conclusion* We who are not patients are thus being put at risk without our consent.

Like the trigger argument, the consent argument supports the additional conclusion that we ought to declare a moratorium on xenografts. This would permit us not only to assess the risk, but to decide whether we want to take it. The power of the argument comes from the idea that clinical trials of xenografts turn us all into research subjects, even though we've never been informed of our risks or consented to participate.

Rickety-Bridge Position

I'm one of many who reject the monkey's-paw view in favor of what I'll call the rickety-bridge position. Because xenografts can save lives, they take us where we want to go, and it would be a mistake to declare a moratorium on them. Yet they are admittedly a rickety and potentially dangerous bridge, and we need to gather data to assess their danger, even as we continue to creep forward.

The factors favoring a moratorium are powerful, but I think three considerations ultimately outweigh them. Before discussing them, I'll state them as the premises of an argument.

LIVES-SAVED ARGUMENT

> *Premise 1* A moratorium on xenografts would result in the death of people who otherwise might be saved.

Premise 2 Patients with diabetes or neurological disorders like Parkinson's disease would be denied the potential benefit of animal-cell implants.

Premise 3 We would reduce only marginally the chance of an epidemic of a novel, AIDS-like infectious disease.

Conclusion By imposing a moratorium, we would be buying only relative safety and paying too high a price in lives and (potential) benefits for it.

Premise 1 While the triggering of an epidemic by a xenograft is a realistic possibility, no one believes it's more than slightly probable. In considering whether to adopt a moratorium, we thus must balance the slender likelihood of a catastrophic plague against the virtual certainty of the death of hundreds (perhaps eventually thousands) of people. I recommend we favor real people who will surely die over those we imagine dying in the remote event of an epidemic.

Those certain to die who otherwise might be saved are people needing the temporary support provided by an animal liver. (Animal hearts have never been used successfully this way, and dialysis has made relying on animal kidneys unnecessary, but the use of an animal liver can sometimes make the difference between life and death.) If surgeons are forbidden by a moratorium to use a pig liver to bridge the gap between the time a patient's liver fails and the time a human donor liver is located, many patients will die. Nor can they be saved by the use of artificial-liver machines, because such machines employ pig liver cells to do their job.

An obvious implication of Premise 1 is that attempting to secure complete safety from an epidemic by imposing a moratorium has to be paid for in human lives.

Premise 2 Premise 2 indicates that death isn't the only human price a moratorium would exact. People with neurological disorders, diabetes, and spinal-cord injuries would be denied any potential benefit of animal-cell transplant therapy. The therapy is now more of a promise than an established treatment, but for some people it offers the only realistic hope of bettering their lives. What's more, a moratorium would be a barrier to further efforts to improve cell-implant therapy, which holds more immediate promise than animal organ transplants.

Premise 3 That viruses repeatedly and unpredictably cross from other species into ours suggests that a moratorium on xenografts would have little value in reducing the chance of an HIV-like epidemic. Viruses cross from one species to another, and we can do little or nothing to prevent it. Species jumping happens often with flu viruses, yet it's a rare occurrence for an alien invader to produce a disease like the English Sweating Sickness or the Spanish Influenza. It's even rarer, fortunately, for an invading virus to cause a disease like AIDS.

Whether we like it or not, our species is inescapably involved in nature's genetic experiments, and it's an illusion to think that by forbidding xeno-grafts we can gain safety from epidemics of novel diseases. The best we can accomplish is to reduce marginally the present likelihood of one occurring, but to achieve even this anemic result, we'd have to pay for it in lost lives and delayed (or abandoned) treatments for diseases needing better therapies.

Reasonable people may differ about whether the cost of a moratorium is worth the protection it provides, but in making that reckoning, everyone needs to consider that a moratorium exacts a price. It's one measured in human lives and suffering and in promising therapies postponed.

CONSENT?

How can a defender of the rickety-bridge view respond to the argument that clinical trials of xenografts put us at risk without our consent? I think we can admit it's true, but not have to agree a moratorium is justified.

No one knows exactly how much risk xenografts expose us to, but we've been exposed to it for a least a century. So far as we can tell, no adverse effects have resulted. It's true one could occur at any moment, but that's been so since the time Emrich Ullmann attached the pig kidney to his patient's blood vessels. Xenografts are merely one of the more-or-less con-stant background risks we face all the time.

This isn't to say we shouldn't take steps to minimize whatever risk xenografts involve. That this should be done is part of the rickety-bridge position. The idea is to preserve and improve lives, while protecting against risk in every reasonable way possible.

Setting Policy

Animal cell implants are facts on the ground, and clinical trials of animal-human organ transplants hover on the horizon. We thus need to decide without delay how we're going to regulate xenotransplant research. The following recommendations would be endorsed, I believe, by everyone favoring continuing clinical trials.

1. Establish a single national agency to regulate xenotransplant research.

   Now the FDA, NIH, and Department of Health and Human Services all have bits of responsibility. But shared responsibility can leave regulatory gaps, allowing researchers to engage in risky experiments. The current HHS Secretary's Xenotransplantation Advisory Subcommittee could be charged with approving and monitoring all clinical trials involving implanting animal materials into humans.

2. Require the regulatory agency to enforce policies to reduce the likelihood that xenografts will trigger an epidemic disease. Mechanisms are already falling into place to transform xenotransplantation research from a freebooting enterprise conducted with minimum supervision to a regulated activity.

   The Subcommittee has framed guidelines regulating research and clinical trials. They provide for protecting patients, monitoring them and health-care workers for disease, and specifying the use of only specially bred animals as donors.

   A National Patient Registry was established in 1998 to keep track of xenograft recipients. Should one develop an infectious disease, her contacts can be quickly identified.

   A Biological Specimen Repository was also set up to store blood and tissue samples taken from donors, recipients, and those exposed to them. The registry and the tissue archive, in cooperation with parallel institutions in other countries, will provide a means of monitoring adverse events. They will also be a source of data for those studying the safety of xenografts.

3. Forbid the use of primates as cell or organ donors.

   Researchers have moved in this direction by using cell implants from pigs only, but no agency has forbidden employing primates as donors. This leaves open the possibility of another Baby Fae case, a transplant using primate organs approved only by a local institutional review board.

   Virologists agree that the main threat of the emergence of a new lethal and communicable disease comes from primate viruses. Hence, the risk of exposing humans to animal cells can be significantly reduced by eliminating primates as donors.

4. Discontinue clinical trials involving animal cells or tissues if another therapy is demonstrated to be at least as successful.

   If, for example, human stem-cell implants turn out to be as effective as pig-cell implants in treating Parkinson's disease, we should stop using pig cells. Any new therapy achieving the same (or better) therapeutic results as an older one and lacking its risks should be preferred.

5. Demonstrate success in primate models before performing animal-to-human xenografts.

Before proceeding with animal-to-human xenografts, most researchers consider it reasonable to require scientists to demonstrate first a significant number of successes in non-human primates. This might be done by showing, for example, that pig organs can function well enough to keep baboons alive for several weeks or months.

6. Continue research into viral transmission.

Animal-to-animal xenografts should be studied to learn more about how viruses are transmitted and activated. We also need to know more about how they mutate and recombine with human genetic material to produce new viruses. Such information is crucial in determining how much danger clinical trials of xenografts pose.

Staying Alert

Xenotransplantation, despite its problems, remains a goal worth pursuing. Yet it's a footbridge so rickety it demands we stay watchful in negotiating it. We must proceed cautiously, taking one step at a time and staying alert to the possibility of impending disaster. We must, above all, be prepared to end clinical trials at the first sign of trouble. That's the time to declare a moratorium.

If we remain realistic and cautious, however, we may be able to get the monkey's paw to grant our wishes without causing a disaster.

But What About Costa Linda?

We might, by monitoring and regulating be able to protect the United States from becoming the source of an epidemic, but infectious diseases know no boundaries.

The country of Costa Linda is fictional, but it can stand for those countries in South and Central America, Africa, Asia, the Middle East, and Eastern Europe, where the regulation of medical research is either slight or non-existent. Medical entrepreneurs in such countries may be free to establish xenotransplantation centers and offer, to those able to pay, services that would be denied to them in North America and Western Europe.

Xenotransplantation, compared to the production of bomb-grade plutonium, is a cottage industry that can be carried out virtually anyplace with relatively modest start-up costs. With the growing pressure to regulate xenotransplantation in developed countries, carrying out animal research has become increasingly expensive, using primates as donors for humans is discouraged, and conducting human trials using animal organs may be postponed for the near future. But surgeons in "xenoshelters" like Costa Linda could, if the political environment is permissive, follow their own rules.

Neither the World Health Organization nor international medical associations has the power to regulate or enforce safety recommendations. They can advise governments and use political persuasion to get their rules adopted, but they can't keep determined people possessing the necessary skills and motivations from performing xenografts on their own terms.

International governmental agreements regulating xenotransplantation are called for. The agreements must contain inspection provisions and penalties for failing to enforce accepted regulations. Biological threats, we now know, must be taken as seriously as nuclear ones.

In Nevil Shute's 1957 novel *On the Beach,* the bomb triggering the worldwide nuclear catastrophe that wipes out the human race is one dropped, not by the United States or Russia, but by a small country in a local war.

Costa Linda poses a similar danger.

11

Grow Your Own Organs

Stem-Cell Engineering and Regenerative Medicine

August 1, 2025: William Osler Hospital

Alice Littlewood was tossing pseudoplasma rockets at the spacecraft zipping across the wholewall display, while her twelve-year-old daughter Cara keyed the remote to guide them into evasive patterns.

"Zapped!" Alice exclaimed as a freighter exploded, producing a dull *whoom!* and erupting into a ball of flames.

Alice waved as she caught sight of me. We'd been introduced in the office of Dr. Samuel Clinewold and chatted briefly on the phone a couple of times. But Alice was scheduled for surgery the next morning, and I wanted to talk to her face-to-face.

We'd made arrangements to meet in her room at Osler, but she was out when I arrived. Dean Bryer, her husband of fifteen years, was sitting in a chair reading a book, and I'd accepted his offer to escort me through the maze of corridors to the hospital's entertainment center.

Dean and I sat down at a table with bottles of juice and watched the match between Alice and Cara. A scattering of people were playing at the other game stations, but the large room was mostly empty.

"She's looking good, don't you think?" Dean asked.

Alice was forty-five, five-nine, slim and willowy, with a long, slender neck. She moved with ease and grace and laughed when she scored a point by blasting one of Cara's ships. She was obviously enjoying life and was the image of health.

Except Alice wasn't healthy. Not really. Between the *whooms* of the explosions and the sizzling noises of rockets, I could hear the mechanical *tick-whoosh* . . . *tick-whoosh* . . . of the left ventricular assist device implanted under her ribs on the left side.

"Thanks for agreeing to talk to me." I shook hands with Alice as she came over to the table. Cara was behind her.

"I'm so excited, I'm glad to have somebody to share it with." Alice turned and kissed her daughter on the cheek. "Go with your dad, and I'll see you later up in the room."

Cara hugged her mother. Dean then took Cara's hand, and they walked out of the entertainment center.

"I had really bad luck last year, as I was telling you." Alice got a bottle of juice out of a cooler and sat down at the table with me. The *tic-whoosh* . . . of her artificial heart blended with the repeated *whoom!* and *zizzz!* of the games.

"Somewhere I picked up a virus, and I was sick as a cat for a couple of weeks. It's nothing terrible, I thought. I'd felt sicker before. But then I didn't seem able to recover. I couldn't shake off the fatigue, and when I tried to start running again, even fast walking set me to gasping and panting."

She paused, recalling. "Then I began to get worried. My feet and ankles swelled, like somebody had filled them up with compressed air. I couldn't walk a block without getting short of breath, then I found I could sleep better propped up in a lounge chair than lying flat in bed."

Alice had stopped doing anything that took much effort for six months. She expected to recover. Her body was simply taking a long time. After all, she wasn't as young as she used to be.

Eventually, at Dean's repeated insistence, Alice made arrangements to consult her internist, Dr. Lawrence Cervando. After examining her, Dr. Cervando ordered a series of laboratory and imaging tests, then, without waiting for the results, sent her to see Dr. Consuelo Tang, a cardiologist.

"That scared me," Alice said. "My dad died of a heart attack when he was fifty, and I've always felt sure I was going to have one too. You might say I was just waiting for it."

Dr. Tang took Alice's medical history and examined her. She listened to Alice's heart with a stethoscope that transmitted data for computer analysis. Dr. Tang then reviewed the laboratory findings and studied the holotomographic images sent to her from the testing center. She accessed her diagnostic program, then gazed for a long time at the information on the screen.

"You have a condition called dilated cardiomyopathy," Dr. Tang said at last. "Your heart is of abnormal size, and it shows signs of serious injury. So far as I can tell, you don't have an active infection, but from what you've told me and from the scarring I see, I suspect your heart was damaged by a viral infection."

"Is there a treatment?"

Alice was even more worried than she had been. Her heart was damaged. What if she died suddenly? Could Dean and Cara manage on their own? Of course they could. But she wouldn't be with them. That's what bothered her most. She'd have to leave her family the way her father had left her and her mother.

"Not a quick fix," Dr. Tang said. "You're in class two congestive heart failure. I can give you some drugs to strengthen your heart's output, but that's not going to fix the basic problem. If the damage wasn't so severe, we could limit ourselves to using cell implants to increase functioning heart tissue." She shook her head. "But that won't fix the problem either. Not really."

"Do this mean you can't do anything?" Alice swallowed, her mouth suddenly dry and tasting of metal.

"Oh, no." Dr. Tang looked surprised. "We can give you a new heart."

"A transplant?"

"Yes, but not from another person."

"What?" Alice felt confused. "An animal heart?"

"Oh, no. We quit using pig organs years ago." Dr. Tang laughed. "You're going to get a heart that's a perfect match. We're going to grow one for you from your own cells."

That had been ten months ago.

The day after getting her diagnosis from Dr. Tang, Alice paid a visit to Osler's Stem-Cell Therapy Unit and had cell samples taken. Dr. Clarence Thompson, the physician at the unit who had met with her, explained that her cells would be cultured, then fused with enucleated eggs. After four days of development, the stem cells would be recovered, placed in a growth medium, and treated with a series of biochemical messengers.

The messengers would program the cells and trigger the growth of tissues. The tissues, bathed in a nutrient medium, would be supported by an absorbable matrix. Sequenced biochemical messengers would then be supplied to direct the growing tissues to develop into a heart. It would ultimately turn into one both anatomically correct and complete, with all tissues and cell types in their proper places.

"We'll be growing several hearts," Dr. Thompson told her. "The process isn't perfect, but maybe out of three or four we'll get one that's perfectly normal."

The growth process took months, though. Before her new heart was fully developed, Alice's original heart began to fail faster than Dr. Tang had anticipated. The drugs she'd been given to strengthen her heartbeat and prevent the buildup of fluids in her body became ineffective. Constantly fatigued, unable to work, panting for breath, Alice felt miserable and depressed.

"I was ready to lie down and die." Alice frowned at the memory. "I felt worthless and more out of this world than in it." "I hate to put you through extra surgery," Dr. Tang told her. "But it's going to be another six months before your heart is large enough to transplant safely, so I suggest you consider letting us give you an artificial heart to bridge the gap."

Alice agreed to talk to the cardiac surgeon.

"These left-ventricular assist devices are so good you could live with one for ten or twenty years," Dr. Clinewold told her. "We don't even recommend transplants for people who are elderly or too frail for surgery. But they aren't as good as your own heart, and you're still a young woman."

"Will I have to stay hooked up to the machine?"

"Oh, no." Dr. Clinewold shook his head. "Your LVAD will be completely implantable. The battery powering it is also implantable and can be recharged through the skin."

I met Alice just after she'd received her LVAD. She'd given me permission to follow her course until she got the transplant.

The LVAD allowed Alice to return to a more-or-less normal life. But she was still aware of being dependent on a machine, and as good as it was, the artificial heart wasn't perfect.

"It alters its rhythm, depending on what I'm doing," Alice told me. "But it's always a few beats behind. And that's more upsetting than you might imagine. You wonder, is my heart working?" She put the palms of her hands together as if praying. "But now I'm going to get my own heart back."

"Is that the way you think of the transplant?" I asked. "As getting your heart back?"

"I do." Alice smiled. "It's going to be my heart Dr. Clinewold sews into place, not a heart from a dead person or some animal. It's a part of me, isn't it? It's like growing new skin, only it's a whole organ."

I didn't see Alice and Dean until three days after the transplant. I knew from talking to Dr. Clinewold that the surgery had gone smoothly. Alice had made a quick recovery, with no complications and no infection. She was being released from Osler that morning, and I met her and Dean in her room.

"I'm delighted," Alice told me. "My heart is working perfectly, and it's so much better than having that hunk of metal pounding away in my chest.

I felt like the crocodile that swallowed the alarm clock in *Peter Pan*. Wherever you were in the house, you could hear me coming." She laughed.

"She's got to take it easy, though," Dean said. "The heart has to be conditioned by starting easy, then built up by increasingly demanding exercise."

"But I don't have to take drugs." Alice looked pleased. "It really is my heart. And I'm back to being myself—my real self."

ALICE LITTLEWOOD isn't a real person. Her story is nothing but science fiction, yet at its core lies the kernel of a real promise. The story expresses the ancient dream of organ transplantation as spare-parts surgery.

We replace, in this vision, the body's diseased or damaged organ by a healthy one, in the way we replace a car's worn-out water pump with a new one. The new organ not only functions normally, it's tolerated by the body of the recipient. We restore what is lost, making bodies as good as new, and maybe even better sometimes.

Xenotransplants could solve most of the ethical and social issues that swarm like angry bees around the current practices of acquiring and distributing transplant organs. (See Chapters 9 and 10.) But xenotransplantation doesn't seem to be standing on the threshold of practical success, and the fear that implanting animal materials into humans may trigger an epidemic of a new and devastating infectious disease may slow, if not halt, its advancement. Besides, there's little hope xenografts could ever be tolerated without using powerful immunosuppressive drugs to damp down the immune system.

The kernel of promise at the core of Alice Littlewood's story is that we may be able to develop a technology for growing organs using a person's own cells. A transplanted organ would then be tolerated without immunosuppressive drugs, because the organ would be, in fact, the recipient's own. Because the heart grown from one of Alice's stem cells isn't immunologically alien to her, it will be tolerated by her body.

Less dramatic, but just as promising, we may be able to avoid the need for transplants in most cases by using stem cells to repair damaged organs. Patching up organs, instead of replacing them, would ease, if not eliminate, the organ shortage.

Stem cells, then, offer the most elegant solutions to the problem of preserving the lives of people who otherwise will die from dozens of end-stage organ diseases. Controlling stem cell will allow us to perform feats that now seem like magic.

Is such stem-cell engineering possible?

Regenerative Medicine

This question became more realistic than speculative in November of 1998 when research groups headed by James Thomson of the University of Wisconsin, Madison and John Gearhart of Johns Hopkins University independently announced they had succeeded in isolating human embryonic stem cells.

This discovery has encouraged researchers to start thinking about developing a sophisticated stem-cell engineering as the basis for a regenerative medicine of almost unimaginable power. Stem cells might be used to cure diseases like Alzheimer's, Huntington's, or Parkinson's that lack an effective treatment. They might provide a cure for diabetes, spinal cord injury, or macular degeneration. Or they might be employed to repair organs like the heart and liver and thus eliminate the need for the majority of transplants.

The most startling possibility is that we might be able to control and orchestrate developmental processes to fabricate (as in Alice Littlewood's case) new vital organs. Replacing a diseased heart, kidney, liver, or lung with a new copy of the patient's own organ would offer significant advantages over a donor transplant.

Regenerative medicine requires harnessing and regulating the body's inherent powers to rebuild itself. Before we can realize this dream, however, we must first acquire much more information about controlling the fundamental biological processes involved in human development and repair.

This means extending our knowledge of the way stem cells operate, but to acquire such knowledge, we must find the means of dealing with what some consider a serious moral impediment to stem-cell research. Those objecting to research using embryonic stem cells have succeeded in getting their views expressed in federal regulations that have become roadblocks to research.

I'll explain later the reasoning behind the moral objections and argue that the roadblocks erected on them should be removed. I maintain that research medicine has an obligation to increase our knowledge of stem cells in order to lay the foundations for regenerative medicine.

PRIMER

The Greek god Proteus was a shape shifter, changing his form from serpent, to lion, to human at will. That the power of stem cells is truly protean is best grasped by considering human development.

The process is triggered at the moment a sperm combines with an egg. The resulting embryo is totipotent, meaning it's capable of turning into a complete individual. All the genetic information needed to achieve this is present in that single cellular package, and given the right circumstances, the events leading to a fully formed child unfold, step by step, in a pre-determined, programmed process.

The embryo begins dividing at fertilization. The single cell, in keeping with its genetic program, turns into two cells. Each remains, to this point, totipotent. If the cells are separated and allowed to develop independently, the emerging individuals will be identical twins.

The embryo, after its initial doubling, continues to divide—four cells, then eight, then sixteen, and so on. After four days of dividing, the embryo consists of a hundred cells that form a hollow sphere called a blastocyst. It's at this stage, in normal reproduction, that the embryo embeds itself in the wall of the uterus and continues the process of becoming a fetus.

The blastocyst's outer layer of cells is called the trophoblast, and it's pro-grammed to form the gestational equipment—the placenta, umbilical cord, and amniotic sac. But parts of the program in the cells of the trophoblast have been shut down. Thus, even if trophoblast cells are put into a uterus, they aren't capable of forming the rest of a human body. The information needed is no longer accessible to them.

But other cells still have this capacity. Inside the blastocyst is a sort of bump called, in the terms of old-fashioned observational biology, the inner cell mass—a cluster of fifteen or twenty cells. These are embryonic stem cells, and (aside from the gestational equipment) they have the capacity to form every type of cell in the human body. Embryonic stem cells are, in the jargon of developmental biology, pluripotent.

The inner cell mass, under normal circumstances, develops into the three germ layers of the embryo: ectoderm, mesoderm, and endoderm. Skin, eyes, and the nervous system emerge from the ectoderm; bone, blood, and muscle tissue (including the heart) develop from the mesoderm. The liver, lungs, and the lining of the stomach and intestines grow out of the endoderm.

Embryonic stem cells, on the way to forming these tissues and organs, continue to divide, and as they do, they branch off or differentiate into a variety of more specialized multipotent cells. These cells eventually give rise to the over two hundred different cell types that make up tissues and organs.

Before embryonic stem cells differentiate, they possess the potential to become any type of multipotent cell. But the multipotent cells are special-ized. Their fate is determined, and when they divide, they produce only cells of the same type. Hemopoietic stem cells, for example, produce red and white blood cells and platelets. Ectodermal stem cells give rise to neurons and skin cells, and mesodermal stem cells produce muscle, cartilage, and bone cells. (This is how they behave, unless we tinker with them. But more about this later.)

Multipotent stem cells are also called *adult* stem cells. Biologists believe all the tissues in the human body—blood, bone, skin, lung, intestine, and so on—are produced by adult stem cells. Yet the cells assumed responsible haven't all been identified. No one has found, for example, stem cells that direct the formation of heart, lung, liver, or pancreatic tissue.

Even so, researchers are confident such cells are there waiting to be discovered. Their confidence, based mostly on animal studies, was recently bolstered by the discovery of neural stem cells. These cells produce all three common cell types making up the brain: astrocytes, oligodendrocytes, and neurons.

Finding neural stem cells was especially satisfying, because the old view was that we're born with all the brain cells we'll ever have, so when they die, we're out of luck. The discovery took some of the bite out of the popular observation that everybody loses ten thousand brain cells a day.

DISCOVERY

Thomson and Gearhart obtained their embryonic stem cells from different sources. Thomson retrieved his from fourteen embryos produced by in vitro fertilization at reproductive medicine clinics but never implanted. Unneeded embryos are typically destroyed by clinics, and Thomson obtained the consent of the couples concerned to use their surplus embryos.

Gearhart found his stem cells in tissue from five- to nine-week aborted fetuses. (The abortion decisions were made prior to Gearhart's request to use the tissue.) Stem cells from the inner-cell mass of the blastocyst migrate to the ovary and testis during development. Known as embryonic germ cells or germ-line cells, they form the sperm and ova and so transmit genetic information to the next generation. Embryonic germ cells are protected from the process that turns embryonic stem cells into adult ones.

The cells Gearhart isolated from the fetal tissue are apparently no different in their potential from the embryonic stem cells Thomson acquired directly from blastocysts.

Thomson succeeded in getting five of his fourteen original clusters of stem cells to grow into colonies. Unlike most colonies of cultured human cells, they've continued to maintain the normal number of chromosomes as they have divided.

Thomson also discovered his colonies possess another important feature. They have a high concentration of telomerase, an enzyme that preserves normal chromosome lengths. The enzyme is found in high concentration in cells biologists call immortal, and thus its abundance in Thomson's colonies suggests the cells have an unlimited potential to go on dividing, producing more and more normal stem cells. This means stem cells can be available virtually off the shelf and in whatever numbers are needed.

ORGAN REPAIR

The first and most immediate therapeutic application of stem cells is likely to be using injections of *adult* stem cells to repair damaged or defective organs. If this turns out to be an effective method of restoring an organ's function, it may be possible to avoid (or at least delay) most organ transplants.

Organ repair offers to reduce the demand for donor organs, yet it also holds the promise of an even more satisfactory result. Those whose organs could be restored by the use of stem cells that are tolerated by their immune system wouldn't have to cope with the problems of rejection.

The most dramatic evidence for the effectiveness of stem cell therapy in promoting organ repair was reported in 2001 by two research groups. Both focused on treating heart damage, but each used different types of stem cells.

A team led by Piero Anversa and Donald Orlic at New York Medical College began with stem cells harvested from the bone marrow of mice. They selected cells that hadn't started to differentiate into the various types of blood cells, ending up with "purified" adult cells. They flagged these cells with a green fluorescent dye so they could keep track of them, then injected them into the deliberately damaged hearts of a group of mice.

The cells began to differentiate. But, astoundingly, instead of producing the blood cells they would have in the bone marrow, they morphed into heart muscle cells (cardiomyocytes), smooth muscle cells that form artery walls, and epithelial cells that line blood vessels. These results demonstrated for the first time that injected stem cells could produce new heart tissue. This was particularly striking, because the stem cells weren't even from the heart.

The tissue formed by the new cells also appeared to work as well as the original tissue. The pumping effectiveness of the left ventricle of the treated mice was measured as forty percent more than that of untreated mice.

A second experiment, equally dramatic, was carried out by Silviu Itescu's group at Columbia University. Itescu isolated from the bone marrow (for the first time) stem cells called angioblasts that are responsible for the development of small blood vessels and showed they could be effective in treating damaged hearts.

When a heart attack occurs, heart cells deprived of oxygen die, but other cells in the region around the dead cells increase to four or five times their normal size to take their place. Eventually, the enlarged cells die and are replaced by scar tissue. Scar tissue doesn't contract, so if a heart is exten-, sively scarred, it may not be able to circulate an adequate amount of blood to keep someone's tissues supplied with oxygen. The person is likely to die and so is in need of a transplant.

Itescu reasoned that if the expanded cells could be supplied with oxygen, they wouldn't die and thus scar tissue wouldn't form to take their place. To test this hypothesis, his team injected angioblasts into the bloodstream of rats with surgically induced heart attacks.

The angioblasts, apparently following a biochemical signal, migrated to the heart. Once there, they produced new blood vessels, and, as Itescu had predicted, this prevented the enlarged cells from dying. Functioning heart cells thus took the place of scar tissue. The left ventricular function of the treated rats improved by fifteen percent, and the increase paralleled the growth of the new blood vessels.

THERAPY

A therapy based on these findings is easy to imagine. In addition to treating those having a heart attack with a clot-busting drug, for example, we might inject them with angioblasts. The angioblasts would migrate to the heart, form new blood vessels, and so prevent scar tissue from forming. The often crippling damage of a heart attack might thus be significantly limited, if not prevented. Those suffering from heart failure might be treated similarly, the new cells compensating for those destroyed by disease.

Could damage to the heart be treated (following the technique of Anversa and Orlic) by injections of stem cells from the bone marrow? Perhaps, if the cells produced new functioning heart tissue. Whether either approach works can only be determined by clinical trials with humans, but it seems quite possible at least one will be successful.

A remarkable aspect of the Anversa-Orlic experiment is its demonstration that stem cells from the bone marrow can behave appropriately when in the heart. This suggests the local biochemical environment is able to supply the differentiation and growth factors needed to trigger the cells to regenerate the types of tissues required.

The therapeutic potential of this is profound. It means it may not be necessary to identify the stem cell responsible for a specific type of tissue in order to develop therapies for replacing or repairing it. Relatively few adult stem cells have been identified, so if bone marrow cells behave in humans the way they do in mice, we'd be able to initiate treatments to repair the heart, even though we haven't identified heart stem cells.

Here are some of the other sorts of organ repairs and tissue replacements researchers consider likely:

Islet cells Growing new insulin-producing cells in the pancreas could cure diabetes.

Brain cells Replacing cells destroyed or damaged in neurological diseases like Parkinson's, Alzheimer's, and Huntington's might reverse the symptoms or delay the onset of disease.

Nerve cells Growing new neural connections might reverse paralysis resulting from spinal cord damage. Paraplegics and quadriplegics might be able to walk again, control the movement of their arms and hands, and regain lost functions.

Blood vessels Growing new blood vessels could treat heart disease, atherosclerosis, and tissue damage resulting from poor circulation.

Bone Producing new bone cells might speed the healing of fractures and reverse damage caused by osteoporosis.

Lung Promoting the growth of new lung tissue might be effective in treating emphysema and obstructive lung diseases.

Cartilage Injecting stem cells (or chondrocytes) into the joints of those suffering from rheumatoid arthritis or osteoarthritis could produce the growth of new cartilage. Cartilage damaged in accidents might also be replaced.

Skin Injecting skin-producing stem cells could speed the healing of wounds and promote the growth of new skin to cover extensive burns.

Blood Injecting stem cells might help cancer patients whose bone marrow has been destroyed or damaged by chemotherapy.

Retina Growing new functioning cells in the retina to replace damaged or defective ones could cure a variety of forms of complete or partial blindness, including macular degeneration.

Liver Treating cirrhosis by injections of stem cells that form new liver tissues might cure diseases now treatable only by a transplant.

Scientists are quick to observe that lists like this are likely to be only partial. We cannot now imagine all the therapeutic possibilities adult stem cells might offer. Because we are made of cells, in principle every disease could be treated by using a sophisticated stem-cell technology.

REJECTION

Stem cells, like other cells, have protein markers on their surface that express their genetic identity. Hence, if donor cells are injected into a recipient, the recipient's immune system may reject them. While stem cells, for reasons not wholly clear, are less likely to trigger an immune response than other cells, rejection does occur. To control it, recipients would now have to be treated with a regimen of the same immunosuppressive drugs used to prevent organ rejection.

But scientists are considering several ways to prevent rejection. One is to remove the protein molecules on the surface of stem cells that mark them as nonself and use them to create colonies of "universal donor" cells. Another possibility is to find protein molecules that will mask a cell's surface proteins. These masked stem cells could then slip past the immune defenses. This technique has been used with some success in preventing transplanted pig organs from triggering hyperacute rejection in primates. (See Chapter 9 for details.)

Another way of getting around the rejection problem is to use a person's own embryonic stem cells. With a jolt of current, an individual's body cell is fused with an egg cell from which the nucleus has been removed. After the embryo forms a blastocyst, the embryonic stem cells are then removed from the inner-cell mass. These recovered cells are genetically identical with the person who contributed the DNA. Hence, they can be injected into that person without provoking an immune response.

A fourth approach is to match stem cells with recipients in the way kidneys are matched. This would require developing and maintaining a bank of stem cell lines. The bank would have to contain a variety of stem cells sufficient for making an immunological match with any potential recipient.

The most elegant solution to the rejection problem, some suggest, would be to implant embryonic stem cells into the bone marrow of a recipient. The recipient would then develop an immune tolerance to the cells, and they could then be transplanted into any of the recipient's organs or tissues without provoking an immune reaction.

It's too early to say which approach is likely to emerge as the best for transforming the potential of stem-cell therapy into a practical reality. Yet few scientists doubt they can make at least one work.

TISSUE ENGINEERING

Years before human stem cells had been identified, scientists were already working with biological materials to construct organs and other body parts to take the place of diseased or damaged ones. The research area is known as *tissue engineering*, and it not only continues to flourish, it's made definite progress in achieving some of its goals.

Perhaps tissue engineering's greatest accomplishment has been the development of skin. In May 1998 the Federal Drug Administration approved a "skin construct" called Apligraf manufactured by Organogenesis, a biotech company.

Apligraf may be the first successful bioartificial organ. It's made up of a dermis and an epidermis, the same two layers that constitute human skin. The dermis is formed by growing fibroblast cells on a collagen gel. The fibroblasts turn the gel into a fibrous matrix, which is then sewn with cells called keratinocytes. When these cells grow, they form the epidermis, and the result is a two-layer swatch of functioning skin.

The materials constituting the skin are natural products. The collagen of the gel is derived from cattle tendons. The fibroblasts and keratinocytes are extracted from the foreskins of circumcised infants. The engineering challenge was to find a way to combine these ingredients to produce a skin substitute as effective as natural skin. This required solving such problems as sterilizing the collagen without destroying it, culturing the cells to keep them alive and reproducing, and then persuading them to grow in uniform layers. This wasn't basic science, but it was basic tissue engineering.

The test for Apligraf was whether it would behave enough like human skin to make it therapeutically effective. Researchers conducted a clinical trial to compare its use in treating leg ulcers caused by leaky veins (venous ulcers) with the standard therapy of covering the wound with moist pressure bandages.

The results were stunning. Some 47 percent of the hardest-to-heal wounds (defined as ones that hadn't healed in at least a year) closed completely when covered with Apligraf. A mere 19 percent closed when treated with conventional therapy.

Apligraf also did more than cover the leg wounds. It apparently supplied growth factors that help speed wound healing—exactly what human skin does. Tests are now underway to determine Apligraf's effectiveness in treating burns and diabetic ulcers and in closing the wounds of reconstructive surgery. Apligraf isn't the only "skin construct" being tested. Several biotech companies are seeking FDA approval for other versions.

TISSUE REPAIRS

The most sophisticated method for engineering tissue is to employ biochemical growth factors to encourage the development of a particular tissue in the location where it's needed. This is a technique that will also play a crucial role in the development of stem-cell engineering.

Bone growth factors (morphogenetic proteins), for example, have the power to speed the healing of fractures and to replace bone that has been destroyed by degenerative diseases. This is a biotechnology that is already known to work. Patients with bone fractures that hadn't healed after nine months, in one study, were treated with bone growth factors and did as well as those who received the standard therapy of bone implants.

Blood vessel growth factors (angiogenetic proteins) have been shown to cause new blood vessels to grow in experimental animals. If we can control angiogenesis, we can treat some forms of heart disease by growing new blood vessels to circumvent the blocked arteries that keep the heart from receiving a sufficient blood supply. A therapy using angiogenesis would reduce the need for transplants.

Researchers are also developing techniques for growing cartilage, heart valves, skeletal muscles, and cardiac muscle. Cosmetic noses can be fashioned by seeding synthetic polymer scaffolds of the right shape with chrondocytes that replace the polymer with cartilage as they grow. External ears can be built from cartilage by similar techniques.

One team of scientists is attempting to develop breast implants by taking tissue from a woman's leg and then growing it on a properly shaped bio-degradable polymer matrix. The resulting breast would be only cosmetic, lacking normal internal structures and capacities. Yet it would be made of the woman's own tissue and thus superior to prostheses and implants.

Tissue engineering has pursued the possibility of repairing tissues in place and made it clear that this therapeutic strategy can be counted on to pay off. The use of stem cells promises to realize the goal of tissue repair to a greater extent than anyone imagined possible. Virtually every tissue might be repaired by the use of stem cells and a combination of growth factors.

DUPLICATE ORGANS

The Mt. Everest of tissue engineering is the construction of complete, functioning internal organs. Because some organs are considerably simpler than others, engineered versions of them may be available before long.

Intestine segments, for example, have been grown in the abdominal cavities of animals, and the same techniques would most likely be successful in humans. This would be a therapeutically significant advance, because the only treatment now available for babies born without intestines (short-bowel syndrome) is a transplant. Like all infant organs, though, intestines are rarely available. Death is then the expected outcome.

The biggest challenge taken on by tissue engineering so far is the construction of a working human liver. The liver is made up of six distinct types of cells arranged in organized groups called lobules. The cells carry out hundreds of biochemical processes, and what each cell does and when depends on its interactions with surrounding cells. The liver is also highly vascular, with all the blood from the body flowing through it. Cells deep inside must be exposed to the blood not only to do their job, but to receive the oxygen they need to stay alive.

The tissue engineers face both regulatory and structural problems. They must learn what factors to use to control the growth of the right variety of liver cells, getting them to grow in the ways they must to perform their physiological functions. They must also promote the growth of blood vessels within the mass of cells. This means getting the cells and blood vessels to arrange themselves into a three-dimensional structure that will function the way a liver does.

Researchers have invested much work in building livers during the last decade. Several groups have shown that layers of liver tissue can be grown using animal cells. So far, however, these tissues have been limited in the tasks they can perform. David Mooney and Antonio Mikos report, for example, that the "liverlike" tissue they've grown on a matrix of synthetic material can perform only single chemical functions. Given the number of functions performed by the human liver, this makes an implantable bio-artificial liver seem a distant dream.

Linda Griffith-Cima at MIT has worked for several years on the structural problems of engineering a liver. Her aim has been to devise a three-dimensional skeleton that attracts the various sorts of liver cells to their proper places and serves as an internal and external structure for the developing organ.

To form the skeleton, Griffith-Cima uses a computer-controlled printing technique to lay down patterns of polymers, then to build them up one layer at a time. The porous structure of the skeleton allows the liver cells to attach themselves to the layers. Her goal is to use specific protein sequences as lures to attract and bind the liver cells to their proper locations. Internal blood vessels must be grown along with the liver tissue to keep it supplied with oxygen.

Tissue engineers are generally optimistic about the prospect of developing a functioning liver. They also believe it may be possible, eventually, to construct kidneys and hearts. No one considers it likely such goals will be achieved in a few years. Even under the most optimistic scenario, donor organs are going to be needed for transplants for several more decades.

Synergy

"With my plates and your paper, we can turn out perfect currency," runs a line from a 1940s counterfeiting movie. The relation between the newly emerging stem-cell engineering and the more established tissue engineering promises a similar synergy. Tissue engineering is paving the way for the even more powerful technology of stem-cell engineering.

Tissue engineering has pioneered techniques for forming tissues and organs, but it has encountered significant limits. The fabrication of three-dimensional functioning organs like the liver, heart, kidneys, and lungs may be possible, but it may take such a long time to solve the problems inherent in their construction that stem-cell engineering may offer swifter success.

Stem-cell engineering, when it comes to growing organs, must rely on the methods devised by tissue engineering. Developing organs need to be sustained in a "bioreactor" or growth chamber that provides them with nutrients, monitors relevant cellular and physiological values, carries off waste products, and supplies the necessary growth factors at the proper time. Tissue engineering hasn't perfected bioreactors by any means, but it has developed the technology beyond its primitive beginnings of cells growing on plates of nutrient agar.

Tissue engineering, in its efforts to construct functional organs and cosmetic body parts, has faced the problems of finding the right materials and methods for constructing three-dimensional frameworks to support and guide cellular growth. While tissue engineering has a long way to go, researchers like Griffth-Cima have made substantial advances.

Stem-cell engineering will require all of tissue engineering's techniques for guiding and monitoring the development of cells, coaxing cells to form layers of tissues, and guiding the development of three-dimensional organ structures. Without the techniques of tissue engineering, the use of stem cells will be limited to tissue and organ repairs.

Organs to Order

Embryonic stem cells have the inherent potential to develop into any kind of tissue and any sort of organ or bodily structure. They encode in their DNA the entire program of information needed to construct the liver, the heart, the left big toe, or even the brain. Given the right circumstances—an embryo's implantation in a uterus—the process of biological development consists of the reading out of this program and the directed formation of the right cells, tissues, and organs in the right order. Step by step, in a predetermined sequence, events occur leading to a fully formed infant.

Birth defects occur when something happens to interfere with the working out of this stored program. Radiation or a virus may alter some of the program's elements. A dietary deficiency may not supply the right molecular materials for the construction directed by the program. Or the stored program itself may contain a mutation that produces a defect or disease.

Stem-cell engineering would make possible a powerful eugenics. (The word is inflammatory, but it's the only one we have.) By manipulating stem cells and using the techniques of in vitro fertilization, we could eliminate many genetic diseases from family lines. We could also use genetic engineering methods to insert genes to make sure our offspring have traits we consider desirable—musical ability, verbal skill, athletic talent.

But if we choose, we can already eliminate genetic diseases by testing and selecting embryos before implanting them. And so far as adding genes to enhance traits is concerned, quite apart from the question of whether it's a good idea, we don't know what genes might be involved in the sorts of complex traits we consider desirable. Trying to improve our children, we would most likely damage them.

The real and immediate interest in stem-cell engineering isn't preventing birth defects or improving our offspring, but producing transplant organs. What would it take, granted the perfection of tissue engineering's bioreactors and biosythetic skeletons, for us to be able to pull this off?

By adding growth factors to cultures, James Thomson was able to induce stem cells to turn into heart, nerve, blood vessel, and other cell types. But Thomson wasn't able to control what types of cells developed from the cultures and in what order they were expressed. Yet this is exactly the control we must possess to develop transplantable hearts and livers from stem cells.

Exercising control requires a knowledge of the host of biochemical factors that signal cells to differentiate. The primordial stem cells must change into adult ones, then these into the variety of cells that make up specific tissues. We must also know the growth factors required to direct the development of the various types and layers of tissues. We must, finally, get the tissues to assemble themselves into functioning organs.

The entire process of directing the growth of new organs requires that we orchestrate biochemical factors and processes. We must be able to initiate the reproduction of cells, turn on the production of growth factors, then turn them off. We must know how to grow a heart instead of a foot. (If we ever acquire such knowledge, we might even be able to grow limb replacements. If lizards can regrow tails, we should be able to regrow new hands or new eyes.)

The problem with this vision is that only a few differentiation and growth factors have been identified so far. We don't know how many are required to grow any organ. Nor (consequently) do we have any idea about what their concentrations should be in a cell culture, when they should be applied, or how long cells and tissues should be exposed to them.

By some estimates, about fourteen thousand genes may be involved in the immensely complicated signal-receptor system governing embryonic development in higher mammals. We haven't identified the genes that encode the information needed to grow the heart, for example, and we don't know how to turn them on and off in the necessary sequence. Until we figure out how to do that, we can't begin orchestrating the development of stem cells to produce working organs.

There is more room for hope than pessimism, however. Not even the leading molecular biologists in the 1950s and '60s guessed that by now we would understand how the information in DNA replicates itself and directs the synthesis of proteins. Also, even the most knowledgeable experts thought it would probably be the middle of the current century before we'd have even a rough draft of the human genome. Instead, we got it in the century's first year. (Or second, some might say.)

Scientists are in the position of somebody like Leonardo who has the idea of an airplane, but no clue about the intermediary steps involved in building one. He doesn't know about steam power, much less internal combustion or jet engines. He sights the top of the mountain above the clouds, but he's still searching for the path leading to it.

Most scientists firmly believe the powerful technology of stem-cell engineering is within our grasp. It may take twenty or even fifty years before we're able to grow replacement organs, but long before we can do that, we'll be able to treat diseases that now cannot be treated at all.

Yet the road toward this goal may be blocked by those who have serious moral objections to research involving embryonic stem cells. These objections depend on the view taken about the nature of the embryo.

Human Embryos

Opinion, public and otherwise, has coalesced around three exclusive views of the status of the human embryo:

A. An embryo is a clump of cells that, although it contains all the genetic information needed to develop into a human, has no special moral status.

B. Because an embryo has the potential to develop into a human, it deserves to be treated with respect.

C. An embryo is a human from the moment an egg and sperm unite and thus has the same claim to life as any other person.

Those holding View A recognize that an embryo has the potential to develop into a fetus, then into a child, but they don't consider potentiality as giving embryos a special moral status. That status, in this view, is acquired only when the potentiality begins to be actualized—namely, when the embryo becomes embedded in a uterus and the stages of development begin to unfold.

View A is reflected in reproductive medicine's use of the term *pre-embryo* to refer to the product of in vitro fertilization. More is required to be an embryo, as the term pre-embryo implies, than the union of two gametes.

Because those holding A see nothing morally special about embryos, they see no reason not to treat them in the casual way we treat other biological products like a kidney or a culture of heart cells. If embryos aren't needed, they can either be discarded or used for research. Destroying embryos to acquire stem cells is not a problem for holders of A.

Those endorsing view B consider the fact that an embryo has the potential to develop into a human as marking it as unique. They regard this potential as a morally relevant property of embryos, one that entitles them to be treated with respect.

Embryos should not (on View B) be produced for trivial purposes. To produce an embryo is to create a potential person, and thus the reason for doing so must be serious. Such a reason might be a couple's need to rely on in vitro fertilization to have a child. This is a worthwhile goal, and the only way to accomplish it involves producing embryos.

The destruction of an embryo, because it prevents a potential person, must also be justified. That an embryo created for use in assisted reproduction is no longer needed may be sufficient. (Others, holding a sterner version of B, may ask for a stronger reason.) To recognize the inherent dignity of the embryo, its destruction should be conducted in a fashion showing respect. An embryo shouldn't, for example, be thrown out with the trash.

Those holding B agree it's morally acceptable to create and destroy embryos for research purposes. Research offers the possibility of making discoveries that may save lives, and saving lives is a serious moral purpose. Destroying an embryo to acquire stem cells for research or treatment is thus morally legitimate. That embryos must be sacrificed to achieve such a purpose may be an unfortunate fact, but it's not a moral wrong.

EMBRYOS AS PERSONS

Those holding View C consider a human embryo to have the same moral status as any other person—a newborn baby, a teenager, a middle-aged woman. One proponent of C, in a letter to a newspaper, describes embryos as "our tiniest citizens," and another calls them "our most vulnerable citizens."

View C is endorsed by the Roman Catholic Church, as well as by a variety of other groups opposed to abortion. The Pontifical Academy for Life's "Declaration on the Production and the Scientific and Therapeutic Use of Human Embryonic Stem Cells" spells out in explicit detail the implications C has for basic research and clinical trials. Granted an embryo is a person, it follows that (as the Pontifical Academy says) the embryo "has the right to its own life." We of course must assert this claim on its behalf, as we would for an unconscious person, because the embryo is unable to assert it for itself.

If an embryo has a right to life, then destroying an embryo is the moral equivalent of killing a person. Holders of C condemn using embryonic stem cells on this ground. Removing stem cells from the blastocyst, in the language of the Pontifical Academy, "critically and irremediably" damages the embryo—i.e., destroys it. This is "a gravely immoral act" and thus one we are prohibited on moral grounds from performing.

What about using stem cells obtained from cultures? If the original cells were acquired by destroying embryos or as a result of abortion, it's morally wrong to use them. Because, as the Pontifical Academy says, "A good end does not make right an action which in itself is wrong," even if stem cells were taken from a culture and used to treat diseases and save lives, using them would not be morally legitimate. The original "illicit act" of destroying an embryo or fetus taints them (and succeeding generations) forever.

Restrictions and Guidelines

Those holding C, the Catholic Church in particular, are implacable foes of research involving human embryos. Their opposition becomes understandable, granted their view that the destruction of an embryo is equivalent to homicide. The equation embryo = fetus = person thus often turns disputes about stem cells into a debate about abortion.

Strong lobbying by abortion opponents led Congress in 1995 to approve an appropriations act including an amendment forbidding the use of federal funds for research in which embryos are created or "destroyed, discarded, or knowingly subjected to risk of injury or death." This is known as the Dickey amendment, and since then it has been attached routinely to legislation appropriating funds for research. Its effect has been to outlaw federal funding for most (some say all) forms of stem-cell research.

The 1998 work by Thomson and Gearhart that led to their recovering and culturing stem cells was supported by private money from the Geron Corporation, a small biotech company. To avoid even the appearance of violating the law, Thomson went so far as to carry out his research in a building separate from the one housing his university laboratory. (Gearhart's research perhaps qualified for federal funding; despite controversy over research involving fetal tissue, it's not prohibited by law.)

The Dickey amendment is seen by most scientists as hampering research so seriously that it may delay for decades the realization of the potential medical benefits of stem-cell engineering. Without federal funding, scientists won't have the support needed for the basic research, and the only work carried out will be relatively small projects funded by private corporations or foundations.

Other countries conduct stem cell research under few restrictions. The British Parliament in 2001, for example, passed laws allowing researchers to produce embryos and acquire stem cells from them. Whatever research advances are made are likely to be achieved by British, European, Israeli, or Australian scientists. The United States may thus lose its leadership position in biotechnology.

Because of concerns about the impact of the Dickey amendment, Harold Varmus, then-Director of the National Institutes of Health, assembled a panel in 1998 to review the question of the legitimacy of doing research with stem cells.

Harriet Raab, the General Counsel for the Department of Health and Human Services, the department responsible for NIH, acting in keeping with the panel's recommendation, notified Varmus in January 1999 that the law against destroying embryos didn't apply to stem cells. A stem cell, the panel had reasoned, isn't an embryo. Lacking the capacity to produce a placenta, it's not totipotent. Thus, a stem cell isn't able to develop into a human, even if were implanted in a uterus.

The NIH issued guidelines for conducting research on stem cells within the bounds of the law. The guidelines hold that federal funds can be used to support stem cell research, "if the cells were derived (without federal funds) from human embryos that were created for purposes of fertility treatment and were in excess of the clinical need of the individuals seeking such treatment." Thus, cell lines grown in colonies like Thomson's are acceptable for use in federally funded research.

John Gearhart, when told this news, reflected the approval of most of the biomedical research community. "This is a very, very big deal," he said.

For those regarding embryos as persons, it was also a very, very big deal, but in a wholly negative way. The National Council of Catholic Bishops condemned the NIH guidelines, claiming that for the first time in American history, the federal government would be sanctioning the destruction of human life for research purposes.

The claim about the status of embryos I've called View C is compatible with the HHS decision that stem cells aren't embryos and are thus morally legitimate subjects of research. But those holding C object to the guidelines on the grounds that they tacitly sanction the destruction of embryos and even promote it by creating a "market" for stem cells. Also, because it's morally wrong to destroy embryos, those who encourage it are complicitous in it and thus deserving of blame.

The issue of supporting stem-cell research with public money shows every sign of remaining a flashpoint of controversy. Just as the abortion issue is not likely to disappear from our society's social and legal agenda, neither is the stem-cell issue.

MOVING ROADBLOCKS

View C, the notion that an embryo has the same moral status as a person, is the source of the pressure to restrict stem-cell research. To move toward settling the issue of pursuing the research with federal funding requires addressing C directly. Three sorts of responses to C are relevant:

1. Showing by argument that C is mistaken;
2. Showing that respecting those holding C doesn't require accepting C as a basis for public policy;
3. Finding a way of achieving the aims of embryonic stem-cell research without destroying embryonic stem cells.

I'll address each response separately.

Flaw? Theologians, Catholic and otherwise, don't claim their view of embryos rests on faith or divine revelation. They hold, rather, that it can be established by rational argument. I consider it important, therefore, to call attention to a flaw in the argument most often used to establish the claim that a human embryo is the moral equivalent of a person.

The argument is put most succinctly by the jurist John T. Noonan:

> The positive argument for conception as the decisive moment of
> humanization is that at conception the new being receives the genetic
> code . . . A being with the human genetic code is man.

"Man" has a serious claim (right) to life; thus, the embryo, a being with the human genetic code, has a serious claim to life.

The same argument lies behind this statement of the Pontifical Academy: "The living human embryo is—from the moment of the union of the gametes—a *human subject.* . . . From this it follows that as a *human individual* it has the *right* to its own life . . ."

The error in all formulations of this argument is the implicit assumption that being human in the biological sense (being a human embryo or possessing the human genetic code) is equivalent to being human in the moral sense.

Ethicists use the phrase "person in the moral sense" to refer to beings entitled to full moral consideration. Aliens from Tau Ceti might be completely different from humans biologically, yet possess characteristics (such as rationality) entitling them to the moral treatment we accord humans. We might sensibly ask whether a computer like HAL in Stanley Kubrick's *2001: A Space Odyssey* is a person in the moral sense and so entitled to moral treatment.

Consider a parallel case. The knowledge that something is a bear doesn't establish, by itself, that the animal is or isn't a person in the moral sense. We need to be told what it takes to qualify to be a person. The criteria need to be spelled out for us, then we need to be shown that a bear either does or doesn't satisfy them.

The argument by Noonan and the Pontifical Academy begs the question of whether a human embryo is a person in the moral sense. This results from the ambiguous use of "person," "humanized," "human person," and "man." The biological information that an embryo is a human embryo doesn't automatically establish that it's a person in the moral sense and thus deserving of moral treatment.

We are owed a second argument, one that spells out criteria for being a person (in the moral sense) and demonstrates that a human embryo satisfies them. We aren't free to give biological answers to moral questions in talking about human embryos any more than we are when talking about bear embryos.

POLICY

Those holding C are serious in regarding the destruction of embryos as the moral equivalent of killing innocent people. I (along with millions of others) believe this view is mistaken, although I don't consider those who hold it to be deluded or duped. The status of the human embryo (like the status of the fetus or HAL) is a matter about which reasonable people can disagree.

We are bound to respect individuals in a pluralistic, democratic society, even when we disagree with them. Respecting them means (in part) not forcing them to renounce their beliefs, not requiring them to be "re-educated" to induce them to change their beliefs, and granting them the freedom to advocate their beliefs and criticize the beliefs of others.

But respecting people doesn't mean we as a society are obliged to adopt their beliefs as a basis for public policy. When the matter at issue is one about which reasonable people can differ and facts alone cannot settle the dispute, we aren't obliged to adopt the view of the minority. Indeed, in such a situation, the view of the majority should prevail.

Those holding C think C should prevail because they believe it is right. They charge that those favoring embryonic stem-cell research support it only because they're motivated by the prospect of securing useful knowledge. Hence, acts of killing (critics say) are countenanced for the sake of a utilitarian aim.

But what holders of C fail to appreciate is that the rest of the world considers C to be wrong. The aim of stem-cell research is definitely utilitarian, but it's an aim we can pursue without causing any significant moral harm. Even though those who accept C hold their view as a matter of conscience, we aren't bound to set aside the general interest of society to satisfy either their conscience or their conception of what is right.

Regenerative medicine promises to bring enormous benefits to our society, but its development depends on perfecting stem-cell engineering. Most of society doesn't consider destroying embryos to resemble killing people in the slightest, much less as equivalent to it. Thus, most of us consider the development of a regenerative medicine that can relieve suffering and save lives to be a purpose sufficiently serious to warrant the destruction of human embryos.

The moral principle that "It's wrong to kill an innocent person" is violated, only if one accepts view C. I've suggested C is wrong, but even if a segment of the population believes it's correct, we don't have to be bound by their decision. In framing policies regulating biomedical research, we need not tie the hands of investigators by forbidding them to destroy human embryos in their work.

A FINESSE?

Is it possible to go forward with stem cell research in a way compatible with C? We could, if so, avoid a confrontation sure to leave a large number of people disturbed and angry.

One possibility is to restrict research to *adult* stem cells. The Pontifical Academy endorses this approach, describing it as representing "a more reasonable and humane method for making correct and sound progress in this new field of research and the therapeutic applications which it promises."

Adult stem cells may indeed offer more possibilities than scientists had first believed. A research group headed by Marc Hedrick presented results in the April 2001 issue of *Tissue Engineering* showing that stem cells could be extracted from body fat and induced to grow different tissues. Depending on what factors were added to the culture medium, the cells were capable of turning into muscle, bone, or cartilage.

Adult stem cells, as earlier work had also shown, seem able to produce a variety of tissue types. Does this mean that, using the right growth factors, any adult stem cell can be made to produce *any* type of tissue? No one knows.

We also don't know much about the possibilities of embryonic stem cells. The only way we can get the information we need to compare the potential powers of adult and embryonic stem cells is to continue research using both. Staking all our therapeutic hopes on adult stem cells on the basis of what we know now is premature.

A second possibility (of avoiding confrontation with C) is to focus research on embryonic stem cells isolated from germline cells recovered from the reproductive tissue of aborted fetuses. If an abortion occurred spontaneously, holders of C have no grounds for objecting to research using the stem cells.

This is the one exception to the general condemnation of embryonic stem-cell research by the National Conference of Catholic Bishops. No embryos are created or destroyed, no abortion is performed, so the stem cells are morally clean.

(But even so you can't please everybody. Some holders of C object that using fetal material is unacceptable, because it would encourage intentional abortions.)

Two considerations limit this possibility. First, stem cells obtained from embryos appear to be identical with those from germline cells, but it may be too soon to declare them identical. At least some additional research is needed to be sure.

Second, acquiring stem cells from embryonic tissue is time-consuming and expensive. Acquiring them from embryos is fast and cheap. Spending the extra time will lengthen the delay in developing treatments, and spending the extra money will restrict the amount of research that can be done.

Whether both these costs are worth paying to accommodate the beliefs of those who accept C is a matter for public discussion. But a discussion is appropriate only after we have compelling evidence that stem cells from both sources are essentially identical. The second possibility, then, isn't at the moment an acceptable one.

The third possibility is to find a new source for pluripotent stem cells. If neither embryos nor fetal tissue was their source, those holding C would have no ground for opposing stem-cell research.

Maybe there is a third source. John Haines, in April 2001, announced that his company, Anthrogenesis Corporation, had succeeded in extracting from human placentas cells it called placental multipotent stem cells. Anthrogenesis scientists believe some of the inner-cell-mass cells of the blastocyst migrate to the placenta, as well as to the ovaries and testis of fetal tissue. No evidence supporting this belief has been offered at this time, however.

The Anthrogenesis scientists have also not demonstrated that the stem cells they isolated are capable of developing into the full range of cells making up the human body. If the placental cells aren't pluripotent, they are likely only adult stem cells, not embryonic stem cells.

If the cells turn out to be embryonic stem cells, those holding C can accept stem-cell research, so long as the cells come from the placenta. But until that time, we must go forward with research using embryonic stem cells. Otherwise, we won't know enough to say whether they possess properties different from those of stem cells from other sources.

The way matters stand, the development of stem-cell engineering requires research on stem cells acquired from embryos. This isn't necessarily the way things will always be, but it's the way they must be for now.

Obligation

What distinguishes the biomedical sciences from pure biology is their implicit commitment to the instrumental goal of gaining knowledge for the purpose of controlling diseases.

The biomedical sciences don't want simply to understand the way the human body works, the way disease occurs, and what happens to it if medicines are given. These questions aren't disinterested or pure. The knowledge sought is *instrumental*, and the reason for seeking it is to use it to control disease. The control may take the form of prevention, treatment, cure, or even elimination.

Regenerative medicine, based on stem-cell engineering, holds the promise of being the most powerful form of disease control the world has ever known. It has the potential (among others) to cure diseases like Parkinson's (for which treatments are ultimately ineffective), diabetes (for which they are effective but imperfect), and Huntington's (for which treatments are nonexistent).

Regenerative medicine, prospectively, has the power to manage effectively, or even cure, virtually every non-infectious disease and disability.

Such a medicine has the potential power to make the blind see and the lame walk. Organs crippled or destroyed by disease could be replaced by ones as good as or better than new. Because they would be copies of the individual's own organs, rejection wouldn't be a problem. Transplant recipients would no longer have to make the devil's bargain of exchanging a life-threatening disease for a chronic disorder.

Transplantation, in the world of regenerative medicine, would advance from its current status as a second-rate (though valuable and effective) medical technology to one as elegant and effective as the prevention of smallpox by vaccination or the cure of wound infections by antibiotics.

Biomedicine's inherent commitment to finding a way to control disease, imposes on biomedical scientists a prima facia obligation to work toward the development of regenerative medicine. This means promoting and pursuing stem-cell research.

If we don't do this, the magic will never happen.

Acknowledgments

"He owes everybody but the post office," my father once said of one of his profligate friends.

That comes close to capturing my feeling about the number of debts I've acquired in writing this book. Physicians, surgeons, social workers, nurses, and scientists, some total strangers, went out of their way to help me. They found time in their overscheduled lives to meet with me, read drafts of chapters, and supply information, advice, and encouragement. Patients and their families also talked with me, sharing their experiences, even though for them the times were often marked by stress, doubt, and fear.

So many people have done me favors I can't acknowledge them all. But I'll mention the few who did the most to shape this book into its final form.

I'm grateful to Kirk Jensen, my editor, for daring to take a chance on a book that departs sharply from the academic format. (How many books contain detailed cases? How many use fiction to raise issues?) Also, his criticisms were perceptive and his suggestions to the point. I appreciate his patience as well. (But then, the book is hardly more than a year late.)

Edward L. Trimble, M.D., a friend of many years, was kind enough to arrange a visiting appointment for me at Johns Hopkins University School of Medicine, where he is on the faculty. I appreciate the unfailing courtesy and helpfulness of the physicians, staff, and patients of Johns Hopkins Hospital. I learned from them all, and I'm particularly grateful to cardiac transplant surgeon Scott Stuart, M.D., for his time.

Jeffrey Lowell, M.D., a transplant surgeon and member of the faculty at Washington University School of Medicine, did much to educate me and improve this book. He arranged for me to attend meetings of a committee evaluating transplant candidates and to talk with recipients. He also read in manuscript more than half the chapters and made detailed comments on them.

Sondra Schlesinger, Ph.D., a virologist and also a member of the faculty of the Washington University School of Medicine, did me the favor of reading my chapters on xenotransplantation and stem cells. She not only kept me from making several factual errors, she led me to rethink and revise my position.

These readers, all of them experts, saved me from a number of blunders, but the remaining ones (whatever they may be) I claim for myself alone. Also, if I didn't always take the advice I was offered, the resulting flaws are my own fault.

My friend Christopher Hoffman, Ph.D., J.D., read drafts of most of the chapters and made a variety of useful suggestions, some of which I actually took. My colleague Thaddeus Metz talked over the ethical issues about stem cells with me and helped me improve my argument. Piers Rawling, another colleague, encouraged me to put into practice my plan of taking a case-based approach to discussing transplant issues.

I also have an institutional debt. During some of the time I worked on this book I was supported by a grant from the University of Missouri Research Board. I'm grateful for the opportunity the grant gave me.

My greatest debt, as has been true for years, is to Miriam Munson. She was my first reader and most gentle critic. Yet her kindness did not extend to my prose. She convinced me to excise large chunks of turgid verbiage, helped make lame sentences run, and demanded I meet a high standard of clarity in both expression and structure. When the reading is easy, thank her, and when it's not, blame me.

I don't think I owe anything to the post office. But should I mention UPS and FedEx?

RONALD MUNSON
University of Missouri-St. Louis
munson@umsl.edu

Notes and References

CHAPTER I: A MODERN LAZARUS

Note Robby Benson, Marge, and the staff and surgeons at Osler are based on real people. But facts about other people and other circumstances have also been folded into this account. Osler Hospital is also a composite, and the dialogue is based on reconstruction, rather than quotation.

Greene, A.C., *Taking Heart*. New York: Simon & Schuster, 1990. A personal account of what it's like to be in heart failure, then get a transplant.

Oz, M., *Healing From the Heart*. New York: Dutton, 1998. Oz is concerned with "complementary medicine," but I am indebted to his discussion of implanting an LVAD and its importance in extending life.

Pizer, H.F., *Organ Transplants: A Patient's Guide*. Cambridge, MA: Harvard University Press, 1991. Information about drugs and what to expect.

Siebert, C., "Carol Palumbo Waits for Her Heart," *New York Times Magazine*, 18 April, 1997, pp. 40–45, 74–81. Siebert's account of the conflict between "organ harvesting" teams is unparalleled; I've followed his sequence of operative events.

United Network for Organ Sharing (UNOS) website, www.unos.org. Statistics on the need and availability of organs, waiting-lists, donors, survival times, and much else can be found here. I have used UNOS statistics throughout the book, unless otherwise noted.

CHAPTERS 2–3: MICKEY MANTLE'S LIVER

Note Mickey Mantle, Jr., died in Dallas on December 20, 2000 from complications of cancer. Two years earlier he had surgery to remove a skin cancer on his neck.

Alexander, S. "They Decide Who Lives, Who Dies," *Life Magazine*, 1962. Reprinted in R. Hunt and J. Arras, *Ethical Issues in Modern Medicine*. Palo Alto, CA: Mayfield, 1977, pp. 409–424. An account of the first attempt in the U.S. to ration access to a life-saving therapy.

Altman, L. K., "Death of a Hero: Mantle's Cancer Most Aggressive His Doctors Had Seen," *New York Times*, 14 August, 1995.

———, "Defending Tough Decisions in a Case Open to Hindsight," *New York Times*, 15 August, 1995.

American Medical Association, Council on Ethical and Judicial Affairs, "Ethical Considerations in the Allocation of Organs and Other Scarce Medical Resources Among Patients," *Archives of Internal Medicine*, 1995, 155: 29–40.

Associated Press, "New Liver Woes for Mantle," 23 June, 1995.

Ballingrud, D., "Debating Who Deserves a Transplant," *St. Petersburg Times*, 8 June, 1995.

Brody, J., "Questions Are Raised on Mantle Transplant," *New York Times*, 2 August, 1995.

Campbell, D.A., et al., "One Center's Experience With Liver Transplantation: Alcohol Use Relapse Over the Long Term," *American Association for the Study of Liver Disease and the International Liver Transplantation Society, Supplement*, 1997, 4: 58–64.

Cohen, C., Benjamin, M., and the Ethics and Social Impact Committee of the Transplant and Health Policy Center, Ann Arbor, Michigan, "Alcoholics and Liver Transplantation," *JAMA*, 1991, 265: 1299–1301.

Courier-Journal (Louisville, KY), "Readers Forum: Special Treatment?," 16 June, 1995.

Dallas Morning News, "A Hero in Death: Mantle Organ Donor Helped Save Six Lives," 7 August, 1995.

DeMaria, N., Colantoni A., and Van Thiel, D., "Liver Transplantation for Alcoholic Liver Disease," *Hepato-Gastroenterology*, 1998, 45: 1364–1368. See p. 1364 for the definition of alcoholism.

Fabrega, E., Crespo, E., J., et al., "Alcoholic Recidivism After Liver Transplantation for Alcoholic Cirrhosis," *Journal of Clinical Gastroenterology*, 1998, 26: 204–206. Presents evidence to show recidivism does not affect compliance.

Foster, P.F., et al., "Prediction of Abstinence From Ethanol in Alcoholic Recipients Following Liver Transplantation," *Hepatology*, 1995, 25: 1469–1477.

Glannon, W., "Responsibility, Alcoholism, and Liver Transplantation," *Journal of Medicine and Philosophy*, 1998, 23: 31–49.

Goodstein, L., "Crying Foul Over Mantle: Liver Transplant Sparks Ethics, Alcoholism Debate," *Washington Post*, 10 June, 1995.

Kolata, G., "Getting on Transplant List is the First of Many Hurdles," *New York Times*, 10 June, 1995.

———, "Transplants, Morality and Mickey," *New York Times*, 11 June, 1995. Arthur Caplan and Mark Siegler on Mantle and alcoholism.

Lucey, M.R., "Alcohol Use After Liver Transplantation in Alcoholics: A Clinical Cohort Follow-Up Study," *Hepatology*, 1997, 25: 1223–1226. Evidence presented to show alcohol use and liver damage is unusual in the first five post-transplant years.

Mantle, M., et al., with Herskowitz, M., *A Hero All His Life*. New York: Harper-Collins, 1996. Part I, "Extra Innings" (pp. 1–33), consists of Mantle's reflections on his alcoholism. Most of the biographical information used here comes from this source.

McCartney, S., *Defying the Gods: Inside the New Frontiers of Organ Transplants*. New York: Macmillan, 1994. An account of the liver transplant program at Baylor on which I have based the one presented here.

McKenna, M.A.J., "Some Exploit Edge in Organ Shopping," *Atlanta Journal and Constitution*, 9 June, 1995.

———, "Mantle's Prognosis Intensifies Debate About Transplants," *Atlanta Journal and Constitution*, 2 August, 1995. Annas, Banja, and Caplan are quoted as skeptical about transplanting patients with liver cancer.

Moss, A.H., and Siegler, M., "Should Alcoholics Compete Equally for Liver Transplantation?" *JAMA*, 1991, 265: 1295–1298. No, the authors argue.

Myerson, A., "Mantle Has Liver Cancer, Needs Treatment," *New York Times*, 8 June, 1995.

———, "Cancer from Mantle's Liver Spreads to Right Lung," *New York Times*, 2 August, 1995.

———, "Mantle Worsens as His Cancer Spreads," *New York Times*, 10 August, 1995.

———, "Mantle's Last Medical Bills," *New York Times*, 20 August, 1995.

Newman, J., UNOS Assistant Director of Communications, personal communication in e-mail from UNOS, 29 June, 2000.

Pageaux, G-P, Michael, J., et al., "Alcoholic Cirrhosis Is a Good Indication for Liver Transplantation, Even for Cases of Recidivism," *Gut: An International Journal of Gastroenterology and Hepatology*, 1999, 45: 421–426. Statistics cited about alcoholics are from this study.

Sullivan, P., and Laslander, M., "Experts: No Favoritism for Yankee Great's Transplant," *Boston Herald*, 9 June, 1995.

Trafford, A., "Mickey Mantle: Tough Call," *Washington Post*, 8 August, 1995.

———, "What's Fair in Transplants?," *Washington Post*, 21 January, 1997.

Ubel, P., "Transplantation in Alcoholics: Separating Prognosis and Responsibility From Social Bias," *Liver Transplantation and Surgery*, 1997, 3: 343–346.

United Network for Organ Sharing, "UNOS Position Statement on Mickey Mantle's Transplant," issued in Richmond, VA, no date (first quoted in newspapers 9 June, 1995).

Washington Post, "Letters: Mickey Mantle, Tough Call," 29 August, 1995.

CHAPTER 4: THAT OTHERS MAY LIVE

Note The story of the Howards and their daughter Claire is based on the case of Baby Gabrielle.

American Medical Association, Council on Ethical and Judicial Affairs, "The Use of Anencephalic Neonates as Organ Donors," *Journal of the American Medical Association*, 1995, 273: 1614–1618. The AMA's initial position.

———, "Reconsideration of AMA Opinion on Anencephalic Neonates as Organ Donors," *Journal of the American Medical Association*, 1996, 275: 443–444. The Council decides to suspend its original opinion.

Associated Press, "Brain-Dead Baby Allowed to Die; No Recipients Found for Organs," 22 February, 1988. Baby John was the first anencephalic infant put on life support under the Loma Linda protocol. When he was declared brain dead after seven days, his liver was refused as unusable by four transplant surgeons; a blood-type match for his heart wasn't located.

Blakeslee, S., "A Baby Born Without Her Brain is Kept Alive to Donate Her Heart," *New York Times*, 19 October, 1987. Baby Gabrielle case.

———, "New Attention Focused on Infant Organ Donors," *New York Times*,

14 December, 1987. Baby Gabrielle case; case of the child of Brenda and
Michael Winner, who wanted their child to be kept on life support until organ
recipients could be located. Only Loma Linda agreed.

————, "No Infants Found for Baby's Organs," *New York Times*, 20 February, 1988.

————, "Infant Transplant Program is Halted to Reassess Issues," *New York
Times*, 19 August, 1988. Closing of the Loma Linda program.

Ethics and Impact Committee, Transplant Policy Center, Ann Arbor, MI
(M. Benjamin, Chair), "Anencephalic Infants as Sources of Transplantable
Organs," *Hastings Center Report*, October/November, 1988, pp. 28–30.

Ferguson, M., "Anencephalic Infants as Organ Donors," *Journal of the American
Medical Association*, 1995, 274: 1786–1787. Argues that because so few people
(estimated at 100 or so) would be helped, the debate is a distraction.

Fost, N., "Organs from Anencephalic Infants: An Idea Whose Time Has Not Yet
Come," *Hastings Center Report*, October/November, 1988, pp. 5–10.

Gorman, C., "A Balancing Act of Life and Death," *Time*, 1 February 1988, p. 49.
Baby Gabrielle and the Loma Linda program.

Kolata, G., "Doomed Babies Are Seen as the Donors of Organs," *New York Times*,
24 May, 1995. Responses to the June 1995 AMA's Council on Ethical and
Judicial Affairs position that anencephalic infants need not be declared dead
to become donors.

Loma Linda University's Protocol Committee, "Modified Medical Management
of Anencephalic Infants for Organ Donation," *BioLaw*, January, 1988, 2:
763–769.

Reuters, "Baby to Be Born as Organ Donor," 9 December, 1987. The child of
Brenda and Michael Winner is accepted into the Loma Linda program.

Shewman, D.A., "Anencephaly: Selected Medical Aspects," *Hastings Center
Report*, October/November, 1988, pp. 11–18.

————, Capron, A.M., Warwick, L.B., Peacock, J., and Schulman, B.L., "The Use
Of Anencephalic Infants as Organ Sources," *Journal of the American Medical
Association*, March, 1989, 26: 1773–1781. Statistics on anencephalics; estimates
that the number of donors would be small, and criticism of proposed revision
of guidelines to permit donors; report on infants under Loma Linda protocol;
Joyce Peabody quoted.

Volpe, J.J., "Brain Death Determination in the Newborn," *Pediatrics*, August,
1987, 80: 293–297.

Walters, J.W., "Loma Linda University's Protocol on Anencephalic Infants as Organ
Donors," *Hastings Center Report*, October/November, 1988, pp. 222–223.

Walters, J.W., and Ashwal, S., "Organ Prolongation in Anencephalic Infants:
Ethical and Medical Issues," *Hastings Center Report*, October/November, 1998,
pp. 19–27. Walters was Chair of the Protocol Committee, January 1986–February 1988. A history of changes in the protocol, as well as data about Leonard
Bailey's transplantation of the heart from Baby Gabrielle into Paul Holc.

Task Force on Brain Death in Children, "Guidelines for the Determination of Brain
Death in Children," *Pediatrics*, August, 1987, 80: 298–300.

CHAPTER 5: KIDNEY FOR SALE

Note The account of the illegal kidney sale is fictional. Annas, G.J., "Life, Liberty,
and Pursuit of Organ Sales," *Hastings Center Report*, February, 1984, pp. 22–23.

Banks, G.J., "Legal and Ethical Safeguards: Protection of Society's Most Vulnerable Participants in a Commercialized Organ Transplantation System," *American Journal of Law and Medicine*, Spring, 1995, 21: 45–110. See pp. 79–81 for a discussion of the "Living Provider Organ Market."

Justice B. Cardoza, Schloendorff v. Society of New York Hospital, 105 N.E. 92, 93, NY, 1914.

Denise, S.H., "Regulating the Sale of Human Organs," *Virginia Law Review*, 1985, 71: 1015–1037. Contains a discussion of Jacobs and his Congressional testimony.

Dinman, B.D., "The Reality and Acceptance of Risk," *JAMA*, 1980, 244: 1226. Statistics on risks of various activities.

Donelly, P.K., et al., "Transplants From Living Donors in the United Kingdom and Ireland: A Centre Survey," *British Medical Journal*, 25 February 1989, 298: 490–493.

Evans, M., "Organ Donation Should Not be Restricted to Relatives," *Journal of Medical Ethics*, 1989, 15: 15–20.

Ganley, P.P., "Living Related Liver Transplantation (LRLT) in Children: Focus on Issues," *Pediatric Nursing*, December, 1995, 21: 523–525.

Gore, A., quoted in D. Lamb, *Organ Transplants and Ethics*, p. 134.

Grouven, U., et al., "Kidney Transplantation From Cadaveric Donors Versus Living Related Donors: Improved Results in the Cyclosporine Era," *Clinical Investigator*, 1993, 71: 621.

Haberal, M., et al., "Living Unrelated Donor Kidney Transplantation Between Spouses," *World Journal of Surgery*, 1992, 16: 1183–1187.

Kass, M., "Organs for Sale? Propriety, Property, and the Price of Progress," *Public Interest*, Spring, 1992, 107: 65–86.

Kinsley, M., "Take My Kidney, Please," *Time*, 13 March, 1989, p. 88.

Kleinman, I., "Ethical Considerations in Living Organ Donation and a New Approach," *Archives of Internal Medicine*, 1992, 152: 1484–1488.

Lamb, D., *Organ Transplants and Ethics*, pp. 134–135. London: Routledge, 1990. Discusses the Jacobs case; quotes the freelance ads and Albert Gore.

Laskow, D.A., et al., "Analysis of 22 Years Experience in Living-Related Transplantation at the University of Alabama in Birmingham," in *Clinical Transplants*, ed. P. Terasaki, pp. 179–191. Los Angeles: UCLA Tissue Typing Laboratory, 1991.

Levey, A.S., Hou, S., Bush, H.L., Jr., "Kidney Transplantation From Unrelated Living Donors: Time to Reclaim a Discarded Opportunity," *New England Journal of Medicine*, 3 April, 1986, 314: 914–916.

Mavrodes, G., "The Morality of Selling Human Organs," *Ethics, Humanism, and Medicine*, 1980, pp. 133–139. New York: Alan R. Liss.

McMaster, P., and Mirza, D.F., "Use of Live Organ Donation: A Necessary Evil," *Transplantation Proceedings*, 1995, 27: 103–105.

Murray, T.H., "The Gift of Life Must Always Remain a Gift," *Discover*, March, 1986, pp. 90–92.

Najarian, J.S., et al., "Twenty Years or More of Follow-Up of Living Kidney Donors," *Lancet*, 1992, 340: 807–810.

Park, K., et al., "A 16-Year Experience With 1275 Primary Living Donor Kidney Transplants: Univariate and Multivariate Analysis and Risk Factors Affecting Graft Survival," *Transplantation Proceedings*, June, 1996, 28: 1578–1579.

Price, D., "The Texture and Content of Living Donor Transplant Laws and Policies," *Transplantation Proceedings*, February, 1996, 28: 378–379.

Radcliffe-Richards, J., et al., "The Case for Allowing Kidney Sales," *Lancet*, 27 June, 1998, 352: 1950–1952.

Rhoads, S.E., "The Sale of Human Body Parts," *Michigan Law Review*, 1974, 72: 1182–1264. See pp. 1219–1220, in particular.

Ross, L.F., Rubin, D.T., et al., "Ethics of a Paired-Kidney-Exchange Program," *New England Journal of Medicine*, 12 June, 1997, 336: 1752–1755.

Seitel, A., "Life Insurance for Kidney Donors: An Update," *Transplantation*, 1988, 45: 819–820.

Sutherland, D.E.R., "Living Related Donors Should Be Used Whenever Possible," *Transplantation Proceedings*, February, 1985, 17: 1503–1509. Statistics on mortality and risks of living donors.

———, "A Positive View of Living Donors for Transplantation," *Clinical Transplants*, 1994, 15: 364–365. Statistics on mortality and risks of living donors.

Terasaki, P.A., et al., "High Survival Rates of Kidney Transplants from Spousal and Living Unrelated Donors," *New England Journal of Medicine*, August 10, 1995, 333: 333–336. Survival rates higher with kidneys from living donors.

Terasaki P., et al., "Organizing a Living Donor Pool: Could the Concept Work?" *Nephrology News and Issues*, February, 1996, 10: 37–38.

Williams, S., et al., "Long-Term Renal Function in Kidney Donors: A Comparison of Donors and Their Siblings," *Annals of Internal Medicine*, 1986, 106: 1–8.

CHAPTER 6: DONORS OF LAST RESORT

American Medical Association, Council on Ethical and Judicial Affairs, "The Use of Minors as Organ and Tissue Donors," *Code of Medical Ethics: Current Opinions with Annotations*, 1996–1997 Edition, pp. 34–36.

Curran, W.J., "A Problem of Consent: Kidney Transplantation in Minors," *New York University Law Review*, May, 1959, 34: 890–898. Quotes from the Marsden decision.

Dwyer, J., and Vig, E., "Rethinking Transplantation Between Siblings," *Hastings Center Report*, September-October, 1995, 25: 7–12.

Fox, R.C., and Swazey, J.P., *The Courage to Fail: A Social View of Organ Transplants and Dialysis*, 2nd Ed. Rev. Chicago: University of Chicago Press, 1978.

Kramer, M.R., and Sprung, C.L., "Living Related Donations in Lung Transplantations," *Archives of Internal Medicine*, 15 September, 1995, 155: 1734–1738.

Moore, F.D., *Transplant: The Give and Take of Tissue Transplantation*. New York: Simon & Schuster, 1972. A historical and scientific account of transplantation by a pioneer in the field, with special attention to the Brigham's patients.

Pescinski. *In Re Guardianship of Pescinski*, 67 WI 2nd 4, 226 NW 2nd (180), 1975. Day quotations on pp. 183–184.

Ross, L.F., "Moral Grounding for the Participation of Children as Organ Donors," *Journal of Law, Medicine, and Ethics* Summer, 1993, 21: 251–257.

Saikewicz, *Superintendent of Belchertown State School, et al. v. Saikewicz*, 370 NE 2d 417 (MA), 1977.

Singer, P. A., Siegler, M., et al., "Ethics of Liver Transplantation with Living Donors," *New England Journal of Medicine*, 31 August, 1989, 321: 620–622.

Starzl, T.E., "Will Live Organ Donations No Longer be Justified?" *Hastings Center Report* April, 1985, 15: 5.

Strunk v. Strunk, 445 S.W.2nd 145 (KY), 26 September, 1969. The quotation of the court opinion is from p. 146.

Sutherland, D.E.R., "A Positive View of Living Donors for Transplantation," *Clinical Transplantation*, 1994, pp. 364–365. Statistics on operative mortality and survival probability of live kidney donors.

Sutherland, D.E.R., Goetz, F.C., and Najarian, J. S., "Pancreas Transplants from Related Donors," *Transplantation*, 1984, 38: 625–633.

Terasaki, P., et al., "High Survival Rates of Kidney Transplants from Spousal and Living Unrelated Donors," *New England Journal of Medicine*, 10 August, 1995, 333: 333–336.

Warshofky, F., *The Rebuilt Man*. New York: Crowell, 1965. See pp. 162–163 for circumstances surrounding the Marsden case.

Williams, R. W., "Consent for Children as Organ Donors," *Hawaii Medical Journal*, April, 1995, 54: 498–500.

CHAPTER 7: KUROSAWA IN CALIFORNIA

Note In a segment of the ABC News program *Turning Point* entitled "Animal Transplants: Madness or Miracle," broadcast in 1997, Teresa Trefagin identified herself as the mother of Baby Fae.

Note The articles by Lawrence K. Altman and Dennis Breo provide the most details about the events and people in this case, and I have drawn upon them in my account.

Adler, J., with Huck, J., and McAlvey, P., "Baby Fae's Heart Gives Out," *Newsweek,* 26 November, 1984, p. 94.

Altman, L.K. "Baboon's Heart Implanted in Infant on Coast," *New York Times*, 28 October, 1984.

———, "Doctors Say Baby with Baboon Heart Is Doing 'Remarkably Well,'" *New York Times*, 29 October, 1984.

———, "Baby with Baboon Heart Better; Surgeons Defend the Experiment," *New York Times*, 30 October, 1984.

———, "Survival Record Is Set by Heart-Implant Baby," *New York Times*, 31 October, 1984.

———, "Cuddling and Hugging Is Parents' Medicine for Thriving Baby Fae," *New York Times*, 1 November, 1984.

———, "Baby Fae Continues to Thrive After 6 Days with Baboon's Heart," *New York Times*, 2 November, 1984.

———, "Baby Fae Was Taken Home to Die Before Surgery," *New York Times*, 3 November, 1984.

———, "Hospital Staff Hears Sermon Hailing Heart-Transplant Baby," *New York Times*, 4 November, 1984.

———, "Confusion Surrounds Baby Fae," *New York Times*, 6 November, 1984.

———, "Baby Fae's Mother Asks Privacy and Repeats Support of Surgery," *New York Times*, 9 November, 1984.

———, "Baboon Transplant Tests Described," *New York Times*, 11 November, 1984.

———, "Baby Fae Put Back on Respirator: Heart and Kidneys Begin to Fail," *New York Times*, 14 November, 1984.

———, "Baby Fae Rallying with 2 New Drugs," *New York Times*, 15 November, 1984.

———, "Baby Fae, Who Received a Heart from Baboon, Dies after 20 Days," *New York Times*, 16 November, 1984.

———, "Baby Fae Dies, but Doctor Sees Gain for Science," *New York Times*, 17 November, 1984.

———, "Learning from Baby Fae," *New York Times*, 18 November, 1984.

———, "The Doctor's World: Surgeon Still Dreams of Baboon Heart for Babies," *New York Times*, 15 December, 1987.

Annas, G.J. "Baby Fae: the 'Anything Goes' School of Human Experimentation," *Hastings Center Report*, 1985, 15: 15–17.

Armstrong, S., "Baby Fae Case Raises Tough Issues," *Christian Science Monitor*, 6 November, 1984.

Associated Press, "Human Heart Not Sought for Baby Fae," 29 October, 1984.

———, "Baby Fae Is Eating Well 9 Days After Transplant," 5 November, 1984.

———, "Baby Fae Requires Additional Drugs: Her System Tries Harder to Reject Baboon Heart," 13 November, 1984.

———, "Baby Fae's Parents Were Sure of Baboon Heart Transplant," 24 November, 1984.

———, "Baby Fae's Parents Say They Wanted Surgery," 27 November, 1984.

Bailey, L.L., Nehlsen-Cannarella, S.L., et al., "Baboon to Human Cardiac Xeno-transplantation in a Neonate," *JAMA*, 20 December, 1985, 254: 3321–3329.

Bazell, R., "Hearts of Gold," *New Republic*, 18 February, 1985, pp. 17–20.

Begley, S., with Gosnell, M., "Crossing the Barrier," *Newsweek*, 12 November, 1984, p. 116.

Berg, M.V., "Baby Fae Doctor Says Baboon Heart Case Enhanced Education," *New York Times*, 5 April, 1987.

Boffey, P.M. "Baby Fae Appears Well After First Sign of Rejecting Baboon Heart," *New York Times*, 12 November, 1984.

———, "Medicine Under Scrutiny," *New York Times*, 20 November, 1984.

Breo, D., "Baby Fae," in *Extraordinary Care*, pp. 212–232. Chicago: Chicago Review Press, 1986. Reprints of Breo's articles from *Medical World News*.

———, "Two Surgeons Who Dared Are Still Chasing Their Dreams," *JAMA*, 24 November, 1989, 262: 2904–2916. Leonard Bailey and William DeVries, the surgeons who implanted the first artificial heart into Barney Clark.

Caplan, A. L. "Ethical Issues Raised by Research Involving Xenografts," *JAMA*, 1985, 254: 3339–3343.

Capron, A. M., "When Well-Meaning Science Goes Too Far," *Hastings Center Report*, 1985, 15: 8–9.

Clark, M., with McAlevey, P., and Sandza, R., "A Baby Gets a Baboon's Heart," *Newsweek*, 5 November, 1984, p. 72.

Clark, M., with Huck, J., et al., "A Breakthrough Transplant?" *Newsweek*, 12 November, 1984, p. 114.

Colen, B.D., "'Miracles' May Leave More Victims Than Heroes," *Los Angeles Times*, 11 December, 1989.

Cummings, J., "Memorial Service Held for Baby Fae," *New York Times*, 18 November, 1984.

Dalton, R., "Animal-Rights Issue Heats Up: As Researchers Agonize, Activists Get Beastly," *San Diego Union-Tribune*, 25 November, 1984.

Dart, J., "Baby Fae's Legacy: High Hope and a Quiet Hero," *Los Angeles Times*, 6 July, 1985.

Dommel, W.F., et al., "Report of the National Institutes of Health Site Visit to Loma Linda University Medical Center for Purposes of Consultation and Review of Institutional Review Board Procedures in Connection with Cardiac Xenograft Transplantation Program," 5 March, 1985. Includes the consent document that Loma Linda never made public.

Eckholm, E., "Baby Death Laid to Wrong Blood Type in Baboon," *New York Times*, 17 October, 1985.

Goodman, E., "No More Baby Faes," *Washington Post*, 24 November, 1984.

Gore, A., Jr. "The Need for a New Partnership," *Hastings Center Report*, 1985, 15: 13.

Gregg, J., "Medical Science or Ghoulish Tinkering?" *San Diego Union-Tribune*, 30 October, 1984.

Hoover, E., "Baby Fae: A Child Who Loved and Lost," *People*, 3 December, 1984, pp. 49–63; second part, 10 December, 1984, pp. 151–160. Some details about Baby Fae's parents and circumstances of the transplant are drawn from these interviews.

Hubbard, L.L. "The Baby Fae Case," *Medicine and Law*, 1987, 6: 385–396.

Jonasson, O., "The Case of Baby Fae," *JAMA*, 20 December, 1985, 254: 3358–3359.

Knoll, E., and Lundberg, G.D., "Informed Consent and Baby Fae," *JAMA*, 20 December, 1985, 254: 3359–3360.

Knox, R.A., "Xenografting: Cross-Species Transplant Researchers Make Strides," *Boston Globe*, 2 September, 1991.

Kushner, T., and Belliotti, R., "Baby Fae: A Beastly Business," *Journal of Medical Ethics*, 1985, 11: 178–183.

Losman, J.G., "The Research Road to Baby Fae and Beyond," *New York Times*, 27 November, 1984.

Macdonald, K., "2nd Baboon-Heart Transplant Eyed: Baby Fae Might Get Another If First Is Rejected," *Washington Post*, 2 November, 1984.

McCormick, R.A., "Was There Any Real Hope for Baby Fae?," *Hastings Center Report*, 1985, 15: 12–13.

Mathews, J., "Baboon Heart Transplant in Baby Defended," *Washington Post*, 29 October, 1984.

———, "Baby with Baboon's Heart Making Steady Progress: No Sign of Rejection as Survival Record Falls," *Washington Post*, 31 October, 1984.

———, "Doctors Cautious on Next Transplant: 'Baby Fae' Stable after Five Days with Baboon Heart," *Washington Post*, 1 November, 1984.

———, "More Rejection Crises Likely for Baby Fae: Lasting Damage to Infant a Possibility," *Washington Post*, 15 November, 1984.

———, "Baby with Baboon Heart Dies: Kidneys Fail 20 Days after Fae's Transplant," *Washington Post*, 16 November, 1984.

———, "Surgeon Hails Infant's Legacy," *Washington Post*, 17 November, 1984.

———, "Head Nurse Shares Memories of Fae: 2000 Gather at Church to Honor Infant and Parents," *Washington Post*, 18 November, 1984.

———, "Infant Survivor of Heart-Repair Operation Overcame Long Odds," *Washington Post*, 23 November, 1984.

———, "Baby Fae's Mother Says Options Explained Late," *Washington Post*, 27 November, 1984.

———, "Colleague Warned Doctor before Baby Fae Implant: More Research Urged on Procedure," *Washington Post*, 27 May, 1985.

The Nation, Editorial: "Baby Fae: A Life," 1 December, 1984, p. 571.

New York Times, Editorial: "The Baboon Heart and Baby Fae," 11 November, 1984.

———, Editorial: "The Life and Death of Baby Fae," 17 November, 1984.

"NIH Approves the Consent for Baby Fae, or Does It?" *Hastings Center Report*, April, 1985, 15: 2.

Preston, T.A., "Baby Fae: The Ethics of Medical Adventurism," *Washington Post*, 14 November, 1984.

———, "Baby Fae—What Does She Mean to Us?," *Medical World News*, 26 November, 1984, p. 84.

Rankin, D., "Personal Finance: The Staggering Cost of a Baby Fae," *New York Times*, 9 December, 1984.

Raspberry, W., "Baby Fae's Life," *Washington Post*, 31 October, 1984.

Redfern, M., "Why Baby Fae Never Stood a Chance," *New Scientist*, 29 November, 1984, p. 7.

Reemtsma, K., "Clinical Urgency and Media Scrutiny," *Hastings Center Report*, 1985, 15: 10–11.

Regan, T., "Use Animal Organs for Human Transplants?" *U.S. News & World Report*, 12 November, 1984, p. 58.

———, "The Other Victim," *Hastings Center Report*, 1985, 15: 9–10.

Richburg, K.B., "Baby Fae Shows 1st Signs of Rejecting Baboon Heart: Doctors Weigh New Transplant Alternatives," *Washington Post*, 12 November, 1984.

Russell, C., and Rensberger, B., "Baby Fae Case Leaves Tremors: Heart Specialists Find Fault with Transplant," *Washington Post*, 17 November, 1984.

Russell, C., with Mathews, J., "Lack of Scrutiny Fueled Baby Fae Controversy: Baboon-Heart Transplant Escaped Preview by National Warning Network," *Washington Post*, 18 November, 1984.

Schaefer, R.A., *Legacy: Daring to Care, the Legacy of Loma Linda*. Loma Linda, CA: Legacy Publishing, 1990.

Schwartz, H.S., "Bioethical and Legal Considerations in Increasing the Supply of Transplantable Organs: From UAGA to 'Baby Fae,'" *American Journal of Law and Medicine*, 1985, 10: 397–437.

Schwartz, J., "FDA Sets Animal-Human Transplant Guidelines: Rules Would Govern Variety of Therapies," *Washington Post*, 21 September, 1996.

Sheldon, R., "The IRB's Responsibility to Itself," *Hastings Center Report* 1985, 15: 11–12.

Silberner, J., "Postmortem in Baby Fae," *Science News*, 21 December, 1985, 128: 390.

Steinbrook, R., "Surgeon Tells of 'Catastrophic' Decision: Baby Fae's Death Traced to Blood Mismatch Error," *Los Angeles Times*, 16 October, 1985.

Sullivan, W., "Medical Experts Disagree on Merits of Baby's Baboon Heart Transplant," *New York Times*, 17 November, 1984.

Trachtman, L.E., "Why Tolerate the Statistical Victim?" *Hastings Center Report*, 1985, 15: 14.

United Press International, "Baby Fae's Parents Are Accepting Bids to Sell Their Story," 7 November, 1984.

Veatch, R.M., "The Ethics of Xenografts," *Transplantation Proceedings*, Supplement 2, 1986, 18: 93–97.

Wasowicz, L., "How Much Is Scientific Lesson Worth? Doctors Debate Baby Fae's Legacy," *Los Angeles Times*, 13 January, 1985.

CHAPTER 8: BUT ARE THEY REALLY DEAD?

Arnold, R.M., and Youngner, S.J., "The Dead Donor Rule," *Kennedy Institute of Ethics Journal*, 1993, 3: 263–278.

Arnold, R.M., Youngner, S.J., et al., eds. *Procuring Organs for Transplant: The Debate Over Non-Heart-Beating Cadaver Protocols*. Baltimore, MD: Johns Hopkins University Press, 1995.

Bernat, J.L., "A Defense of the Whole-Brain Concept of Death," *Hastings Center Report*, 1998, 28: 14–23.

Cole, D., "Statutory Definitions of Death and the Management of Terminally Ill Patients Who May Become Organ Donors After Death," in R.M. Arnold, et al., eds., *Procuring Organs for Transplant*, pp. 69–89.

DeVita, M.A., and Snyder, J.V., "Development of the University of Pittsburgh Medical Center Policy for the Care of Terminally Ill Patients Who May Become Organ Donors After Death Following the Removal of Life Support," *Kennedy Institute of Ethics Journal*, 1993, 3: 131–143.

————, "Reflections on Non-Heart-Beating Organ Donation: How Three Years of Experience Affects the University of Pittsburgh's Ethics Committee's Actions," *Cambridge Quarterly of Health Care Ethics*, 1996, 5: 285–299. Discussion of the use of drugs that do not benefit the patient.

Institute of Medicine, *Non-Heart-Beating Organ Transplantation: Medical and Ethical Issues in Procurement*. Washington, DC: National Academy Press, 1997.

Kolata, G., "Controversy Erupts Over Organ Removals," *New York Times*, 13 April, 1997.

Lynn, J., "Are the Patients Who Become Organ Donors Under the Pittsburgh Protocol for 'Non-Heart-Beating Donors' Really Dead?," in R.M. Arnold et al., eds., *Procuring Organs for Transplant*, pp. 91–102. See pp. 96–97 for anecdotal estimate of resuscitation times.

Pernick, M.S., "Brain Death in a Cultural Context: The Reconstruction of Death, 1967–1981," in S.J. Youngner, et al., eds., *Definition of Death*, pp. 3–33. Historical review; particularly useful for background to the Harvard criteria.

President's Commission for the Study of Ethical Problems in Medicine and Biomedical and Behavioral Research, *Defining Death: A Report on the Medical, Legal, and Ethical Issues in the Determination of Death*. Washington, DC: U.S. Government Printing Office, 1981.

Report of the Ad Hoc Committee of the Harvard Medical School to Examine the Definition of Brain Death, "A Definition of Irreversible Coma," *JAMA* 1968, 205: 337–340.

Report of the Medical Consultants on the Diagnosis of Death to the President's Commission for the Study of Ethical Problems in Medicine and Biomedical and Behavioral Research, in *Defining Death*, pp. 65–539.

United Network for Organ Sharing, "Donors Recovered in the U.S.: 1992–1999." Based on UNOS Scientific Registry data as of January 1, 2000.

Veatch, R.M., "The Impending Collapse of the Whole-Brain Definition of Death," *Hastings Center Report*, 1993, 23: 18–24.

Youngner, S.J., Arnold, R.M., and Schapiro, R., eds., *The Definition of Death: Contemporary Controversies*. Baltimore, MD: Johns Hopkins University Press, 1999. See articles by Baruch A. Brody, James L. Bernat, Chris Pallis, Robert M. Veatch, and Norman Fost on different concepts of death and their difficulties.)

CHAPTERS 9–10: XENOTRANSPLANTATION

Advisory Group on the Ethics of Xenotransplantation (Great Britain), *Animal Tissue into Humans*. London: Stationery Office, 1997.

Bach, F.H., Fishman, J.A., Daniels, N., et al., "Uncertainty in Xenotransplantation: Individual Benefit versus Collective Risk," *Nature Medicine*, February, 1998, 4: 141–144. The possibility of the wisdom of a moratorium is raised.

Butler, D., "Last Chance to Stop and Think on Risks of Xenotransplants," *Nature*, 22 January, 1998, 391: 320–324.

Cooper, D.K.C., and Lanza, R.P., *Xeno: The Promise of Transplanting Animal Organs into Humans*. New York: Oxford University Press, 2000. I relied on this work for my account of recent efforts to make xenotransplantation work.

de Bousingen, D.D., "Europe Supports Moratorium on Xenotransplantation," *Lancet*, 1999, 353: 476.

Fink, J.S., "Transplantation in Parkinson's Disease," *Artificial Organs*, 1997, 21: 199–202.

Food and Drug Administration, "Guidance for Industry: Public Health Issues Posed by the Use of Nonhuman Primate Xenografts in Humans," 5 September, 2000, http:www.fda.gov//cber/gdlns/xenoprim.txt.

Frassier, S.D., "The Not So Good Old Days: Working with Pituitary Growth Hormone in North America: 1956 to 1985," *Journal of Pediatrics*, Supplement, 1997, 131: 1–4.

Government of Great Britain, *The Government Response to "Animal Tissue into Humans," the Report of the Advisory Group on the Ethics of Xenotransplantation*. London: Stationery Office, 1997.

Hanson, M.J., "The Seductive Sirens of Medical Progress: The Case of Xenotransplantation," *Hastings Center Report*, September-October, 1995, pp. 5–6.

Institute of Medicine, Committee on Xenograft Transplantation, *Xenotransplantation: Science, Ethics, and Public Policy*. Washington, DC: National Academy Press, 1996.

Kuman, P.D., "Xenotransplantation in the New Millennim: Moratorium or Cautious Experimentation," *Perspectives in Biology and Medicine*, Summer, 2000, 43: 562–576.

Logan, J.S., and Sharma, A., "Potential Use of Genetically Modified Pigs as Organ Donors for Transplantation into Humans," *Clinical and Experimental Pharmacology and Physiology*, 1999, 26: 1020–1025.

Morgan, F., "Babe the Magnificent Organ Donor? The Perils and Promises Surrounding Xenotransplantation," *Journal of Contemporary Health Law and Policy*, 1997, 14: 127–160.

Salomon, D.R., Ferguson, R.M., and Helderman, J.H., "Correspondence: Xenotransplantation: Proceed With Caution," *Nature*, 5 March, 1998, 392: 11–12.

Schwartz, J., "FDA Sets Animal-Human Transplant Guidelines: Rules Would Govern Variety of Therapies," *Washington Post*, 21 September, 1996.

United States Public Health Service, "Draft Guidelines on Infectious Diseases in Xenotransplantation," 61 *Federal Register*, 1996, at 49: 920–921.

Weiss, R.A., "Xenotransplantation," *British Medical Journal*, 1998, 317: 931–934.

———, "Xenotransplants and Retroviruses," *Science*, 20 August, 1999, 285: 1221–1222.

Xenotransplantation on the Web, "A Selection of Resources on Xenotransplantation, Including People, Events, and an Online Library," www.xenotransplant.
ineu.org/xenotransans/index.htm.

CHAPTER 11: GROW YOUR OWN ORGANS

Associated Press, "Study Finds Gene Injections Can Restore Muscle in Mice,"
14 December, 1998.
Begley, S., "From Human Embryos, Hope for 'Spare Parts,'" *Newsweek*,
16 November, 1998, p. 73.
Boheler, K.R., and Fiszman, M.Y., *Cells, Tissues, Organs*, 1999, 165: 237–245.
Boyce, N., "U.S. Paves the Way for Embryonic Stem Cell Transplants,"
New Scientist, 30 January, 1999, p. 6.
Capron, A.M., "At Law: Good Intentions," *Hastings Center Report*, March-April,
1999, pp. 26–27. See for an account of steps leading to the 1999 NIH guide-
lines.
Cohen, P., "Grow Your Own Organs," *New Scientist*, 30 January, 1999, p. 6.
French, A.J., Greenstein, J., et al., "Current and Future Prospects for Xenotrans-
plantation," *Reproduction, Fertility, and Development*, 1998, 19: 683–696.
Grady, D., "Fat Is Good Source of Stem Cells, a Study Says," *New York Times*,
10 April, 2001. Claims of Marc H. Hedric's group.
Hall, S.S., "The Recycled Generation: Stem-Cell Research Holds the Promise of an
Endless Supply of New Body Parts," *New York Times Magazine*, 30 January,
2000, pp. 30–35, 46, 74–76. Discusses use of enucleated cow cells and human
cells.
Han, S.S.W., and Fischer, I., "Neural Stem Cells and Gene Therapy: Prospects for
Repairing the Injured Spinal Cord," *JAMA*, 3 May, 2000, 283: 2300–2301.
Lemonick, M.D., "The Biological Mother Lode," *Time*, 16 November, 1998,
pp. 96–97.
Lenoir, N., "Europe Confronts the Embryonic Stem Cell Research Challenge,"
Science, 25 February, 2000, 287: 1425–1426.
Mooney, D.J., and Mikos, A.G., "Growing New Organs," *Scientific American*,
April, 1999, pp. 60–65. Excellent account of the basic accomplishments and
aims of tissue engineering from which I have drawn information.
National Bioethics Advisory Commission, *Ethical Issues in Human Stem Cell
Research: Executive Summary*; Vol. I, *Report and Recommendations*; Vol. II,
Commissioned Papers; Vol. III, *Religious Perspectives*; September, 1999,
Rockville, MD. See also www.bioethics.gov.
National Institutes of Health, "Stem Cells: A Primer," May, 2000, www.nih.gov/
news/stemcell/primer/htm.
———, "National Institutes of Health Guidelines for Research Using Human
Pluripotent Stem Cells," 24 August, 2000, www.nih.gov/news/stemcell/
stemcellguidelines/htm.
Noonan, J.T., Jr., "An Almost Absolute Value in History," in R. Munson,
Intervention and Reflection, 6th ed., pp. 83–86. Belmont, CA: Wadsworth
Publishing, 2001.
Parenteau, N., "Skin: The First Tissue Engineered Products, The Organogenesis
Story," *Scientific American*, April, 1999, pp. 83–84.

Pedersen, R.A., "Embryonic Stem Cells for Medicine," *Scientific American*, April, 1999, pp. 69–73.

Pollack, A., "Neural Cells Grown in Labs Raise Hopes on Brain Disease," *New York Times*, 30 May, 2000.

Pontifical Academy of Life, "Declaration on the Production and the Scientific and Therapeutic Use of Human Embryonic Stem Cells." Issued at Vatican City: 25 August, 2000. A four-page statement by the Roman Catholic Church.

Reuters, "Scientists Say Cell Treatment Can Reverse Diabetes in Mice," 28 February, 2000.

Service, R.F., "Designer Tissues Take Hold," *Science*, 13 October, 1995, 27: 230–232.

Shamblott, M., et al., "Derivation of Pluripotent Stem Cells from Cultured Human Primordial Germ Cell," *Proceedings of the National Academy of Science*, November, 1998, 95: 13726–13731.

Stolberg, S.G., "Decisive Moment on Parkinson's Fetal-Cell Transplants," *New York Times*, 20 April, 1999.

———, "Stem Cell Research Advocates in Limbo: Abortion Opponents Have Urged Bush to Cut Off Money of Projects," *New York Times*, 19 January, 2001.

Thomson, J., et al., "Embryonic Stem Cell Lines Derived from Human Blastocysts," *Science*, 6 November, 1998, 282: 1145–1147.

Wade, N., "Primordial Cells Fuel Ethical Debate," *New York Times*, 10 November, 1998. I'm indebted to Wade's reports on the most recent research.

———, "Human-Cow Hybrid Cells Are Topic of Ethics Panel," *New York Times*, 16 November, 1998.

———, "Panel told of Vast Benefits of Embryo Cells," *New York Times*, 3 December, 1998.

———, "Experiment Offers Hope for Tissue Repair," *New York Times*, 22 January, 1999.

———, "Advisory Panel Votes for Use of Embryonic Cells in Research," *New York Times*, 19 June, 1999.

———, "Embryo Cell Research: A Clash of Values," *New York Times*, 2 July, 1999.

———, "Cancer Society Quits Group on Cell Research," *New York Times*, 29 July, 1999.

———, "Mouse Cells Are Converted Into Specialized Brain Cells," *New York Times*, 30 July, 1999.

———, "Stem Cells Yield Promising Results," *New York Times*, 31 March, 2001.

———, "Findings Deepen Debate on Using Embryonic Stem Cells," *New York Times*, 3 April, 2001. Political disputes restrict embryonic stem cell research.

———, "Company Says It Can Derive Stem Cells from the Placenta," *New York Times*, 6 April, 2001.

Wright, S.J., "Human Embryonic Stem-Cell Research: Science and Ethics," *American Scientist*, August, 1999, 87: 352–361. Includes a sketch of the history of federal regulation of stem cells.

Index